Endocrinology Research and Clinical Developments Series

THYROID HORMONES: FUNCTIONS, RELATED DISEASES AND USES

Endocrinology Research and Clinical Developments Series

Estrogens: Production, Functions and Applications
James R. Bartos (Editor)
2009. ISBN: 978-1-60741-086-7

Thyroid Hormones: Functions, Related Diseases and Uses
Francis S. Kuehn and Mauris P. Lozada (Editors)
2009. ISBN: 978-1-60741-080-5

Endocrinology Research and Clinical Developments Series

Thyroid Hormones: Functions, Related Diseases and Uses

Francis S. Kuehn
and Mauris P. Lozada
Editors

Nova Biomedical Books
New York

For permission to use material from this book please contact us:
Telephone 631-231-7269; Fax 631-231-8175
Web Site: http://www.novapublishers.com

Library of Congress Cataloging-in-Publication Data

Thyroid hormones : functions, related diseases, and uses / [edited by] Francis S. Kuehn and Mauris P. Lozada.
p. ; cm.
Includes bibliographical references and index.
ISBN 978-1-60741-080-5 (hardcover : alk. paper)
1. Thyroid hormones. I. Kuehn, Francis S. II. Lozada, Mauris P.
[DNLM: 1. Thyroid Hormones. WK 202 T5495 2009]
QP572.T5T566 2009
612.4'4--dc22 2009011429

Published by Nova Science Publishers, Inc. ✦ New York

Contents

Preface

The thyroid is one of the largest endocrine glands in the body. The thyroid controls how quickly the body burns energy, makes proteins, and how sensitive the body should be to other hormones. It participates in these processes by producing thyroid hormones, principally thyroxine and triiodothyronine. These hormones regulate the rate of metabolism and affect the growth and rate of function of many other systems in the body. The thyroid also produces the hormone calcitonin, which plays a role in calcium homeostasis. As discussed in this book, both excess and deficiency of thyroxine can cause disorders. Thyrotoxicosis or hyperthyroidism, a cause of Graves Disease, is caused by an excess of circulating free thyroxine, free triiodothyronine, or both. Hypothyroidism is the case where there is a deficiency of thyroxine, triiodiothyronine, or both. Clinical depression can sometimes be caused by hypothyroidism. This book presents a wide variety of research on the role of thyroid hormones and their effects.

Chapter I - Thyroid hormone (TH) is indispensable for brain development. Lack of sufficient TH in the neonatal period causes serious damage to neural cells leading to mental retardation and abnormal development of virtually all organ systems, a syndrome termed cretinism. To exert their effect in the brain, the TH must cross brain barriers: i.e. the blood-brain barrier (BBB) and the blood – cerebrospinal fluid (CSF) barrier formed by the brain capillary endothelial cells and choroid plexus epithelial cells, respectively. It has become increasingly clear that the TH flux into and out of brain by saturable transport mechanisms through a number of transporters, e.g. organic anion transport polypeptide (OATP), monocardoxylate transport (MCT), L-type amino acid transporter (LAT) and a number of ATP-binding cassette (ABC) transporter superfamily such as P-gp, MRP, BCRP. OAPT1C1 and MCT8 demonstrate a high degree of specificity towards to the TH and are the main transporters for the TH entry into brain. When mutations in MCT8 in humans are associated with severe psychomotor retardation and elevated T_3 level. On the other hand, P-gp exports the TH from brain to blood. Nevertheless, the vast majority of TH in the serum is bound to proteins, including thyroxine binding protein (TBG), transthyretin (TTR), serum albumin, and a number of lipoproteins, which roles in TH transport have recently attracted attention. These TH binding proteins maintain the large extrathyroidal pool of TH which ensure a constant supply of TH to the brain, protect the brain against abrupt changes in TH production and degradation and iodine deficiency. The binding proteins in CSF help evenly distribute

TH within the brain and prevent its loss. In conclusion, the TH homeostasis in brain is precisely controlled by a number of TH transporters in brain barriers and the TH binding proteins which act as storage molecules to buffer the TH level.

Chapter II - The assessment of the thyroid function has become a regular procedure in clinical practice as part of the check-up for routine health care. The diagnosis of thyroid dysfunction (TD) is initially accomplished on the basis of altered serum hormone levels: thyrotropin (TSH), thyroxine (T4), and triiodothyronine (T3). As our ability to detect ever more subtle degrees of TD has improved (with highly sensitive and specific assays), we are now dealing with a new medical problem. In clinical practice there are an increased number of subjects with a subtle deviation of serum TSH levels as the only alteration. This new group of patients has what is known as *subclinical* thyroid disease. Therefore TD is classified as: 1) *clinical* (TSH and thyroid hormones out of normal range) and 2) *subclinical* (isolated TSH alteration). Epidemiological studies have demonstrated that subclinical TD occurs more frequently than clinical TD. However, the management of subclinical TD is controversial and has been the subject of recurrent debates between thyroidologists. In line with this disagreement, there is no consensus on the TSH, free T4 and free T3 cutoff values at which treatment should be initiated in patients with subclinical TD.

In the background of this discussion are the limitations of the current diagnostic methods for detecting thyroid disease. In other words, it is difficult to define what normality is in this regard. From a physiological point of view we already know that normality (physiological homeostasis) is not equivalent to equality (the same) with regard to serum TH levels. The limitations of the diagnostic procedures are obvious to the extent that they cannot separate healthy outliers from those subjects who really have the disease. Serum TH levels alone do not explain the variability and severity of symptoms observed in patients with TD. Therefore nowadays, it is not possible to determine which patients with subclinical TD will develop the typical complications of clinical dysfunction and which will see their mild elevations in TSH be auto-resolved.

Almost all corporal organs and systems are influenced by the metabolic activity of thyroid hormones (TH). Advances in physiology and molecular medicine have improved our understanding of the consequences of hormone action in target cells. A highly elaborate multi-step system regulates not only the synthesis of TH but their tissue action as well. Currently we are able to determine to some extent the cellular TH activity in different organs, which should be reflected in different biological markers. The ability to determine the activity of TH on target tissues will enable us to administrate the adequate supplementation dose of T4 more accurately, only to patients who need it, avoiding over-treatment.

Chapter III - Thyroid hormone (L-3, 3',5-triiodothyronine, T_3) exerts important actions on cellular energy metabolism, being mitochondria the major target for its calorigenic effects. Acceleration of O_2 consumption by T_3 is due to transcriptional activation of respiratory genes in target tissues such as liver, leading to increased production of reactive oxygen species (ROS) and the consequent depletion of antioxidant mechanisms. The increase in ROS generation primarily occurs at mitochondrial and other subcellular sites of hepatocytes, concomitantly with a higher respiratory burst activity of Kupffer cells, which act as redox signals regulating important cellular functions such as protein activity and gene expression. Indeed, ROS produced at the Kupffer-cell level activate redox-sensitive transcription factors such as nuclear factor-κB (NF-κB), signal transducer and activator of transcription 3 (STAT3), and activating protein 1 (AP-1), as evidenced by the abolishment of the T_3-induced DNA binding capacity of these proteins by pre-treatment with antioxidants or the Kupffer-cell inactivator $GdCl_3$. Up-regulation of gene expression by T_3 is also accomplished in Kupffer cells, leading to an enhancement in the synthesis and release of the cytokines tumor necrosis factor-α (TNF-α) and interleukin (IL)-1 and IL-6. The TNF-α response elicited by T_3 correlates with the activation of the IκB kinase complex (IKK), which ultimately triggers NF-κB DNA binding with the consequent expression of the NF-κB-responsive genes encoding for inducible nitric oxide synthase, manganese superoxide dismutase, the anti-apoptotic protein Bcl-2, and the type I acute-phase protein haptoglobin. T_3-induced IL-6 signaling T_3 involves the Janus kinase (JAK)-STAT3 pathway up-regulating the expression of both type I (haptoglobin) and type II (β-fibrinogen) acute-phase proteins. In addition to these actions, T_3-dependent TNF-α and IL-6 responses trigger liver cyclin-dependent kinase-2 expression and cellular proliferation, which may be associated with c-jun N-terminal kinase (JNK) and AP-1 activation or with JAK and STAT3 activation, respectively. These data indicate that T_3-induced calorigenesis also triggers non-genomic effects leading to an expression pattern representing adaptive mechanisms to re-establish redox homeostasis and promote cell survival under conditions of ROS toxicity. This redox signaling in T_3 action has been shown to be associated with significant protection against ischemia-reperfusion liver injury. Thus, T_3 administration represents a novel preconditioning strategy with clinical potential. The latter view is of particular importance considering that, with the exception of ischemic preconditioning, all the other protecting strategies studied have not been transferred to clinical application. Noteworthy, T_3 is a widely used and well-tolerated therapeutic agent that has either no important adverse effects or minimal side-effects that can be readily controlled.

Chapter IV - Thyroid hormones are used for treatment of patients with depressive disorders. In order to find genetic and molecular factors defining the sensitivity to thyroid hormones, the effects of chronic thyroxine (T4) treatment (2 mg/l, 60 days, in drinking water) on locomotor activity, anxiety-related, depressive-like behavior and freezing reaction (catalepsy) as well as on the 5-HT_{1A} and 5-HT_{2A} serotonin receptors in the brain were investigated in catalepsy-resistant AKR/J and catalepsy-prone ASC/Icg (Antidepressant Sensitive Catalepsy) strains. The latter was selectively bred for the high predisposition to catalepsy from intercross between CBA/Lac and AKR/J parental strains. In AKR mice T4 increased predisposition to catalepsy and locomotion in the open field test compared with the respective controls, but did not affect forced swim immobility. In contrast, in ASC mice T4 significantly decreased predisposition to catalepsy and immobility time in the forced swim test without any effect on locomotion in the open field. No influence of T4 on anxiety-related behavior in mice of these strains was shown. T4 treatment significantly increased head-twitch response to 5-HT_{2A} receptor agonist, DOI (1 mg/kg, ip) and the receptor mRNA level in the cortex in AKR, but not in ASC mice. Although the hormone did not affect 5-HT_{1A} receptor mRNA level in the hippocampus and midbrain of ASC mice, a marked attenuation of hypothermic effect of 5-HT_{1A} receptor agonist, 8-OH-DPAT (1 mg/kg, ip) in the T4-treated ASC was found. It was suggested that the cortical 5-HT_{2A} receptor mediated the T4-induced activation of locomotion, while the 5-HT_{1A} receptor was involved in the anticataleptic and antidepressant effects of the hormone. The results indicate that hereditary predisposition to catalepsy can predict behavioral effect of chronic T4 treatment in mice.

Chapter V - Thyroid hormones are major hormones regulating development and energy expenditure in mammals and avian species. They modulate the transcription of target genes by interacting with intracellular thyroid receptors that bind to thyroid hormone response elements (TRE) located on DNA. Mitochondria are also reported to be targets of thyroid hormones, with early or delayed effects occurring through several pathways. In mammals, a direct short-term activation of enzymes involved in the respiratory chain results in higher rates of mitochondrial oxidative phosphorylation and the generation of reactive oxygen species (ROS). Additional long-term effects are mediated through changes in the mitochondrial coupling of oxidative phosphorylation, partly via a mechanism involving uncoupling proteins (UCP) and increasing proton leak. Moreover, triiodothyronine is reported to regulate fatty acid utilization, through the activation of enzymes involved in β-oxidation. Part of the mechanisms regulated by these hormones is dependent on the coordinated stimulations of the transcription of the nuclear and mitochondrial genomes. The present review focuses on the central role of thyroid hormones in the regulation of mitochondrial oxidations in light of the recent data obtained in mammals and birds.

Chapter VI - The etiology of Graves' ophthalmopathy (TAO), representing the most common extrathyroidal manifestation of Graves'disease (GD), is multifactorial. In spite of majority of GD patients having some evidence of ocular involvement, only a minority (3-5%) develops severe TAO. Graves' ophthalmopathy is an autoimmune disease of the orbit involving both the retroorbital connective tissue and the extraocular muscles, but its pathogenesis is still incompletely understood. Multiple genetic (class II HLA genes and cytotoxic T lymphocyte associated-4 regions), environmental (smoking, stress, and iodine uptake), and endogenous factors are involved in the pathogenesis of GD (the thyroid cell itself appears to play a major role in the disease progression through the expression of a number of immunologically active peptides such as adhesion molecules, cytokines, CD40, and complementary regulatory proteins). Examination of retroorbital tissues in the initial inflammatory phase of TAO reveals an accumulation of hydrophilic glycosaminoglycans, increased fat volume, marked T and B lymphocytic infiltration, and presence of many pro-inflammatory cytokines and growth factors. Peripheral blood levels of pro-inflammatory cytokines released from T and B lymphocytes or by the thyroid follicular cells (IFNγ, IL-1β, IL-2, sIL-2R TNFα, IL-6, IL-6R) and antibodies of TSH receptor (TRAb) secreted from B lymphocytes are markers of the immune system activity. Updated the efficacy of the new anti-cytokine and anti-lymphocyte treatment of the Graves' ophthalmopathy has been revived. In this revieved study the positive results of anti-B lymphocyte (anti-CD20; rituximab] and anti-TNFα monoclonal antibodies (infliximab; etanercept) administration as new therapeutic options in the treatment of patients with active TAO were described.

Chapter VII - Graves ophthalmopathy (GO) is the most common cause of orbital inflammation and proptosis in adults. There is however, no agreement on its management. Corticosteroids and external beam orbital radiation (XRT) have been used to treat active inflammation. Other immunomodulatory agents, including azathioprine, cyclosporine, intravenous immunoglobulin (IVIG), and plasmapheresis have not proved to be effective. Newer agents including anti-CD20 monoclonal antibodies (rituximab) and TNF blockers hold potential therapeutic value but have not been formally investigated. Moreover, the lack of standard study design, treatment protocols, and outcome measures limits comparison of studies. Despite these limitations, there is evidence that the combination of corticosteroids and orbital radiation therapy is more effective than corticosteroids alone in the treatment of moderate to severe GO. In order to evaluate the management of GO, the design and funding of a multi-center trial is required.

Chapter VIII - We report a retrospective study of thyroid function in seven infants whose mothers had Graves' disease and hyperthyroidism during the gestational period due to onset, relapse, instability, or poor compliance. Three infants showed transient central hypothyroidism, one of whom had short-term neonatal thyrotoxicosis before central hypothyroidism. These infants had TRAb $< 50\%$ and TSAb $< 400\%$ at birth, and maternal hyperthyroidism appeared before 32 weeks gestation. Three other infants had neonatal Graves' disease until 1, 2 and 3 months of age, respectively, with TRAb $> 70\%$ and TSAb $> 700\%$ at birth, and maternal hyperthyroidism appeared after 28 weeks gestation. One infant whose mother had hyperthyroidism until 10 weeks gestation was euthyroid after birth. These cases suggest that passage of thyroid hormones from mother to fetus occurs when the maternal level of thyroid hormones is high. Maternal hyperthyroidism before 32 weeks gestation and relatively high autoantibodies in the neonate are related to development of central hypothyroidism. In addition, maternal hyperthyroidism after 28 weeks gestation may not be related to development of central hypothyroidism.

Chapter IX - The role of thyroid hormone (T3) in astrocyte morphogenesis is clearly demonstrated. T3 regulates several aspects of astrocyte differentiation and maturation, including the production of cytoskeleton, extracellular matrix (ECM) molecules and growth factors. T3 induces astrocytes to secrete a combination of growth factors including fibroblast growth factor-2 (FGF2) and epidermal growth factor (EGF) that act autocrinally influencing different aspects of astrocyte and neuronal differentiation and function. In addition, T3 alters the expression and organization of the glial fibrillary acidic protein (GFAP) and the ECM proteins laminin and fibronectin, and regulates the expression of the proteoglycans syndecans, thus producing a high-quality substrate for neuronal differentiation. In fact, T3-treated astrocytes promote neural growth and neuritogenesis. Indeed, and indirect mechanism of thyroid hormone on neuronal development mediated by astrocytes has been proposed. Moreover, an important and additional role of T3 in regulating glutamate uptake by cerebellar astrocytes was recently demonstrated. This effect is promoted by the up regulation of astrocytic glutamate transporters GLAST and GLT-1 that result in glial and neuronal protection against glutamate toxicity. Therefore, T3 is involved in the control of most facets of functional neural networks, a large amount of them mediated by the improvement of astrocytic microenvironment.

Chapter X - Amiodarone is a benzofuranic derivative, iodine-rich drug widely used for treatment of cardiac tachyarrhythmias. It often leads to transient changes in thyroid function tests, either due to the high iodine content of the drug or due to the direct toxic effect of the drug. The prevalence of amiodarone induced thyroid dysfunction depends on dietary iodine intake, age and sex of the patient and also presence of underlying thyroid disorder. Thyroid dysfunction occurs in about 15% of patients treated with amiodarone (Amiodarone induced hypothyroidism (AIH) or Amiodarone induced thyrotoxicosis (AIT)).

AIH is commoner in iodine sufficient areas and in patients with a background of Hashimoto's thyroiditis and is related to failure to escape from the acute Wolff Chaikoff effect. It may develop as early as 2 weeks or as late as 3 years following initiation of amiodarone therapy. Treatment of AIH consists of levothyroxine replacement, while continuing amiodarone therapy.

AIT is more complex and there are two varieties namely AIT type I and AIT type II. AIT type I is commoner in iodine deficient areas and typically occurs with underlying thyroid disease (due to Jod Basedow phenomenon). There is some benefit in stopping amiodarone in such a scenario and treating with thionamides with or without potassium perchlorate. AIT type II on the other hand is commoner in iodine sufficient areas and occurs due to the direct toxic effect of amiodarone on thyroid follicular cells. Withdrawal of amiodarone with or without glucorticoids is useful. Mixed forms are best treated with a combination of thionamides, potassium perchlorate and glucocorticoid. Thyroidectomy is contemplated in resistant cases. Radio-iodine is usually of little benefit due to low thyroidal radioiodine uptake.

Thyroid function tests should be performed at baseline prior to initiation of amiodarone therapy. Clinicians should also note presence of any goiter and document any history of autoimmune disorders. Thereafter thyroid function tests need to be repeated at 3-6 month interval initially and thereafter annually for at least a year following withdrawal of therapy. This is of utmost importance to detect amiodarone induced thyroid problems.

A significant proportion of patients on amiodarone are also on Warfarin and it is important to realize that amiodarone as well as thyroid dysfunction alters the pharmacokinetics of warfarin. Therefore adjustments of warfarin dosage have to be made accordingly.

A newer drug, namely dronedarone is currently under review. As dronedarone does not contain iodine it is hoped that it will have the same benefits but not the ill effects on thyroid function.

Chapter XI - Experimental evidence for the physiological effects of secondhand smoke is limited although it affects millions of people globally and its prevalence is increasing, despite currently adopted anti-smoking measures. As early as adolescence, exposure to tobacco products increases the risk for developing cardiovascular disease (1) highlighting the necessity to understand the secondhand smoke effects on human health. Recent evidence demonstrated that a 1-hour secondhand smoke exposure to bar/restaurant levels is accompanied by statistically significant increases in triiodothyronine (T_3) and free thyroxine (fT_4) levels of healthy adult non-smokers (2). These increases of thyroid hormone levels effects affected metabolism with a 6% increase in resting energy expenditure and were not attributed to an anterior pituitary response (i.e., thyroid stimulating hormone secretion), but to the – probably short-term – effects of a different mechanism. Interestingly, further work in this area revealed that the same secondhand smoke exposure is accompanied by a decrease in gonadal hormones in both sexes as well as marked increases in thyroid hormone secretion and interleukin-1β production in men (3). The less pronounced alterations in thyroid hormone secretion of women suggested the involvement of estrogens which are known to influence serum total T_4 and T_3 concentrations by increasing the glycosylation of thyroxine-binding globulin – a protein heavily involved in T_4 and T_3 binding – and by slowing its clearance from the blood. Analogously, the statistically significant decrease in the T_3:fT_4 ratio following the secondhand smoke exposure in men as well as the inverse association between testosterone and T_3 suggested the involvement of androgens, which are known to decrease the glycosylation of thyroxine-binding globulin. These results were not limited to extrathyroidial processes, as fT_4 levels were not significantly influenced by changes in the serum concentrations of binding proteins, reflecting purely functional thyroid state. Therefore, the observed effects of gonadal hormones may also indicate a down-regulating effect on thyroid gland hormonogenesis. Based on these results and data from chronic active smoking, it was suggested that chronic passive smoking (lifestyle incorporating frequent exposures to passive smoke) may have clinical implications such as thyroid and gonadal abnormalities particularly in males. In this light, this chapter reviews current knowledge on the effects of secondhand smoke on the thyroid in an attempt to unravel the underlying mechanisms associated with the increase in thyroid hormone secretion following exposure to secondhand smoke.

In: Thyroid Hormones: Functions, Related Diseases and Uses ISBN: 978-1-60741-080-5
Editors: F. S. Kuehn, M. P. Lozada

Chapter I

Thyroid Hormone Transport across Blood-Brain Barriers

***R.L. Chen*[1], *J.E. Preston1 and W. Zheng*[2]**
[1]Pharmaceutical Science Division, King's College London, London, UK
[2]School of Health Sciences, Purdue University, West Lafayette, IN 47907-2051, USA.

Abstract

Thyroid hormone (TH) is indispensable for brain development. Lack of sufficient TH in the neonatal period causes serious damage to neural cells leading to mental retardation and abnormal development of virtually all organ systems, a syndrome termed cretinism. To exert their effect in the brain, the TH must cross brain barriers: i.e. the blood-brain barrier (BBB) and the blood – cerebrospinal fluid (CSF) barrier formed by the brain capillary endothelial cells and choroid plexus epithelial cells, respectively. It has become increasingly clear that the TH flux into and out of brain by saturable transport mechanisms through a number of transporters, e.g. organic anion transport polypeptide (OATP), monocardoxylate transport (MCT), L-type amino acid transporter (LAT) and a number of ATP-binding cassette (ABC) transporter superfamily such as P-gp, MRP, BCRP. OAPT1C1 and MCT8 demonstrate a high degree of specificity towards to the TH and are the main transporters for the TH entry into brain. When mutations in MCT8 in humans are associated with severe psychomotor retardation and elevated T_3 level. On the other hand, P-gp exports the TH from brain to blood. Nevertheless, the vast majority of TH in the serum is bound to proteins, including thyroxine binding protein (TBG), transthyretin (TTR), serum albumin, and a number of lipoproteins, which roles in TH transport have recently attracted attention. These TH binding proteins maintain the large extrathyroidal pool of TH which ensure a constant supply of TH to the brain, protect the brain against abrupt changes in TH production and degradation and iodine deficiency. The binding proteins in CSF help evenly distribute TH within the brain and prevent its loss. In conclusion, the TH homeostasis in brain is precisely controlled by a number of TH transporters in brain barriers and the TH binding proteins which act as storage molecules to buffer the TH level.

Abbreviations

ABC, ATP-binding cassette;
ALB, albumin;
BCB, blood – CSF barrier;
BCH, 2-aminoendobicyclo-[2,2,1]-heptane-2-carboxylic acid;
BCRP, breast cancer resistance protein;
BBB, blood-brain barrier;
CSF, cerebrospinal fluid;
CNS, central nervous system;
CP, choroid plexuses;
D_1-D_3, iodothyronine deiodinases;
ECM, extracellular matrix;
HDL, High density lipoprotein;
LAT, large neutral amino acid transporter;
LDL, Low density lipoprotein;
MCT, monocarboxylate transporters;
MDR, multidrug resistance;
MRP, multidrug resistance-related protein;
NTCP, Na+ / taurocholate cotransporting polypeptide;
OATP, organic anion transporting polypeptide;
P-gp, glycoprotein;
rT_3, reverse T_3;
T_3, tri-iodothyronine;
T_4, thyroxine;
TJ, tight junctions;
TTR, transthyretin;
SCH, subclinical hypothyroidism;
SLC, solute carrier;
TAT, aromatic amino acids transporter;
TBG, thyroxine-binding protein;
TTR, transthyretin;
V-C, ventricle-cistern;
ZO, zonula occludens proteins.

1. Thyroid Hormone

Thyroid hormones (TH) including both thyroxine (T_4) and tri-iodothyronine (T_3) are tyrosine – based hormones produced by the thyroid gland. The majority of TH is released in the form of T_4, which is 40 times higher than T_3 (90mM vs 2 mM) in plasma [1]. Both T_4 and T_3 are hydrophobic molecules, with T_3 being more hydrophobic than T_4 due to its relative lack of an ionised phenolic group [2]. However, it is T_4 rather than T_3 that is transported from the bloodstream to cells [2]. T_4, which is considered to act as prehormone, can either be converted to T_3 by deiodination of its outer ring, or inactivated to reverse T_3 (rT_3) by inner-ring deiodination [3]. These reactions are catalysed by three iodothyronine deiodinases (D_1-D_3) with different tissue distribution and substrate specificity [4,5]. In the brain, deiodinase D_2 is responsible for converting T_4 to T_3 [6,7], while D_3 is responsible for inactivation of T_4 to rT_3 and T_3 to T_2 [8,9]. TH exerts its biological activities mostly at the genomic level through an interaction with specific nuclear receptors. Binding of T_3 (the principal bioactive form of TH) to its receptor induces the release of corespressors and the recruitment of coactivators resulting in the stimulation of gene transcription [10-12]. The TH actions are now understood to involve novel extranuclear (nongenomic) mechanisms in a variety of cells including those of central nervous system (CNS) [13], in which T_3 influences ion fluxes across plasma membrane channels and the PI3K/Akt pathway [14,15]. The TH acts on the body to stimulate oxygen consumption and thermogenesis, accelerate protein, lipid, carbohydrate and bone mineral turnover, affect protein synthesis and how human cells use energetic compounds, increase the contractility of skeletal and cardiac muscles and body's sensitivity to catecholamines (such as adrenaline) [16-18]. The TH is indispensable to proper development and differentiation of all cells of the human body [3]. Lack of sufficient TH results in abnormal development of virtually all organ systems, a syndrome termed cretinism (a form of mental deficiency together with deficits in skeletal growth) [19,20]. In particular, hypothyroidism in the neonatal period causes serious damage to neural cells leading to severe mental retardation, neurological deficits and hearing impairment [3,21]. In adulthood, TH is important for neuronal regeneration after injury [22] and is related to high-level cognition [23]. Abnormal plasma TH found in ageing [24-26] and subclinical hypothyroidism (SCH) patients [27,28] is a risk factor for dementia. Working memory is impaired in SCH patients and could be restored after thyroxine treatment [29]. To exert their effect in the brain, the TH must cross barriers between blood and brain comprising the blood-brain barrier (BBB), blood – cerebrospinal fluid (CSF) barrier (BCB) and the arachnoid membrane. The entry of TH via the BBB appears to be the preferred route for the overall distribution of TH in the brain accounting for 80% of the T_4 in the brain [30], whereas the rest is uptaken via the BCB [31] that is necessary to provide circumventricular areas with sufficient amounts of TH [32].

2. Blood-Brain Barriers

The BBB is composed of endothelial cells that line the cerebral vasculature, their capillary basement membranes, the astrocyte end-feet, and pericytes [33]. Cerebral vascular endothelial cells differ from other endothelial cells in the body for their richer and tighter junctions and relative less fenestrae and pinocytotic vesicles [34-36]. The highly developed tight junctions (TJ) between adjacent endothelial cells are formed by a complex of integral membrane proteins [claudin (1, 5, and 12) [37], occludin [38,39], and junctional adhesion molecules [40], and a number of cytoplasmic accessory protein including zonula occludens proteins (ZO) [41-44], cingulin [45]. The end-feet of astrocytes contribute to the barrier permeability and almost completely cover the outer surface of the microvascular basement membranes [46]. Between the endothelium and astrocyte end-feet, is the extracellular matrix (ECM) containing type IV collagen, laminin, and fibronectin, which supports the microvessels and regulates cell survival, growth, and differentiation [47]. At the BCB, TJs are formed between the epithelial cells rather than the endothelia, of the four choroid plexuses (CPs) in the cerebral ventricles. BCB epithelial TJs are different to those of BBB endothelial cells, containing claudin-2 rather than claudin-5 [48]. In addition, the ZOs are relatively short and concentrated close to the apical (CSF) side of the CP [49]. Functionally, the BCB is leakier to ions compared to BBB, as measured by the electrical resistance, which is 26-80 Ω cm^2 in the choroidal epithelium compared to 1462 Ω cm^2 in the cerebral endothelium [50-52]. Besides its barrier function, the CP avidly secretes CSF and synthesizes a number of proteins, many for secretion into CSF, e.g. transthyretin (TTR), vasopressin, transforming growth factor β, IGF – II [49]. The TJs normally prevent free exchange of solutes between blood and brain or CSF [53], except for small lipid-soluble molecules <400 Da which can cross the barriers unassisted via diffusion [54]. Hydrophilic molecules generally cross the endothelial wall via transcellular transport mechanisms, classified into five main categories: carrier-mediated transport, ion transport, active efflux transport, receptor-mediated transport, and caveolae-mediated transport [55].

3. Thyroxine Transporters

For their lipophilicity and relatively small mass (molecular weight of about 700 Da), the transport of TH across cell membranes has originally thought to be a passive diffusion process. However, this notion ignores the highly polar nature of the alanine side chain which is a formidable obstacle for membrane passage of TH [56]. Saturable TH entries to BBB and BCB are shown by a number of studies [57-61] including us [62-66]. It has become increasingly clear that saturable transport mechanisms involving numerous transporters may mediate both TH influx and efflux [67-69]. The first TH transporters were identified at the molecular level were the liver-specific Na^+ / taurocholate cotransporting polypeptide (NTCP) [70] and the organic anion transporting polypeptide 1a1 (Oatp 1a1) [70]. Thereafter other transporters such as monocarboxylate transporters (MCT), amino acid "L" and "T" transporters and fatty acid translocase were recognized to be involved in TH transport in the body [71]. Among them, OATP1C1, MCT8, MCT10 demonstrate a high degree of specificity towards to TH [72]. These transporters distribute differently among different tissues to transport TH (Table 1) [67]. Except NTCP, fatty acid translocase, MCT10, all the others exist in the brain barriers (Figure 1) [73].

3.1. Organic Anion Transport Polypeptide (OATP)

Organic anion transport polypeptides (human: OATPs, rodents: Oatps) form a super-family of sodium-independent transport systems for a number of amphipathic organic compounds including TH [74]. In human, there are 11 different OATPs [75]. Four different OATPs (1A2, 1C1, 2B1 and 3A1) have been found in endothelial cells of BBB and epithelial cells of CP, all except OATP2B1 involve in transporting of TH [76-79]. OATP1A2 is a glycoprotein of 670 amino acids and exhibits a molecular mass of 60 kDa in brain [76].

Table 1. Characteristics of thyroid hormone transporters

Protein	Gene	Species	Tissue distribution	Iodothyroxine transport
NTCP	SLC10A1	human	liver	T_4,T_3,rT_3,T_2
NTCP	SLC10A1	rat		
OATP1A1	SLCO1A1	rat	liver, kidney, CP	T_4,T_3,rT_3,T_2
OATP1A2	SLCO1A2	human	brain, kidney, liver	T_4,T_3,rT_3,T_2
OATP1A4	SLCO1A4	rat	liver, brain, retina	T_4,T_3,rT_3,T_2
OATP1A5	SLCO1A5	rat	liver, kidney, retina	T_4,T_3
OATP1B1	SLCO1B1	human	liver	T_4,T_3
OATP1B2	SLCO1B2	rat	liver	T_4,T_3
OATP1B3	SLCO1B3	human	liver	T_4,T_3
OATP1C1	SLCO1C1	human	brain, cochlea	T_4,T_3,rT_3
OATP1C1	SLCO1C1	rat	brain,	T_4,T_3,rT_3
OATP4A1	SLCO4A1	human	multiple	T_4,T_3,rT_3
OATP4A1	SLCO4A1	rat	multiple	T3, (T_4,rT_3,NT)
OATP4C1	SLCO4C1	human	kidney, other	T_4,T_3
OATP4C1	SLCO4C1	rat		T_3, (T_4,NT)
OATP6B1	SLCO6B1	rat	testis	T_3, T_4
OATP6C1	SLCO6C1	rat	testis	T_3, T_4
LAT1	SLC7A5	human	multiple, tumours	T_4,T_3,rT_3,T_2
LAT1	SLC7A5	rat		
LAT2	SLC7A8	human	multiple, tumours	T_4,T_3,rT_3,T_2
LAT2	SLC7A8	rat		
MCT8	SLC16A2	human	brain, liver, kidney heart, thyroid eye, pituitary, other	T_4,T_3,rT_3,T_2
MCT8	SLC16A2	rat		
MCT10 (TAT1)	SLC16A10	human	skeletal muscle, kidney heart, placenta, intestine	T_3, T_4
MCT10 (TAT1)	SLC16A10	rat	liver, placenta, intestine	T_3, T_4

When expressed in *Venopus laevis* oocytes, it transported T_4, T_3 and reverse T_3 (rT_3) with K_m value for T_4 transport 8.0 μM and for T_3 transport 6.5 μM [80]. OAPT1C1 is a protein of 712 amino acids and has the highest affinity for TH in OAPTs [75]. It transports T_4 with an K_m value of 90.4 nM and rT_3 127.7 nM [77]. It is almost exclusively expressed in brain capillaries and may be crucial for the transport of the pre-hormone T_4 across the BBB [77]. The OATP3A family has one human gene (*SLCO3A1*), which is expressed as two splice variants [79]. OATP3A1_v1 is a protein of 710 amino acids while OATP3A1_v2 is a shorter variant which lacks 18 amino acids at the C-terminal end [79]. Both of them are expressed in epithelial cells of CP and transport TH, with the former locating at the basolateral plasma membrane while the latter at the apical and/or sub-apical membranes [79].

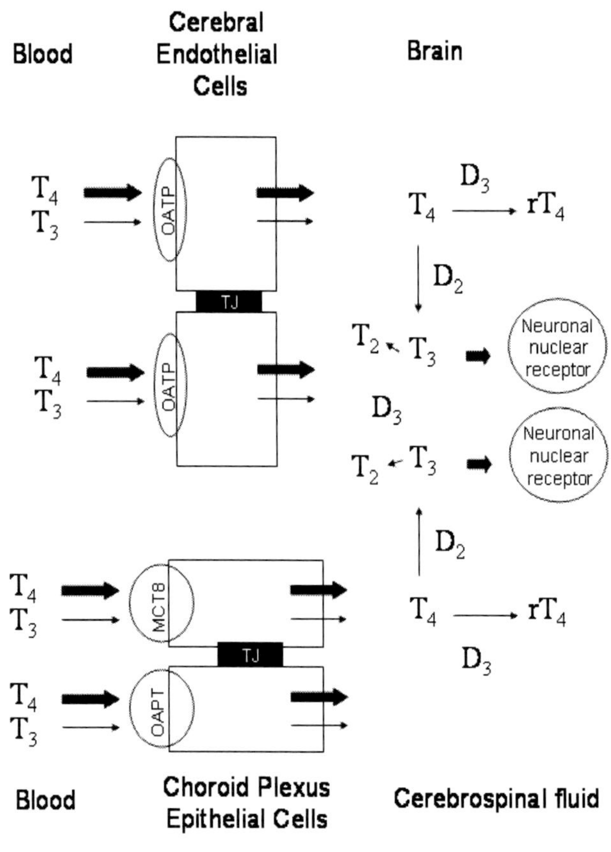

Figure 1. TH is transported through the BBB (OATP) or BCB (OATP and MCT8). In most cases the transport could be bi-directional, although only one direction is shown.

3.2. Monocarboxylate Transport (MCT)

The MCT family comprises up to 14 members, some of which are involved in the transport of important substrates for the brain such as lactate and pyruvate. Among them, MCT8 and MCT10 have been shown to facilitate TH transport in an active and specific way [81]. MCT8 highly expressed in the CP [82], as well as in neurons of the neocortex, hippocampus, basal ganglia et al, all regions known to be sensible to TH [83]. MCT8 has been shown to act as a specific transporter for T_4 and T_3, and displays slightly higher affinity for T_3 [84]. The significance of MCT8 is further confirmed when mutations in MCT8 in humans known as the Allen-Herndon-Dudley syndrome [85-88]. The syndrome affects boys from an early age as the gene coding for MCT8 is located on the X chromosome and consists of severe developmental delay and neurological damage [89,90]. These patients presented low total and free T_4, high total and free T_3, and low rT_3 [91,92]. The accumulation of T_3 in blood could be assumed as its poor uptake in cells [30]. In MCT8-null mice, there were significantly higher T_3 (to 205% of control values) and less T_4 (to 34% of control values) in serum, which mimic abnormal TH concentrations in the Allen-Herndon-Dudley syndrome patients' serum [93]. CNS development is only partially affected in these mice which were indistinguishable from their wild-type or heterozygous littermate [93]. The authors suggest "that the neuronal MCT8 deficiency might well be compensated for by other TH transporters more prominent in mice than in humans, thereby protecting MCT8-null mice from the neurological deficits observed in humans" [93]. In MCT family, MCT10 shares most homology with MCT8: the amino acid identity between them is 49% [94]. MCT10 transports both TH[81] and aromatic amino acids [95-99]. MCT10 is also called the T-type amino acid transporter [81]. MCT10 is more effective for cellular efflux than in the uptake of these ligands [94,100].

3.3. Amino Acid Transporters

As TH is built from two tyrosine residues, it is reasonable to suggest that amino acid transporters may also be involved in the transport of TH. A variety of cells, e.g. cardiomyocytes [101], astrocytes [102], rat pituitary cells [103], erythrocytes [95,96], show competition between T_3 uptake and neutral amino acids such as leucine and tryptophan, suggesting that the TH uptake may involve System L and System T amino acid transporters [104]. System L is a Na^+-independent, 2-aminoendobicyclo-[2,2,1]-heptane-2-carboxylic acid (BCH) sensitive, bi-directional large neutral amino acid transporter (LAT) responsible for the transport of large and small neutral amino acid [105,106]. Four proteins that induce system L activity has recently been identified as LAT1-4 [107-109]. The first two (LAT1, LAT2) are members of the SLC (solute carrier) 7 family [110-113]. The proteins form heteromeric complexes via a disulfide bond with the heavy chain of 4F2 antigen (4F2hc, SLC3A2) or CD98 [110,111], a protein essential for the functional expression of LAT1 and LAT2 at the plasma membrane [112,113]. LAT3 and LAT4 showing the biochemical properties of System L have a monomeric structure and do not require 4F2hc to express functional activity [108,109]. LAT1 is a ubiquitous plasma membrane transporter with a high affinity for large neutral amino acids with Km values in the μM range [106,113,114]. In the brain, LAT1 expression is found predominantly in the endothelial cells forming the BBB [115-117]. LAT2 had less affinity for large neutral amino acids with Km values in the mM range [114] but displays a broader substrate selectivity range than LAT1, accepting also some smaller amino acids such as alanine and glycine [113]. LAT2 was also found in rat brain endothelia cells [114]. To our knowledge, there is not any report on LAT3 and LAT4 in brain endothelial cells. Both T_4 and T_3 are substrates for LAT1 and LAT2 with a slight preference for T_3 [118,119]. System T is a plasma membrane amino acid transport system mediating the Na^+-independent transport of aromatic amino acids (TAT) [105]. In 1990s, specific interaction between cellular uptake of T_3 and Tryptophan in a number of tissues were observed [95-99]. Recently one such TAT termed "TAT1" that is a predicted 514-amino-acid protein with 12 putative transmembrane domains has been characterized in rats and humans [120,121]. TAT1 is also known as MCT10 (SLC16A10), because of its homology with other members of the MCT [81,122]. TAT1 is expressed strongly in intestine, placenta and liver in rat, whereas in humans skeletal muscle and kidney are the major sites of the expression with lower amounts in heart, placenta, intestine [120,121], and is not found in BBB or BCB [94].

4. TH Efflux System

In addition to the entry into brain, the export of TH from brain is also an important factor in the regulation of TH homeostasis in the CNS. The ligand accumulation in the brain after crossing BBB and BCB can be restricted by a number of mechanisms including passive efflux from parenchyma into the CSF by bulk flow, degradation [123], and active efflux transport including mechanisms dependent on the ATP-binding cassette (ABC) transporter superfamily [124]. ABC transporters are known to play a crucial role in the development of multidrug resistance (MDR) [124]. Of them, P-glycoprotein (P-gp), multidrug resistance-related protein (MRP) 1-6 and breast cancer resistance protein (BCRP) are expressed at BBB and BCB [125]. P-gp also called ABCB1 or MDR1 is a 170 kDa plasma membrane protein [126]. P-gp is responsible for the efflux of many drugs and its absence in Mdr1a knock out mice results in elevated drug levels in many tissues especially in the brain [124,127,128]. MRP has many functional similarities with P-gp (e.g. overlapping substrate specificities) even they posses 15% amino acid homology [124]. BCRP, also called ABCG2, has similar tissue distribution with that of P-gp [129]. At BBB, BCRP is more strongly expressed than P-gp or MRP1 [130]. The role of P-gp and other MRPs in the transport of xenobiotics from the CSF to blood also has been reported [131]. Verapamil, which is a potential but not special inhibitor of P-gp [132] [133], significantly reduced TH export from rat FRTL-5 thyroid cells and mouse NIH-3T3 cells [134]. Direct evidence the P-gp exports TH from cells was later found in mdr1 cDNA transfected cell line-MDCKII-MDR [135]. In brain, we reported the existence of a saturable efflux mechanism for TH [65], which was sensitive to number of ligands such as verapamil, probenecid, BCH but not indomethacin in rabbit ventricle-cistern (V-C) perfusion [66]. P-gp has been suggested to be located at the luminal (blood) side of the BBB [136] and at the apical or subapical (CSF) face of the CP [131,137]. The accumulation of T_4 in both brain tissues and the CP after verapamil administration in our study is consistent with the suggestion that P-gp transfers substrates from brain to blood and from the CP into the relatively large volume of the CSF [124]. P-gp could therefore contribute to the maintenance of the high level of T_4 in the CSF [138] by 'recycling' T_4. In contrast, the mrp1 inhibitor indomethacin does not have any effect on T_4 accumulation in the CP, reinforcing the notion that P-gp is a main efflux transport protein in the brain [66]. Probenecid, a prototypical inhibitor of OATP at BBB and BCB [139], is also able to reduce the TH efflux from the brain suggesting a role for OATP transport in the TH efflux which are known to be expressed on both sided of the CP [140]. BCH, a typical inhibitor of amino acid transport "L" system at BBB and BCB [114-116], reduced T_4 leaving the perfusate and increased T_4 accumulation in CP indicating that the TH efflux from the ventricles competes with "L" system (unpublished results).

5. The Roles of Thyroxine Binding Proteins

So far we have considered free TH transport across brain barriers via a number of transporters. However, the vast majority of TH in the serum are bound to proteins, including serum albumin (ALB), transthyretin (TTR), thyroxine-binding protein (TBG) and a number of lipoproteins [2]. In human, only about 0.04 % T_4 and 0.19 % T_3 are free in the plasma [141] and free TH concentrations are in picomolar range. Thyroxine has different affinities for the plasma binding proteins, which shield the molecules from their hydrophobic environment. TTR and TGB have similar affinities to T_4 (ca 5-9 x 10^{-8}M) [142], while ALB has the lowest affinity to T_4 (ca 7 x 10^{-5}M) (Table 2). The affinity for T_3 is reported to be the same order of magnitude, but in each case is slightly lower than that for T_4, being approximately 5 x 10^{-8} M for TBG, 1 x 10^{-7} M for TTR, and 1 x 10^{-5} M for ALB [142]. In plasma, ALB is the most abundant protein at 640 μM (40,000 mgL^{-1}) with TTR 4.6 μM and TBG 0.27 μM [143]. TBG is estimated to carry 65% of bound T_4, and 80% of T_3, whereas TTR carries 15% of T_4, and 9% of T_3 and ALB has 20% of T_4 and 11% of T_3 [144]. Schreiber et al estimated that in humans approximately 1 in 30,000 molecules of plasma ALB has 1 T_4 molecule bound to it, compared to 1 in 300 molecules of TTR and 1 in 3 molecules of TBG [145]. In CSF, the total protein is approximately 250 times less than in blood. ALB is still the most abundant protein in CSF at 2.3 μM (155 mgL^{-1}). But TTR assumes more important in CSF since it is around 200 times more abundant that TGB compared to about 20 times in plasma. Therefore the main binding proteins for the TH in CSF are TTR and ALB although both in lower concentrations compared to plasma (Table 2) [146].

These TH binding proteins maintain the large extrathyroidal pool of TH which can be librated with great rapidity for entry into cells, ensure a constant supply of TH to the cells and tissues by preventing urinary loss [149], protect the organism against abrupt changes in TH production and degradation and iodine deficiency [150]. Liver perfusion studies suggest that these binding proteins facilitate an even distribution of ^{125}I-T_4 and prevent the initial loss of T_4 [151]. Exposure to polychlorinated biphenyls which are potential ligands for TTR having 50-fold greater affinity than T_4 [142] alter TH homeostasis mostly decreasing serum levels of TH, particularly T_4 [152]. Since wide fluctuations in binding protein concentrations do not influence the thyroid functional status of the individual to any large degree [153], their function is open to speculation.

Table 2. Some properties and metabolic parameters of the principal TH binding protein in serum and CSF

	TBG	TTR	ALB
Molecular weight (kDa)	54	55	66.6
Structure	monomer	tetramer	monomer
Carbohydrate content (%)	20	-	-
Number of binding sites for TH	1	2	several
Association constant, Ka (M^{-1})			
For T_4 [142]	5-9x10^8	5-9x10^8	7x10^5
For T_3 [142]	5x10^8	1x10^7	1x10^5
Concentration (μM/mg.L^{-1})			
In serum [143]	0.27/16	4.6/176	640/40,000
In CSF [146]	0.0028/0.166	0.42/14.7	2.3/155
Relative distribution of TH (%)			
In serum			
T_4 [144]	65	15	20
T_3 [144]	80	9	11
In CSF			
T_4 [147]	-	80	-
In vivo survival			
Half-life (days) [148]	5	2	15
Degradation rate (mg.day^{-1}) [148]	15	650	17,000

5.1. Thyroxine-Binding Protein (TBG)

TBG is a 54 kDa glycoprotein synthesized in the liver and consists of a coding polypeptide chain of 415 amino acids [154]. TGB is the main TH transport protein in serum binding most TH due to its highest affinity although it has the least concentration in serum [155]. TBG concentration in the serum of normal adults range from 11 to 21 mg.L^{-1} (Table 2), 140-260 μg T_4.L^{-1} in terms of maximal T_4-binding capacity. Depending on species, TBG binds 60-90% of serum T_4 [152]. The TBG molecule has a single iodothyronine binding site with affinity slightly higher for T_4 than for T_3 [156]. TBG deficiency in humans does not interfere with euthyroid status suggesting that TTR is also important for T_4 transport in humans [157]. Variable amounts of TBG, though much smaller than those in serum, have been detected in amniotic fluid [158], CSF [159] and urine [160].

5.2. Transthyretin (TTR)

TTR is a highly conserved tetrameric protein of 55 kDa consisting of 4 identical subunits of 127 amino acids each with a central cleft which is the binding site for the TH [161]. TTR usually binds only one T_4 molecule because the binding affinity of the second site is greatly reduced through a negative cooperative effect [162]. The TTR tetramer can bind four molecules of retinal binding proteins that do not interfere with T_4 binding, and vice versa [163]. TTR is synthesized mainly in the liver and its concentration in serum is 176 $mg.L^{-1}$ (Table 2) corresponding to a maximal binding capacity of approximately 300 μg $T_4.dl^{-1}$. Changes in TTR concentration have relatively little effect on the serum concentration of serum iodothyronine [164,165]. There is a distinct reciprocal relationship between TGB and TTR concentration related to gender, age, glucocorticoids, estrogen and androgens [166-169].

TTR is also present in the CP and retina [145], and in the cytoplasm of ependymal cells of brain ventricles, within in contact with the apical membrane and cilia [170]. The CP contains 10 times more TTR mRNA in per gram of tissue than liver and secretes TTR at rate 13 times greater than liver [171,172]. TTR production accounts for at least 20% of all protein synthesised by the CPs in the rat [173]. TTR contributes approximately 50% of all secreted proteins into the CSF[172], and about 6% of total protein in CSF (~15 μg TTR mL^{-1} of CSF) [174], where it binds 80% of T_4 [147]. The secretion of TTR by the CP into CSF has been suggested to play a key role in the transfer of T_4 from the blood to the CSF, as a unidirectional secretion of TTR to the CSF may drive TH across BCB [175]. Dickson et al [58] proposed a model for T_4 transport from the bloodstream into CSF based on partitioning of T_4 between CP and surrounding fluid. This suggestion was supported by the results of *in vivo* studies in which ^{125}I-T_4 was injected intra-peritoneally into rats, and the transfer was reduced by addition of flavanoid EMD 21388, which could block the binding T_4 to TTR and subsequent T_4' entry in the CSF [31]. In an *in vitro* study, Southwell et al [176] suggested that T_4 might bind to TTR within the CP cells or with CSF, and the transport of T_4 is related to the concentration of TTR. Zheng et al [177] demonstrated that deposition of lead (Pb) in rat CP was associated with a significant reduction in TTR concentration in CSF and altered T_4 transport across the BCB. In a follow-up study on humans [178], he has shown that Pb exposure was associated with diminished TTR levels in the CSF and TTR was required for TH transport in the CSF and suggested that high levels of Pb in the environment could lead to mental retardation in young children. The effect of TTR on TH efflux from the CNS has been studied by us. In *in situ* CP perfusion, T_4 transport from CSF into blood was significantly reduced with TTR in a dose-dependent manner [179]. In *in vivo* V-C perfusion experiments, the binding of TTR to T_4 in the CSF compartment was also observed to prevent T_4 removal from CSF [65]. In addition, increased T_4 uptake into brain tissues were seen, probably due to elevated T_4 in CSF providing a concentration gradient favouring tissue uptake, and / or TTR-receptor mediated uptake and internalisation [180].

Despite a number of studies indicting the importance of TTR in TH transport in brain, mice lacking the TTR gene maintain normal functioning of thyroid glands in the face of significant reduction in total serum T_4 concentration [181,182]. Using the same model it was found that TTR was not essential for TH to reach the brain [183-186]. Alternatively, a number of researchers have supported the concept behind the involvement of TTR in the transport of TH, arguing that an alternative mechanism for T_4 transport may take over in TTR-null mice [178,187].

5.3. Albumin (ALB)

ALB is a 66.5 kDa protein composing 585 amino acids synthesized by the liver, contributing more than half of the total protein content in serum. As a result, it is the principal contributor to the maintenance of the colloid osmotic pressure [188]. ALB associates with a wide variety of substances including hormones and drugs possessing a hydrophobic region, and thus the association of TH to ALB can be viewed as non-specific. Of the several iodothyronine binding sites on the ALB molecule only one has a relatively high affinity for T_4 and T_3. Serum ALB has been suggested to have a key role in carrier-mediated TH transport through BBB in rat [189], which involves enhanced dissociation of TH from ALB as a result of transient conformation changes about the ligand binding site due to interaction of the serum protein with the surface of the microcirculation, possibly via surface receptors [190]. Similarly, ALB is reported markedly to stimulate T_3 uptake by MCT8 overexpressed in Xenopus oocytes [84]. However, even the most marked fluctuations of serum ALB concentration, including analbuminemia, have no significant effects in TH levels due to its low affinity [191]. In CSF, ALB has a similar role to TTR to maintain T_4 in isolated brain tissue incubation studies however higher concentrations of ALB were needed in order to exact a similar effect with TTR [179].

5.4. Lipoproteins

Lipoproteins binds T_4 and to some extent T_3, and the affinity for T_4 binding is similar to that of TTR [192,193]. These proteins are estimated to transport roughly 3% of the total T_4 and perhaps as much as 6% of the total T_3 in serum [194]. High density lipoprotein (HDL) is the major lipoprotein carrier for TH in human plasma, which account for ca 91% and 78% of the total lipoprotein binding of T_4 and T_3 respectively [195]. HDL do facilitate TH exit from hepatocytes and fibroblasts in a manner of non-specific and non-receptor mediated resembling cholesterol efflux [196]. At physiological levels, the magnitude of the effect of HDL is comparable to that of the three major plasma transport proteins [196]. Low-density lipoprotein (LDL) carries $< 1\%$ of total circulating T_4, and facilitates T_4 entry into LDL receptor competent human fibroblasts [197]. This is different from the three major proteins and HDL which prevent T_4 entry into fibroblasts in a dose-dependent fashion [192]. Because LDL receptors are ubiquitously expressed in the body, the implication is that LDL delivers T_4, in addition to cholesterol, to peripheral cells [196].

6. Conclusion

TH entry into CNS involves a variety of overlapping, but distinct transport mechanisms which serve to emphasize the importance of maintaining adequate TH in the brain. The system is robust so that knocking-out of one of the transport mechanisms the animals do not show any neurological disturbance. TH binding proteins could either be as storage molecules to buffer TH levels or chelators to reduce free TH. By working in coordination with each other, these proteins maintain TH brain homeostasis in brain in the face of plasma fluctuations and changing demand.

References

[1] Yen PM: Physiological and molecular basis of thyroid hormone action. *Physiol. Rev.* 2001;81:1097-1142.

[2] Hulbert AJ: Thyroid hormones and their effects: a new perspective. *Biol. Rev. Camb. Philos. Soc.* 2000;75:519-631.

[3] Heuer H: The importance of thyroid hormone transporters for brain development and function. *Best Pract. Res. Clin .Endocrinol. Metab.* 2007;21:265-276.

[4] Bianco AC, Salvatore D, Gereben B, Berry MJ, Larsen PR: Biochemistry, cellular and molecular biology, and physiological roles of the iodothyronine selenodeiodinases. *Endocr. Rev.* 2002;23:38-89.

[5] Kohrle J: Iodothyronine deiodinases. Methods Enzymol 2002;347:125-167.

[6] Guadano-Ferraz A, Obregon MJ, St Germain DL, Bernal J: The type 2 iodothyronine deiodinase is expressed primarily in glial cells in the neonatal rat brain. *Proc. Natl. Acad. Sci. U S A* 1997;94:10391-10396.

[7] Guadano-Ferraz A, Escamez MJ, Rausell E, Bernal J: Expression of type 2 iodothyronine deiodinase in hypothyroid rat brain indicates an important role of thyroid hormone in the development of specific primary sensory systems. *J. Neurosci.* 1999;19:3430-3439.

[8] Tu HM, Legradi G, Bartha T, Salvatore D, Lechan RM, Larsen PR: Regional expression of the type 3 iodothyronine deiodinase messenger ribonucleic acid in the rat central nervous system and its regulation by thyroid hormone. *Endocrinology* 1999;140:784-790.

[9] Bianco AC, Kim BW: Deiodinases: implications of the local control of thyroid hormone action. *J. Clin .Invest.* 2006;116:2571-2579.

[10] Oppenheimer JH, Schwartz HL, Mariash CN, Kinlaw WB, Wong NC, Freake HC: Advances in our understanding of thyroid hormone action at the cellular level. *Endocr. Rev.* 1987;8:288-308.

[11] Brent GA, Williams GR, Harney JW, Forman BM, Samuels HH, Moore DD, Larsen PR: Effects of varying the position of thyroid hormone response elements within the rat growth hormone promoter: implications for positive and negative regulation by 3,5,3'-triiodothyronine. *Mol. Endocrinol.* 1991;5:542-548.

[12] Yen PM, Ando S, Feng X, Liu Y, Maruvada P, Xia X: Thyroid hormone action at the cellular, genomic and target gene levels. *Mol. Cell Endocrinol.* 2006;246:121-127.
[13] Davis PJ, Leonard JL, Davis FB: Mechanisms of nongenomic actions of thyroid hormone. *Front Neuroendocrinol.* 2008;29:211-218.
[14] Sen L, Sakaguchi Y, Cui G: G protein modulates thyroid hormone-induced Na(+) channel activation in ventricular myocytes. *Am. J. Physiol. Heart Circ. Physiol.* 2002;283:H2119-2129.
[15] Hiroi Y, Kim HH, Ying H, Furuya F, Huang Z, Simoncini T, Noma K, Ueki K, Nguyen NH, Scanlan TS, Moskowitz MA, Cheng SY, Liao JK: Rapid nongenomic actions of thyroid hormone. *Proc. Natl. Acad. Sci. U S A* 2006;103:14104-14109.
[16] Silva JE: Thyroid hormone control of thermogenesis and energy balance. *Thyroid* 1995;5:481-492.
[17] Oppenheimer JH: Evolving concepts of thyroid hormone action. *Biochimie* 1999;81:539-543.
[18] Flamant F, Gauthier K, Samarut J: Thyroid hormones signaling is getting more complex: STORMs are coming. *Mol. Endocrinol.* 2007;21:321-333.
[19] Gruters A, Krude H: Update on the management of congenital hypothyroidism. *Horm. Res.* 2007;68 Suppl. 5:107-111.
[20] Kratzsch J, Pulzer F: Thyroid gland development and defects. Best Pract Res Clin. Endocrinol. Metab. 2008;22:57-75.
[21] Williams GR: Neurodevelopmental and neurophysiological actions of thyroid hormone. *J. Neuroendocrinol.* 2008;20:784-794.
[22] Zou L, Burmeister LA, Styren SD, Kochanek PM, DeKosky ST: Up-regulation of type 2 iodothyronine deiodinase mRNA in reactive astrocytes following traumatic brain injury in the rat. *J. Neurochem.* 1998;71:887-890.
[23] Bulens C: Neurologic complications of hyperthyroidism: remission of spastic paraplegia, dementia, and optic neuropathy. *Arch. Neurol.* 1981;38:669-670.
[24] Loosen PT: Effects of thyroid hormones on central nervous system in aging. *Psychoneuroendocrinology* 1992;17:355-374.
[25] Prinz PN, Scanlan JM, Vitaliano PP, Moe KE, Borson S, Toivola B, Merriam GR, Larsen LH, Reed HL: Thyroid hormones: positive relationships with cognition in healthy, euthyroid older men. *J. Gerontol. A Biol. Sci. Med. Sci.* 1999;54:M111-116.
[26] Volpato S, Guralnik JM, Fried LP, Remaley AT, Cappola AR, Launer LJ: Serum thyroxine level and cognitive decline in euthyroid older women. *Neurology* 2002;58:1055-1061.
[27] Kalmijn S, Mehta KM, Pols HA, Hofman A, Drexhage HA, Breteler MM: Subclinical hyperthyroidism and the risk of dementia. The Rotterdam study. *Clin. Endocrinol.* (Oxf) 2000;53:733-737.
[28] Smith CL, Granger CV: Hypothyroidism producing reversible dementia. A challenge for medical rehabilitation. *Am. J. Phys. Med. Rehabil.* 1992;71:28-30.
[29] Zhu DF, Wang ZX, Zhang DR, Pan ZL, He S, Hu XP, Chen XC, Zhou JN: fMRI revealed neural substrate for reversible working memory dysfunction in subclinical hypothyroidism. *Brain* 2006;129:2923-2930.

[30] Bernal J: The significance of thyroid hormone transporters in the brain. *Endocrinology* 2005;146:1698-1700.

[31] Chanoine JP, Alex S, Fang SL, Stone S, Leonard JL, Korhle J, Braverman LE: Role of transthyretin in the transport of thyroxine from the blood to the choroid plexus, the cerebrospinal fluid, and the brain. *Endocrinology* 1992;130:933-938.

[32] Dratman MB, Crutchfield FL, Schoenhoff MB: Transport of iodothyronines from bloodstream to brain: contributions by blood:brain and choroid plexus:cerebrospinal fluid barriers. *Brain Res.* 1991;554:229-236.

[33] Dejana E: Endothelial cell-cell junctions: happy together. *Nat. Rev. Mol. Cell Biol.* 2004;5:261-270.

[34] Wolburg H, Lippoldt A: Tight junctions of the blood-brain barrier: development, composition and regulation. *Vascul. Pharmacol.* 2002;38:323-337.

[35] Hawkins BT, Davis TP: The blood-brain barrier/neurovascular unit in health and disease. *Pharmacol. Rev.* 2005;57:173-185.

[36] Kniesel U, Wolburg H: Tight junctions of the blood-brain barrier. *Cell. Mol. Neurobiol.* 2000;20:57-76.

[37] Furuse M, Fujita K, Hiiragi T, Fujimoto K, Tsukita S: Claudin-1 and -2: novel integral membrane proteins localizing at tight junctions with no sequence similarity to occludin. *J. Cell Biol.* 1998;141:1539-1550.

[38] Furuse M, Hirase T, Itoh M, Nagafuchi A, Yonemura S, Tsukita S, Tsukita S: Occludin: a novel integral membrane protein localizing at tight junctions. *J. Cell Biol.* 1993;123:1777-1788.

[39] Ando-Akatsuka Y, Saitou M, Hirase T, Kishi M, Sakakibara A, Itoh M, Yonemura S, Furuse M, Tsukita S: Interspecies diversity of the occludin sequence: cDNA cloning of human, mouse, dog, and rat-kangaroo homologues. *J. Cell Biol.* 1996;133:43-47.

[40] Martin-Padura I, Lostaglio S, Schneemann M, Williams L, Romano M, Fruscella P, Panzeri C, Stoppacciaro A, Ruco L, Villa A, Simmons D, Dejana E: Junctional adhesion molecule, a novel member of the immunoglobulin superfamily that distributes at intercellular junctions and modulates monocyte transmigration. *J. Cell Biol.* 1998;142:117-127.

[41] Stevenson BR, Siliciano JD, Mooseker MS, Goodenough DA: Identification of ZO-1: a high molecular weight polypeptide associated with the tight junction (zonula occludens) in a variety of epithelia. *J. Cell Biol.* 1986;103:755-766.

[42] Haskins J, Gu L, Wittchen ES, Hibbard J, Stevenson BR: ZO-3, a novel member of the MAGUK protein family found at the tight junction, interacts with ZO-1 and occludin. *J. Cell Biol.* 1998;141:199-208.

[43] Jesaitis LA, Goodenough DA: Molecular characterization and tissue distribution of ZO-2, a tight junction protein homologous to ZO-1 and the Drosophila discs-large tumor suppressor protein. *J. Cell Biol.* 1994;124:949-961.

[44] Balda MS, Anderson JM: Two classes of tight junctions are revealed by ZO-1 isoforms. *Am. J. Physiol.* 1993;264:C918-924.

[45] Citi S, Sabanay H, Kendrick-Jones J, Geiger B: Cingulin: characterization and localization. *J. Cell Sci.* 1989;93 (Pt 1):107-122.

[46] Abbott NJ, Ronnback L, Hansson E: Astrocyte-endothelial interactions at the blood-brain barrier. *Nat. Rev. Neurosci.* 2006;7:41-53.

[47] Begley DJ, Brightman MW: Structural and functional aspects of the blood-brain barrier. *Prog .Drug Res*. 2003;61:39-78.

[48] Wolburg H, Wolburg-Buchholz K, Liebner S, Engelhardt B: Claudin-1, claudin-2 and claudin-11 are present in tight junctions of choroid plexus epithelium of the mouse. *Neurosci. Lett.* 2001;307:77-80.

[49] Redzic ZB, Segal MB: The structure of the choroid plexus and the physiology of the choroid plexus epithelium. *Adv. Drug Deliv. Rev.* 2004;56:1695-1716.

[50] Zeuthen T, Wright EM: Epithelial potassium transport: tracer and electrophysiological studies in choroid plexus. *J. Membr. Biol.* 1981;60:105-128.

[51] Butt AM, Jones HC, Abbott NJ: Electrical resistance across the blood-brain barrier in anaesthetized rats: a developmental study. *J. Physiol.* 1990;429:47-62.

[52] Zheng W, Zhao Q, Graziano JH: Primary culture of choroidal epithelial cells: characterization of an in vitro model of blood-CSF barrier. *In Vitro Cell Dev. Biol. Anim.* 1998;34:40-45.

[53] Ohtsuki S, Terasaki T: Contribution of carrier-mediated transport systems to the blood-brain barrier as a supporting and protecting interface for the brain; importance for CNS drug discovery and development. *Pharm. Res.* 2007;24:1745-1758.

[54] Pardridge WM: Brain drug development and brain drug targeting. *Pharm. Res.* 2007;24:1729-1732.

[55] Zlokovic BV: The blood-brain barrier in health and chronic neurodegenerative disorders. *Neuron* 2008;57:178-201.

[56] Lai CS, Korytowski W, Niu CH, Cheng SY: Transverse motion of spin-labeled 3,3',5-triiodo-L-thyronine in phospholipid bilayers. *Biochem. Biophys. Res. Commun.* 1985;131:408-412.

[57] Banks WA, Kastin AJ, Michals EA: Transport of thyroxine across the blood-brain barrier is directed primarily from brain to blood in the mouse. *Life Sci.* 1985;37:2407-2414.

[58] Dickson PW, Aldred AR, Menting JG, Marley PD, Sawyer WH, Schreiber G: Thyroxine transport in choroid plexus. *J. Biol. Chem.* 1987;262:13907-13915.

[59] Francon J, Chantoux F, Blondeau JP: Carrier-mediated transport of thyroid hormones into rat glial cells in primary culture. *J. Neurochem.* 1989;53:1456-1463.

[60] Goncalves E, Lakshmanan M, Pontecorvi A, Robbins J: Thyroid hormone transport in a human glioma cell line. *Mol. Cell Endocrinol.* 1990;69:157-165.

[61] Beslin A, Chantoux F, Blondeau JP, Francon J: Relationship between the thyroid hormone transport system and the Na(+)-H+ exchanger in cultured rat brain astrocytes. *Endocrinology* 1995;136:5385-5390.

[62] Preston JE, Segal MB: Saturable uptake of [125I]L-triiodothyronine at the basolateral (blood) and apical (cerebrospinal fluid) sides of the isolated perfused sheep choroid plexus. *Brain Res.* 1992;592:84-90.

[63] Segal MB, Preston JE: The uptake of thyroxine by the isolated perfused choroid plexus of the sheep. *Adv. Exp. Med. Biol.* 1993;331:285-288.

[64] Preston J, Wilson M, Chen R: Aging of the choroid plexus and CSF system: implications for neurodegeneration. in Zheng W, Chodobski A (eds): The blood-cerebrospinal fluid barrier. New York: Taylor and Francis Group, 2005, vol 14, 361-376.

[65] Kassem NA, Deane R, Segal MB, Preston JE: Role of transthyretin in thyroxine transfer from cerebrospinal fluid to brain and choroid plexus. *Am. J. Physiol. Regul. Integr. Comp. Physiol.* 2006;291:R1310-1315.

[66] Kassem NA, Deane R, Segal MB, Chen R, Preston JE: Thyroxine (T4) transfer from CSF to choroid plexus and ventricular brain regions in rabbit: contributory role of P-glycoprotein and organic anion transporting polypeptides. *Brain Res.* 2007;1181:44-50.

[67] Hennemann G, Docter R, Friesema EC, de Jong M, Krenning EP, Visser TJ: Plasma membrane transport of thyroid hormones and its role in thyroid hormone metabolism and bioavailability. *Endocr. Rev.* 2001;22:451-476.

[68] Friesema EC, Jansen J, Milici C, Visser TJ: Thyroid hormone transporters. *Vitam. Horm.* 2005;70:137-167.

[69] Jansen J, Friesema EC, Milici C, Visser TJ: Thyroid hormone transporters in health and disease. *Thyroid* 2005;15:757-768.

[70] Friesema EC, Docter R, Moerings EP, Stieger B, Hagenbuch B, Meier PJ, Krenning EP, Hennemann G, Visser TJ: Identification of thyroid hormone transporters. *Biochem. Biophys. Res. Commun.* 1999;254:497-501.

[71] van der Putten HH, Friesema EC, Abumrad NA, Everts ME, Visser TJ: Thyroid hormone transport by the rat fatty acid translocase. *Endocrinology* 2003;144:1315-1323.

[72] Visser WE, Friesema EC, Jansen J, Visser TJ: Thyroid hormone transport in and out of cells. *Trends Endocrinol. Metab.* 2008;19:50-56.

[73] Abe T, Suzuki T, Unno M, Tokui T, Ito S: Thyroid hormone transporters: recent advances. *Trends Endocrinol. Metab.* 2002;13:215-220.

[74] Hagenbuch B, Meier PJ: Organic anion transporting polypeptides of the OATP/ SLC21 family: phylogenetic classification as OATP/ SLCO superfamily, new nomenclature and molecular/functional properties. Pflugers Arch 2004;447:653-665.

[75] Hagenbuch B: Cellular entry of thyroid hormones by organic anion transporting polypeptides. *Best Pract .Res. Clin. Endocrinol. Metab.* 2007;21:209-221.

[76] Gao B, Hagenbuch B, Kullak-Ublick GA, Benke D, Aguzzi A, Meier PJ: Organic anion-transporting polypeptides mediate transport of opioid peptides across blood-brain barrier. *J. Pharmacol. Exp. Ther.* 2000;294:73-79.

[77] Pizzagalli F, Hagenbuch B, Stieger B, Klenk U, Folkers G, Meier PJ: Identification of a novel human organic anion transporting polypeptide as a high affinity thyroxine transporter. *Mol. Endocrinol.* 2002;16:2283-2296.

[78] Lee W, Glaeser H, Smith LH, Roberts RL, Moeckel GW, Gervasini G, Leake BF, Kim RB: Polymorphisms in human organic anion-transporting polypeptide 1A2 (OATP1A2): implications for altered drug disposition and central nervous system drug entry. *J. Biol. Chem.* 2005;280:9610-9617.

[79] Huber RD, Gao B, Sidler Pfandler MA, Zhang-Fu W, Leuthold S, Hagenbuch B, Folkers G, Meier PJ, Stieger B: Characterization of two splice variants of human

organic anion transporting polypeptide 3A1 isolated from human brain. *Am. J. Physiol. Cell Physiol.* 2007;292:C795-806.

[80] Fujiwara K, Adachi H, Nishio T, Unno M, Tokui T, Okabe M, Onogawa T, Suzuki T, Asano N, Tanemoto M, Seki M, Shiiba K, Suzuki M, Kondo Y, Nunoki K, Shimosegawa T, Iinuma K, Ito S, Matsuno S, Abe T: Identification of thyroid hormone transporters in humans: different molecules are involved in a tissue-specific manner. *Endocrinology* 2001;142:2005-2012.

[81] Visser WE, Friesema EC, Jansen J, Visser TJ: Thyroid hormone transport by monocarboxylate transporters. *Best. Pract. Res. Clin. Endocrinol. Metab.* 2007;21:223-236.

[82] Heuer H, Maier MK, Iden S, Mittag J, Friesema EC, Visser TJ, Bauer K: The monocarboxylate transporter 8 linked to human psychomotor retardation is highly expressed in thyroid hormone-sensitive neuron populations. *Endocrinology* 2005;146:1701-1706.

[83] Bernal J: Action of thyroid hormone in brain. J Endocrinol Invest 2002;25:268-288.

[84] Friesema EC, Ganguly S, Abdalla A, Manning Fox JE, Halestrap AP, Visser TJ: Identification of monocarboxylate transporter 8 as a specific thyroid hormone transporter. *J. Biol. Chem.* 2003;278:40128-40135.

[85] Allen W, Herndon C, Dudley F: Some examples of the inheritance of mental deficiency: apparently sex-linked idiocy and microcephaly. *Am. J. Mental. Defic.* 1944;48:325-334.

[86] Dumitrescu AM, Liao XH, Best TB, Brockmann K, Refetoff S: A novel syndrome combining thyroid and neurological abnormalities is associated with mutations in a monocarboxylate transporter gene. *Am. J. Hum. Genet.* 2004;74:168-175.

[87] Friesema EC, Grueters A, Biebermann H, Krude H, von Moers A, Reeser M, Barrett TG, Mancilla EE, Svensson J, Kester MH, Kuiper GG, Balkassmi S, Uitterlinden AG, Koehrle J, Rodien P, Halestrap AP, Visser TJ: Association between mutations in a thyroid hormone transporter and severe X-linked psychomotor retardation. *Lancet* 2004;364:1435-1437.

[88] Schwartz CE, May MM, Carpenter NJ, Rogers RC, Martin J, Bialer MG, Ward J, Sanabria J, Marsa S, Lewis JA, Echeverri R, Lubs HA, Voeller K, Simensen RJ, Stevenson RE: Allan-Herndon-Dudley syndrome and the monocarboxylate transporter 8 (MCT8) gene. *Am. J. Hum. Genet.* 2005;77:41-53.

[89] Schwartz CE, Stevenson RE: The MCT8 thyroid hormone transporter and Allan-Herndon-Dudley syndrome. *Best. Pract. Res. Clin. Endocrinol. Metab.* 2007;21:307-321.

[90] Jansen J, Friesema EC, Kester MH, Milici C, Reeser M, Gruters A, Barrett TG, Mancilla EE, Svensson J, Wemeau JL, Busi da Silva Canalli MH, Lundgren J, McEntagart ME, Hopper N, Arts WF, Visser TJ: Functional analysis of monocarboxylate transporter 8 mutations identified in patients with X-linked psychomotor retardation and elevated serum triiodothyronine. *J. Clin. Endocrinol. Metab.* 2007;92:2378-2381.

[91] Kakinuma H, Itoh M, Takahashi H: A novel mutation in the monocarboxylate transporter 8 gene in a boy with putamen lesions and low free T4 levels in cerebrospinal fluid. *J. Pediatr.* 2005;147:552-554.

[92] Herzovich V, Vaiani E, Marino R, Dratler G, Lazzati JM, Tilitzky S, Ramirez P, Iorcansky S, Rivarola MA, Belgorosky A: Unexpected peripheral markers of thyroid function in a patient with a novel mutation of the MCT8 thyroid hormone transporter gene. *Horm. Res.* 2007;67:1-6.

[93] Trajkovic M, Visser TJ, Mittag J, Horn S, Lukas J, Darras VM, Raivich G, Bauer K, Heuer H: Abnormal thyroid hormone metabolism in mice lacking the monocarboxylate transporter 8. *J. Clin. Invest.* 2007;117:627-635.

[94] Friesema EC, Jansen J, Jachtenberg JW, Visser WE, Kester MH, Visser TJ: Effective cellular uptake and efflux of thyroid hormone by human monocarboxylate transporter 10. *Mol. Endocrinol.* 2008;22:1357-1369.

[95] Zhou Y, Samson M, Osty J, Francon J, Blondeau JP: Evidence for a close link between the thyroid hormone transport system and the aromatic amino acid transport system T in erythrocytes. *J. Biol. Chem.* 1990;265:17000-17004.

[96] Zhou Y, Samson M, Francon J, Blondeau JP: Thyroid hormone concentrative uptake in rat erythrocytes. Involvement of the tryptophan transport system T in countertransport of tri-iodothyronine and aromatic amino acids. *Biochem. J.* 1992;281 (Pt 1):81-86.

[97] Kemp HF, Taylor PM: Interactions between thyroid hormone and tryptophan transport in rat liver are modulated by thyroid status. *Am. J. Physiol.* 1997;272:E809-816.

[98] Powell KA, Mitchell AM, Manley SW, Mortimer RH, Mortimer RH: Different transporters for tri-iodothyronine (T(3)) and thyroxine (T(4)) in the human choriocarcinoma cell line, JAR. *J. Endocrinol.* 2000;167:487-492.

[99] Ritchie JW, Collingwood CJ, Taylor PM: Effect of hypothyroidism on pathways for iodothyronine and tryptophan uptake into rat adipocytes. *Am. J. Physiol. Endocrinol.* Metab 2001;280:E254-259.

[100] Ramadan T, Camargo SM, Summa V, Hunziker P, Chesnov S, Pos KM, Verrey F: Basolateral aromatic amino acid transporter TAT1 (Slc16a10) functions as an efflux pathway. *J. Cell Physiol.* 2006;206:771-779.

[101] Everts ME, Verhoeven FA, Bezstarosti K, Moerings EP, Hennemann G, Visser TJ, Lamers JM: Uptake of thyroid hormones in neonatal rat cardiac myocytes. *Endocrinology* 1996;137:4235-4242.

[102] Blondeau JP, Beslin A, Chantoux F, Francon J: Triiodothyronine is a high-affinity inhibitor of amino acid transport system L1 in cultured astrocytes. *J. Neurochem.* 1993;60:1407-1413.

[103] Yan Z, Hinkle PM: Saturable, stereospecific transport of 3,5,3'-triiodo-L-thyronine and L-thyroxine into GH4C1 pituitary cells. *J. Biol. Chem.* 1993;268:20179-20184.

[104] Taylor PM, Ritchie JW: Tissue uptake of thyroid hormone by amino acid transporters. *Best .Pract. Res. Clin. Endocrinol. Metab.* 2007;21:237-251.

[105] Christensen HN: Role of amino acid transport and countertransport in nutrition and metabolism. *Physiol. Rev.* 1990;70:43-77.

[106] Omidi Y, Barar J, Ahmadian S, Heidari HR, Gumbleton M: Characterization and astrocytic modulation of system L transporters in brain microvasculature endothelial cells. *Cell Biochem. Funct.* 2008;26:381-391.

[107] Weissbach L, Handlogten ME, Christensen HN, Kilberg MS: Evidence for two Na+-independent neutral amino acid transport systems in primary cultures of rat hepatocytes. Time-dependent changes in activity. *J. Biol. Chem.* 1982;257:12006-12011.

[108] Babu E, Kanai Y, Chairoungdua A, Kim DK, Iribe Y, Tangtrongsup S, Jutabha P, Li Y, Ahmed N, Sakamoto S, Anzai N, Nagamori S, Endou H: Identification of a novel system L amino acid transporter structurally distinct from heterodimeric amino acid transporters. *J. Biol .Chem.* 2003;278:43838-43845.

[109] Bodoy S, Martin L, Zorzano A, Palacin M, Estevez R, Bertran J: Identification of LAT4, a novel amino acid transporter with system L activity. *J. Biol. Chem.* 2005;280:12002-12011.

[110] Mastroberardino L, Spindler B, Pfeiffer R, Skelly PJ, Loffing J, Shoemaker CB, Verrey F: Amino-acid transport by heterodimers of 4F2hc/CD98 and members of a permease family. *Nature* 1998;395:288-291.

[111] Kanai Y, Segawa H, Miyamoto K, Uchino H, Takeda E, Endou H: Expression cloning and characterization of a transporter for large neutral amino acids activated by the heavy chain of 4F2 antigen (CD98). *J. Biol. Chem.* 1998;273:23629-23632.

[112] Pineda M, Fernandez E, Torrents D, Estevez R, Lopez C, Camps M, Lloberas J, Zorzano A, Palacin M: Identification of a membrane protein, LAT-2, that Co-expresses with 4F2 heavy chain, an L-type amino acid transport activity with broad specificity for small and large zwitterionic amino acids. *J. Biol. Chem.* 1999;274:19738-19744.

[113] Segawa H, Fukasawa Y, Miyamoto K, Takeda E, Endou H, Kanai Y: Identification and functional characterization of a Na+-independent neutral amino acid transporter with broad substrate selectivity. *J. Biol. Chem.* 1999;274:19745-19751.

[114] Kido Y, Tamai I, Uchino H, Suzuki F, Sai Y, Tsuji A: Molecular and functional identification of large neutral amino acid transporters LAT1 and LAT2 and their pharmacological relevance at the blood-brain barrier. *J. Pharm. Pharmacol.* 2001;53:497-503.

[115] Boado RJ, Li JY, Nagaya M, Zhang C, Pardridge WM: Selective expression of the large neutral amino acid transporter at the blood-brain barrier. *Proc. Natl. Acad .Sci. U S A* 1999;96:12079-12084.

[116] Kageyama T, Nakamura M, Matsuo A, Yamasaki Y, Takakura Y, Hashida M, Kanai Y, Naito M, Tsuruo T, Minato N, Shimohama S: The 4F2hc/LAT1 complex transports L-DOPA across the blood-brain barrier. *Brain Res.* 2000;879:115-121.

[117] Duelli R, Enerson BE, Gerhart DZ, Drewes LR: Expression of large amino acid transporter LAT1 in rat brain endothelium. *J. Cereb. Blood Flow Metab.* 2000;20:1557-1562.

[118] Ritchie JW, Peter GJ, Shi YB, Taylor PM: Thyroid hormone transport by 4F2hc-IU12 heterodimers expressed in Xenopus oocytes. *J. Endocrinol.* 1999;163:R5-9.

[119] Friesema EC, Docter R, Moerings EP, Verrey F, Krenning EP, Hennemann G, Visser TJ: Thyroid hormone transport by the heterodimeric human system L amino acid transporter. *Endocrinology* 2001;142:4339-4348.
[120] Kim DK, Kanai Y, Chairoungdua A, Matsuo H, Cha SH, Endou H: Expression cloning of a Na+-independent aromatic amino acid transporter with structural similarity to H+/monocarboxylate transporters. *J. Biol. Chem.* 2001;276:17221-17228.
[121] Kim DK, Kanai Y, Matsuo H, Kim JY, Chairoungdua A, Kobayashi Y, Enomoto A, Cha SH, Goya T, Endou H: The human T-type amino acid transporter-1: characterization, gene organization, and chromosomal location. *Genomics* 2002;79:95-103.
[122] Halestrap AP, Meredith D: The SLC16 gene family-from monocarboxylate transporters (MCTs) to aromatic amino acid transporters and beyond. *Pflugers Arch* .2004;447:619-628.
[123] Ghersi-Egea JF, Leninger-Muller B, Suleman G, Siest G, Minn A: Localization of drug-metabolizing enzyme activities to blood-brain interfaces and circumventricular organs. *J. Neurochem.* 1994;62:1089-1096.
[124] Begley DJ: ABC transporters and the blood-brain barrier. *Curr. Pharm. Des.* 2004;10:1295-1312.
[125] Loscher W, Potschka H: Blood-brain barrier active efflux transporters: ATP-binding cassette gene family. *NeuroRx* 2005;2:86-98.
[126] Ling V: Multidrug resistance: molecular mechanisms and clinical relevance. Cancer *Chemother. Pharmacol.* 1997;40 Suppl:S3-8.
[127] Schinkel AH, Smit JJ, van Tellingen O, Beijnen JH, Wagenaar E, van Deemter L, Mol CA, van der Valk MA, Robanus-Maandag EC, te Riele HP, et al.: Disruption of the mouse mdr1a P-glycoprotein gene leads to a deficiency in the blood-brain barrier and to increased sensitivity to drugs. *Cell* 1994;77:491-502.
[128] Weiss J, Dormann SM, Martin-Facklam M, Kerpen CJ, Ketabi-Kiyanvash N, Haefeli WE: Inhibition of P-glycoprotein by newer antidepressants. *J. Pharmacol. Exp. Ther.* 2003;305:197-204.
[129] Schinkel AH, Jonker JW: Mammalian drug efflux transporters of the ATP binding cassette (ABC) family: an overview. *Adv. Drug Deliv. Rev.* 2003;55:3-29.
[130] Eisenblatter T, Huwel S, Galla HJ: Characterisation of the brain multidrug resistance protein (BMDP/ABCG2/BCRP) expressed at the blood-brain barrier. *Brain Res.* 2003;971:221-231.
[131] Rao VV, Dahlheimer JL, Bardgett ME, Snyder AZ, Finch RA, Sartorelli AC, Piwnica-Worms D: Choroid plexus epithelial expression of MDR1 P glycoprotein and multidrug resistance-associated protein contribute to the blood-cerebrospinal-fluid drug-permeability barrier. *Proc. Natl. Acad. Sci. U S A* 1999;96:3900-3905.
[132] Mickisch GH, Kossig J, Keilhauer G, Schlick E, Tschada RK, Alken PM: Effects of calcium antagonists in multidrug resistant primary human renal cell carcinomas. *Cancer* Res 1990;50:3670-3674.
[133] Barnes KM, Dickstein B, Cutler GB, Jr., Fojo T, Bates SE: Steroid treatment, accumulation, and antagonism of P-glycoprotein in multidrug-resistant cells. *Biochemistry* 1996;35:4820-4827.

[134] Cavalieri RR, Simeoni LA, Park SW, Baxter JD, Scharschmidt BF, Ribeiro RC, Lomri N: Thyroid hormone export in rat FRTL-5 thyroid cells and mouse NIH-3T3 cells is carrier-mediated, verapamil-sensitive, and stereospecific. *Endocrinology* 1999;140:4948-4954.

[135] Mitchell AM, Tom M, Mortimer RH: Thyroid hormone export from cells: contribution of P-glycoprotein. *J. Endocrinol.* 2005;185:93-98.

[136] Miller DS, Bauer B, Hartz AM: Modulation of P-glycoprotein at the blood-brain barrier: opportunities to improve central nervous system pharmacotherapy. *Pharmacol. Rev.* 2008;60:196-209.

[137] Baehr C, Reichel V, Fricker G: Choroid plexus epithelial monolayers--a cell culture model from porcine brain. *Cerebrospinal Fluid Res.* 2006;3:13.

[138] Hagen GA, Solberg LA, Jr.: Brain and cerebrospinal fluid permeability to intravenous thyroid hormones. *Endocrinology* 1974;95:1398-1410.

[139] Graff CL, Pollack GM: Drug transport at the blood-brain barrier and the choroid plexus. Curr Drug Metab 2004;5:95-108.

[140] Gao B, Meier PJ: Organic anion transport across the choroid plexus. *Microsc .Res. Tech.* 2001;52:60-64.

[141] Mendel CM, Cavalieri RR, Gavin LA, Pettersson T, Inoue M: Thyroxine transport and distribution in Nagase analbuminemic rats. *J. Clin. Invest.* 1989;83:143-148.

[142] Lans MC, Spiertz C, Brouwer A, Koeman JH: Different competition of thyroxine binding to transthyretin and thyroxine-binding globulin by hydroxy-PCBs, PCDDs and PCDFs. *Eur. J. Pharmacol.* 1994;270:129-136.

[143] Bartalena L, Robbins J: Thyroid hormone transport proteins. *Clin. Lab. Med.* 1993;13:583-598.

[144] Schussler GC: The thyroxine-binding proteins. *Thyroid* 2000;10:141-149.

[145] Schreiber G: The evolutionary and integrative roles of transthyretin in thyroid hormone homeostasis. *J. Endocrinol.* 2002;175:61-73.

[146] Braverman LE, Utiger RD: Werner and Ingbar's the Thyroid: A Fundamental and Clinical Text. Lippincott Williams and Wilkins, 2005.

[147] Herbert J, Wilcox JN, Pham KT, Fremeau RT, Jr., Zeviani M, Dwork A, Soprano DR, Makover A, Goodman DS, Zimmerman EA, et al.: Transthyretin: a choroid plexus-specific transport protein in human brain. The 1986 S. Weir Mitchell award. *Neurology* 1986;36:900-911.

[148] Hayashi Y RS: Genetic abnormalities of thyroid hormone transport serum proteins. . in Weintraub B (ed): Molecular endocrinology: Basic concepts and clinical correlations. New York: Raven Press, 1995, 371-387.

[149] Chan V, Besser GM, Landon J: Effects of oestrogen on urinary thyrosine excretion. *Br. Med. J.* 1972;4:699-701.

[150] Refetoff S, Robin NI, Fang VS: Parameters of thyroid function in serum of 16 selected vertebrate species: a study of PBI, serum T4, free T4, and the pattern of T4 and T3 binding to serum proteins. *Endocrinology* 1970;86:793-805.

[151] Mendel CM: Modeling thyroxine transport to liver: rejection of the "enhanced dissociation" hypothesis as applied to thyroxine. *Am. J. Physiol.* 1989;257:E764-771.

[152] Cheek AO, Kow K, Chen J, McLachlan JA: Potential mechanisms of thyroid disruption in humans: interaction of organochlorine compounds with thyroid receptor, transthyretin, and thyroid-binding globulin. *Environ. Health Perspect.* 1999;107:273-278.

[153] Refetoff S: Inherited thyroxine-binding globulin abnormalities in man. *Endocr. Rev.* 1989;10:275-293.

[154] Hayashi Y, Mori Y, Janssen OE, Sunthornthepvarakul T, Weiss RE, Takeda K, Weinberg M, Seo H, Bell GI, Refetoff S: Human thyroxine-binding globulin gene: complete sequence and transcriptional regulation. *Mol. Endocrinol.* 1993;7:1049-1060.

[155] Mannavola D, Vannucchi G, Fugazzola L, Cirello V, Campi I, Radetti G, Persani L, Refetoff S, Beck-Peccoz P: TBG deficiency: description of two novel mutations associated with complete TBG deficiency and review of the literature. *J. Mol. Med.* 2006;84:864-871.

[156] Hocman G: Human thyroxine binding globulin (TBG). *Rev. Physiol. Biochem. Pharmacol.* 1981;91:45-89.

[157] Larsson M, Pettersson T, Carlstrom A: Thyroid hormone binding in serum of 15 vertebrate species: isolation of thyroxine-binding globulin and prealbumin analogs. *Gen. Comp. Endocrinol.* 1985;58:360-375.

[158] Burman KD, Read J, Dimond RC, Strum D, Wright FD, Patow W, Earll JM, Wartofsky L: Measurement of 3,3',5'-Triiodothyroinine (reverse T3), 3,3'-L-diiodothyronine, T3 and T4 in human amniotic fluid and in cord and maternal serum. *J. Clin. Endocrinol. Metab.* 1976;43:1351-1359.

[159] Hagen GA, Elliott WJ: Transport of thyroid hormones in serum and cerebrospinal fluid. *J. Clin. Endocrinol. Metab.* 1973;37:415-422.

[160] Gavin LA, McMahon FA, Castle JN, Cavalieri RR: Detection of a thyroxine-binding protein physicochemically similar to serum thyroxine-binding globulin in normal human urine. *J. Clin. Endocrinol. Metab.* 1979;48:843-847.

[161] Sunde M, Richardson SJ, Chang L, Pettersson TM, Schreiber G, Blake CC: The crystal structure of transthyretin from chicken. *Eur. J. Biochem.* 1996;236:491-499.

[162] Irace G, Edelhoch H: Thyroxine-induced conformational changes in prealbumin. *Biochemistry* 1978;17:5729-5733.

[163] van Jaarsveld PP, Edelhoch H, Goodman DS, Robbins J: The interaction of human plasma retinol-binding protein and prealbumin. *J. Biol. Chem.* 1973;248:4698-4705.

[164] Woeber KA, Ingbar SH: The contribution of thyroxine-binding prealbumin to the binding of thyroxine in human serum, as assessed by immunoadsorption. *J. Clin. Invest.* 1968;47:1710-1721.

[165] Braverman LE, AvRuskin T, Cullen MJ, Vagenakis AG, Ingbar SH: Effects of norethandrolone on the transport and peripheral metabolism of thyroxine in patients lacking thyroxine-binding globulin. Observations on the physiological role of thyroxine-binding prealbumin. *J. Clin. Invest.* 1971;50:1644-1649.

[166] Braverman LW, Dawber NA, Ingbar SH: Observations concerning the binding of thyroid hormones in sera of normal subjects of varying ages. *J. Clin. Invest.* 1966;45:1273-1279.

[167] Braverman LE, Foster AE, Ingbar SH: Sex-related differences in the binding in serum of thyroid hormones. *J. Clin. Endocrinol. Metab.* 1967;27:227-232.

[168] Braverman LE, Ingbar SH: Effects of norethandrolone on the transport in serum and peripheral turnover of thyroxine. *J. Clin. Endocrinol. Metab.* 1967;27:389-396.

[169] Oppenheimer JH, Werner SC: Effect of prednisone on thyroxine-binding proteins. *J. Clin. Endocrinol. Metab.* 1966;26:715-721.

[170] Kuchler-Bopp S, Ittel ME, Dietrich JB, Reeber A, Zaepfel M, Delaunoy JP: The presence of transthyretin in rat ependymal cells is due to endocytosis and not synthesis. *Brain. Res.* 1998;793:219-230.

[171] Dickson PW, Schreiber G: High levels of messenger RNA for transthyretin (prealbumin) in human choroid plexus. *Neurosci. Lett.* 1986;66:311-315.

[172] Dickson PW, Aldred AR, Marley PD, Bannister D, Schreiber G: Rat choroid plexus specializes in the synthesis and the secretion of transthyretin (prealbumin). Regulation of transthyretin synthesis in choroid plexus is independent from that in liver. *J. Biol. Chem.* 1986;261:3475-3478.

[173] Fung WP, Thomas T, Dickson PW, Aldred AR, Milland J, Dziadek M, Power B, Hudson P, Schreiber G: Structure and expression of the rat transthyretin (prealbumin) gene. *J. Biol. Chem.* 1988;263:480-488.

[174] Chen RL, Athauda SB, Kassem NA, Zhang Y, Segal MB, Preston JE: Decrease of transthyretin synthesis at the blood-cerebrospinal fluid barrier of old sheep. *J. Gerontol. A Biol. Sci .Med. Sci.* 2005;60:852-858.

[175] Schreiber G, Aldred AR, Jaworowski A, Nilsson C, Achen MG, Segal MB: Thyroxine transport from blood to brain via transthyretin synthesis in choroid plexus. *Am. J. Physiol.* 1990;258:R338-345.

[176] Southwell BR, Duan W, Alcorn D, Brack C, Richardson SJ, Kohrle J, Schreiber G: Thyroxine transport to the brain: role of protein synthesis by the choroid plexus. *Endocrinology* 1993;133:2116-2126.

[177] Zheng W, Blaner WS, Zhao Q: Inhibition by lead of production and secretion of transthyretin in the choroid plexus: its relation to thyroxine transport at blood-CSF barrier. *Toxicol. Appl. Pharmacol.* 1999;155:24-31.

[178] Zheng W, Lu YM, Lu GY, Zhao Q, Cheung O, Blaner WS: Transthyretin, thyroxine, and retinol-binding protein in human cerebrospinal fluid: effect of lead exposure. *Toxicol .Sci.* 2001;61:107-114.

[179] Chen RL, Kassem NA, Preston JE: Dose-dependent transthyretin inhibition of T4 uptake from cerebrospinal fluid in sheep. *Neurosci. Lett.* 2006;396:7-11.

[180] Divino CM, Schussler GC: Receptor-mediated uptake and internalization of transthyretin. *J. Biol .Chem.* 1990;265:1425-1429.

[181] Episkopou V, Maeda S, Nishiguchi S, Shimada K, Gaitanaris GA, Gottesman ME, Robertson EJ: Disruption of the transthyretin gene results in mice with depressed levels of plasma retinol and thyroid hormone. *Proc. Natl. Acad. Sci. U S A* 1993;90:2375-2379.

[182] Palha JA, Episkopou V, Maeda S, Shimada K, Gottesman ME, Saraiva MJ: Thyroid hormone metabolism in a transthyretin-null mouse strain. *J. Biol. Chem.* 1994;269:33135-33139.

[183] Palha JA, Hays MT, Morreale de Escobar G, Episkopou V, Gottesman ME, Saraiva MJ: Transthyretin is not essential for thyroxine to reach the brain and other tissues in transthyretin-null mice. *Am. J. Physiol.* 1997;272:E485-493.

[184] Palha JA, Fernandes R, de Escobar GM, Episkopou V, Gottesman M, Saraiva MJ: Transthyretin regulates thyroid hormone levels in the choroid plexus, but not in the brain parenchyma: study in a transthyretin-null mouse model. *Endocrinology* 2000;141:3267-3272.

[185] Palha JA, Nissanov J, Fernandes R, Sousa JC, Bertrand L, Dratman MB, Morreale de Escobar G, Gottesman M, Saraiva MJ: Thyroid hormone distribution in the mouse brain: the role of transthyretin. *Neuroscience* 2002;113:837-847.

[186] Sousa JC, de Escobar GM, Oliveira P, Saraiva MJ, Palha JA: Transthyretin is not necessary for thyroid hormone metabolism in conditions of increased hormone demand. *J. Endocrinol.* 2005;187:257-266.

[187] Schreiber G, Richardson SJ, Prapunpoj P: Structure and expression of the transthyretin gene in the choroid plexus: a model for the study of the mechanism of evolution. *Microsc. Res. Tech.* 2001;52:21-30.

[188] Peters T, Jr.: Serum albumin. *Adv. Protein. Chem.* 1985;37:161-245.

[189] Pardridge WM: Carrier-mediated transport of thyroid hormones through the rat blood-brain barrier: primary role of albumin-bound hormone. *Endocrinology* 1979;105:605-612.

[190] Pardridge WM: Plasma protein-mediated transport of steroid and thyroid hormones. *Am. J. Physiol.* 1987;252:E157-164.

[191] Hollander CS, Bernstein G, Oppenheimer JH: Abnormalities of thyroxine binding in analbuminemia. *J. Clin. Endocrinol. Metab.* 1968;28:1064-1066.

[192] Benvenga S, Robbins J: Lipoprotein-thyroid hormone interactions. *Trends Endocrinol. Metab.* 1993;4:194-198.

[193] Freeman T, Pearson JD: The use of quantitative immunoelectrophoresis to investigate thyroxine-binding human serum proteins. *Clin. Chim. Acta* 1969;26:365-368.

[194] Refetoff S: Thyroid Disease Manager. In Chapter 3a. Thyroid hormone serum transport proteins: structure, Properties, Genes and Transcriptional Regulation. 2007.

[195] Benvenga S, Robbins J: Altered thyroid hormone binding to plasma lipoproteins in hypothyroidism. *Thyroid* 1996;6:595-600.

[196] Benvenga S, Robbins J: Thyroid hormone efflux from monolayer cultures of human fibroblasts and hepatocytes. Effect of lipoproteins and other thyroxine transport proteins. *Endocrinology* 1998;139:4311-4318.

[197] Benvenga S, Robbins J: Enhancement of thyroxine entry into low density lipoprotein (LDL) receptor-competent fibroblasts by LDL: an additional mode of entry of thyroxine into cells. *Endocrinology* 1990;126:933-941.

In: Thyroid Hormones: Functions, Related Diseases and Uses ISBN: 978-1-60741-080-5
Editors: F. S. Kuehn, M. P. Lozada

Chapter II

Markers of Thyroid Function

Juan Carlos Galofré*, Amelia Marí, Rosa Maria Príncipe and Javier Salvador

Department of Endocrinology. Clinica Universitaria
University of Navarra. Pamplona. Spain

Abstract

The assessment of the thyroid function has become a regular procedure in clinical practice as part of the check-up for routine health care. The diagnosis of thyroid dysfunction (TD) is initially accomplished on the basis of altered serum hormone levels: thyrotropin (TSH), thyroxine (T4), and triiodothyronine (T3). As our ability to detect ever more subtle degrees of TD has improved (with highly sensitive and specific assays), we are now dealing with a new medical problem. In clinical practice there are an increased number of subjects with a subtle deviation of serum TSH levels as the only alteration. This new group of patients has what is known as *subclinical* thyroid disease. Therefore TD is classified as: 1) *clinical* (TSH and thyroid hormones out of normal range) and 2) *subclinical* (isolated TSH alteration). Epidemiological studies have demonstrated that subclinical TD occurs more frequently than clinical TD. However, the management of subclinical TD is controversial and has been the subject of recurrent debates between thyroidologists. In line with this disagreement, there is no consensus on the TSH, free T4 and free T3 cutoff values at which treatment should be initiated in patients with subclinical TD.

In the background of this discussion are the limitations of the current diagnostic methods for detecting thyroid disease. In other words, it is difficult to define what normality is in this regard. From a physiological point of view we already know that normality (physiological homeostasis) is not equivalent to equality (the same) with regard to serum TH levels. The limitations of the diagnostic procedures are obvious to the extent that they cannot separate healthy outliers from those subjects who really have the disease. Serum TH levels alone do not explain the variability and severity of

---

* Address for correspondence: Dr Juan C Galofré, Department of Endocrinology, Clinica Universitaria Universidad de Navarra, Avda. Pio XII, 36, 31008 Pamplona (Spain), Tel: +34 948 255 400, E-mail: jcgalofre@unav.es.

symptoms observed in patients with TD. Therefore nowadays, it is not possible to determine which patients with subclinical TD will develop the typical complications of clinical dysfunction and which will see their mild elevations in TSH be auto-resolved.

Almost all corporal organs and systems are influenced by the metabolic activity of thyroid hormones (TH). Advances in physiology and molecular medicine have improved our understanding of the consequences of hormone action in target cells. A highly elaborate multi-step system regulates not only the synthesis of TH but their tissue action as well. Currently we are able to determine to some extent the cellular TH activity in different organs, which should be reflected in different biological markers. The ability to determine the activity of TH on target tissues will enable us to administrate the adequate supplementation dose of T4 more accurately, only to patients who need it, avoiding over-treatment.

I. Introduction

Thyroid hormones (TH) have a fundamental role in the metabolism and are active in every body organ and system, being essential for the correct function of all tissues. Thyroid dysfunction (TD) is currently diagnosed by the determination of Thyroid Stimulating Hormone (TSH) and thyroid hormone serum levels. Thyroid follicular cells secrete two hormones: thyroxin (T4) and triiodothyronine (T3) (1). The finding of a serum TSH concentration out of the normal range indicate the need of investigate the T3 and T4 serum levels. By definition T4 and T3 are within the normal range in subclinical TD. However, this approach, although its great practical value, has obvious limitations (2). It is not possible to assess the action of the hormones on the tissues or their peripheral biological effects.

Fortunately, over the recent years, the sensitivity of the diagnostic tests has been significantly improved, allowing the determination of plasma TSH and HT levels beyond what routine clinical practice requires. However, the principles for diagnosing thyroid diseases have barely changed over the past twenty years, in clear dissonance with the rapid progress experienced during this time by the molecular medicine (3-5). It was in the 80s when Evans and Vennstrom, by cloning the thyroid hormone receptors (TR), introduced the molecular age in the study of the thyroid. Despite the dramatic changes in this area, we are still unable to evaluate the impact of the variations of plasma HT at molecular level on target tissues. Moreover, we cannot distinguish when these variations are a systemic defense response mechanism or when correspond to pathological situations that should be treated. This limitation is not just a theoretical consideration. As a result of it, in many cases, we cannot determine the variability of each patient's response to a specific hormone situation. Therefore this problem is not an academic speculation, but a practical challenge in the daily clinical practice (6-9).

II. Current Methods for the Evaluation of Thyroid Function

1. The Laboratory

The results of various investigations carried out to obtain a diagnosis of TD have to be referred to its clinical context. The clinician should be aware of the limitations of each finding and the situations that may determine the presence of false positive or negative values. The appropriate choice of the test and its interpretation requires knowing the biochemistry and physiology of the thyroid.

At present, we do not have reliable methods to determine the action of TH on the tissues in a direct way. Therefore, the diagnosis is based on the measurement of plasma levels of the pituitary hormone that regulates the activity of the thyroid (TSH) and on the consequences of the actions of this hormone after stimulation in the gland: the serum concentration of T3 and T 4.

A. The Value of the Determination of TSH

TSH is secreted by pulses and follows a circadian rhythm as other pituitary hormones (10). This behavior is due to several factors, being many of them still not well known (11). It has been well described the positive regulation of the hypothalamic factor (TRH). There are other hormones with influence in the secretion of TSH like prolactin (PRL) and growth hormone (GH) that present a similar circadian rhythm as TSH, with increased levels at night and a nadir in the morning. Interestingly, both serotonin and somatostatin negatively regulate TSH, PRL and GH. However, differences exist between the pattern of secretion of PRL and TSH although both have in common their positive response to the TRH stimulus (12). TSH secretion curve shows a specular image to that of cortisol. It is known that cortisol negatively regulates TSH secretion, but it is unclear weather it has a direct influence on the TSH circadian rhythm (13). It is interesting that TSH rhythm runs parallel to leptin. Therefore both hormones have been related, especially in normal subjects and in those with leptin deficiency (14). Apparently only TSH rhythm is affected by serotonin, melatonin or alfa-adrenergic factors but these hormones do not interfere with TSH secretion. There exists a correlation between the rhythm of TSH and the rhythms of gonadotropins, which would support the existence of a common stimulating hypothalamic factor.

There are many cytokines and growth factors that influence on TSH secretion, which adds extra complexity to its regulation. In addition, stress, temperature, iatrogenic factors, nutritional status (15) and the presence of disease can also affect the secretion of TSH (16). Thus, the determination of TSH serum levels alone is not enough to discover rare diseases like the syndrome of resistance to TH or a secondary hypothyroidism (17,18), and has limitations in the diagnosis of other more common situations like low T3 syndrome or the in the assessment of thyroid function during pregnancy (19).

Nowadays we know the TSH stimulatory effect on the follicular cell, but other biological properties of TSH are still poorly explored. Interestingly TSH receptors have been described in other cells like white blood cells, adipocytes, fibroblasts, myocytes, etc. (20-21). It is well known that TH (T3 and T4) have a negative feedback on the TSH secretion. The TSH serum level follows an exponential pattern in relation to the values of T4. In this context it is important to notice that during the day TSH has significant variations in its plasma concentration while T3 and T4 barely change. The great difference in the half-life of these three hormones adds an extra complication in the regulation of Pituitary-Thyroid axis system. TSH half-life ranges around 15 - 30 minutes, while T3 half life is 24 hours. T4 life is much longer, lasting in serum more than a week. Additionally the physiological night TSH surge is blunted in primary hypothyroidism, although the average of TSH serum level is higher during the day when compared with normal subjects. It has also been described that the pulses breadth extent of the pulses of TSH is increased whereas the frequency remains unchanged (22).

The biological meaning of the TSH pulsatile secretion on the follicular cell can be explained by the variation in the response to different concentrations of TSH. The TSH receptor (TSH-R) has seven transmembrane segments with an extracellular aminoterminal end and intracytoplasmic carboxiterminal end. The extracellular domain, which contains 398 residues, is responsible for the high affinity of TSH to its receptor.

There is still one more element that contributes to the TSH relative value as an isolated indicator of thyroid function. The current biochemical tests are highly sensitive and have specificity over 90% for the thyroid function diagnosis, but they are not free from some degree of indetermination. The newest immunometric assays have an intra-assay coefficient of variation lower than 5% when TSH values are close or over 0.5 mU/L. Nevertheless this percentage rises to 15-50% when the values fall between 0.002 and 0.1 mU/mL. Moreover, these tests evaluate the immunogenic property of the hormone but not its bioactivity, and it is known that there are differences between these two parameters, especially in the case of hypothyroidism, where the pattern of glycosylation of the TSH is modified (23).

B. The Value of the Determination of Thyroid Hormones

The measurement of thyroid hormones serum levels is influenced by a number of factors. For instance, the determination of the hormonal free fraction may prevent the influence of the transport proteins. Moreover, as sated before, the information provided by TH blood levels may not translate the action of the hormone in the cell. Some examples of these facts are the low T3 syndrome, the alterations in the proteins transport, the thyroid hormone resistance syndrome, the subclinical dysfunction and the secondary hypothyroidism. Besides all this frequent situations, there are some drugs frequently used in clinical practice that can affect T3 and T4 levels (24). In addition, any process that affects the metabolism will be reflected by an adjustment in TH, although thyroid function may not be modified. The most common situation is the so-called Euthyroid Sick Syndrome (or low T3). The assays for to T3 and T4 measurements are not free of errors or intra-assay variations.

2. Subclinical Thyroid Dysfunction

The incidence of subclinical thyroid disease is significantly higher than overt dysfunction (25). Its diagnostic and therapeutic approach is not free of controversy, particularly in subjects that have slight increases in the value of TSH (3).

Subclinical hypothyroidism affects 10% of the population (7,26). The importance and potential causes of this entity are the subject of ongoing debate (4,5). The pathophysiological alteration of this situation is currently unknown, but the most accepted opinion is that in the majority of cases exists an autoimmune component. The natural history of the disease is variable, but tends to be benign (27).

Various categories of subjects can cause subclincal TD. 1) Patients with a previous history of thyroid disease (undertreated hypothyroidism or overtreated hyperthyroidism) that require therapeutic adjustments. 2) Outliers, which are clinically euthyroid despite they have the TSH serum levels beyond the reference range. These subjects are healthy and not require treatment. In most cases are seronegative (negative autoabtibodies). 3) Subclinical hypothyroidism, with no previous history of thyroid disease: these patients are at risk of develop overt thyroid disease in the future and probably require treatment. Generally are seropositive, but in some cases coexist a mild or incipient DT without an autoimmune component (5).

In clinical practice it is not possible differentiate subjects from group 2 and 3. For that reason, some patients with mild disease may remain untreated when they could probably benefit from treatment. On the other hand, in some situations, L-thyroxine may be administered to healthy subjects. At present, we do not have the method to differentiate these two groups. Therefore it may be difficult to avoid the complications associated with untreated subclinical hypothyroidism, while sometimes thyroid hormone can be administered to healthy patients who do not require the treatment causing unnecessary harm. A TSH level in the upper limit of the reference range can probably reflect a real dysfunction that causes true biological repercussion in some subjects (group 3), whereas the same value can be normal for other subjects, without pathological significance (group 2).

There is an overlapping between patients with real DT and normal outlier subjects. The difference between both groups could only be established by measuring the hormone action at cellular level or with parameters capable of detecting the inability of the thyroid gland to respond to an increased demand of T3 or T4. This idea is supported by the frequent clinical observation that some patients treated with L-T4 do not improve the psychological, mild psychiatric symptoms or the well-being sensation, despite the TSH levels reach the normal range. This treatment apparent lack of effectiveness can be attributed to several factors as the difficulty in losing weight, the lack of circadian rhythm of TSH, the inappropriate T3 supply, or alterations in the hypothalamic-pituitary sensitivity. Unfortunately, the lack of reliable data that could provide information on the tissue thyroid hormone impregnation makes impossible to establish the cause (28). For these reasons it is understandable that the indication to treat patients with subclinical thyroid dysfunction is controversial. The main reason pro treat these patients is preventing the progress toward clinical hypothyroidism, which improves the lipid profile reducing the cardiovascular risk. However, there is controversy about the usefulness of the treatment in the case of reverting dyslipidemia (29). Reasons against treatment can also be argue. Such are the risk of overdosing with its negative side effects (mainly osteopenia and atrial fibrillation). Probably, as previously discussed, this disagreement expresses the present impossibility to perform a correct diagnosis.

There is a remarkable controversy about the degree of complications derived from subclinical TD. This is because the results of different studies show conflicting data. The main disagreements are based on the importance of dyslipidemia (29-33), or the degree of heart disease associated to subclinical TD (34-38). This disparity of point of views probably reflects the limitation to discriminate the diverse entities that make up this disorder.

The previous data suggest, at least, that the limits of TSH normal values of should be revised. Nowadays, there are an increased number of clinicians that consider that the current TSH normal range is no longer useful and establish the pathological cutoff at a lower level. This measure would improve the sensitivity of TSH for detecting thyroid dysfunction, lowering however its specificity and increasing the margins of the debate (4,5,39).

The high prevalence of the thyroid disease justify, in opinion of some experts, the advice of testing thyroid function to every woman over 35 (and repeat it every 5 years), pregnant women and in men over 65 years (1,8). However, this diagnostic effort would not be able to differentiate the groups of subjects that have been previously described.

3. Clinical Diagnosis Indexes

In the mid fifties of the last century, the limited sensitivity of the tests used to determine the thyroid hormone serum levels, forced the clinicians to look for alternatives to adjust the diagnosis of their patients. Based on their clinical experience, they succeeded in designing scales of severity for each type of thyroid dysfunction. Somehow, they face with the same problem we have today, and they solved it in accordance to the tools at their disposal. Thus, in the classical manuals of Endocrinology, we can find a variety of clinical indexes with which it was intended to establish the severity of TD. At that time the methods for biochemical analysis of hormones were not sensitive enough. These clinical parameters have gradually fallen into disuse. However, it is likely that they could recover their usefulness at the present moment, since we see that the determination of a isolated serum hormone value does not reflect its tissue action. Therefore an auxiliary method able to inform us of the activity of these hormones is needed. The identification of these metabolic parameters may help in the diagnosis and orientate the response to treatment.

The Crooks index (40) has proven, since its publication in 1959, to be a good method for evaluating the thyroid hyperfunction. Ten years later the same authors published a scale of assessment of hypothyroidism (41). The delay between the publishing of the two indices is eloquent and reflects upon the difficulty in translating to numerical parameters a proteoform disease such as hypothyroidism. The method was not fully useful, that is why thirty years later Zulewski et al (42) published their proposal to improve it. This new scale reaches acceptable levels of correlation with TSH serum levels. Unfortunately its major limitation is the lack of consistency in assessing subclinical hypothyroidism.

Overall the clinical-diagnose Indexes are useful but lack the necessary sensitivity and specificity. They are not able to distinguish between clinical and subclinical disease. Their limitations are more pronounced in the assessment of hypothyroidism than hyperthyroidism. However they can be used to detect the systemic implications of hormonal action and probably as a complementary method to the biochemical evaluation.

The Index of Crooks et al (40) (Wayne (43) uses the same as Crooks) evaluate a number of parameters that correlate with the serum levels of total T4 and T3. The index provides a numerical scale according to the symptoms or signs observed in the patient (Table 1). The sum of points separate the subjects in euthyroid (<11 points) and hyperthyroid (> 19 points). The method is not clear for subjects who fall between 11 and 19 points. The implementation of this scale to assess hyperthyroid patients with Graves' disease provides a result of 24.3 +/- 4.6 points. It has also been seen that after the β-blockade the score is reduced to 14.3 +/- 5.9. The application to euthyroid subjects yield a score of 4.7 +/- 2.2. It is interesting to note that subjects with subclinical hyperthyroidism have differences when compared with controls. Similarly, the administration of β blockers agents lowers the score in hyperthyroid patients, showing their therapeutic effect. The Index has also provided data showing that hyperthyroid symptoms significantly change over age: the adrenergic symptoms are more prevalent in older age, while tachycardia, fatigue and weight loss are more frequent at younger age.

As previously mentioned, hypothyroidism can be evaluated thanks to the indexes of Billewicz et al (41) (Table 2) or even better, with the posterior modification done by Zulewski et al (42) (Table 3). The method woks in similar way: points are added or subtracted according to the presence of symptoms and signs, providing an overall assessment at the end. Its application depicts acceptable levels of correlation with the serum TSH values (62%), although are less sensitive than the Indexes for hyperthyroidsm. Unfortunately there are important inaccuracies when are used in patients with subclinical hypothyroidism. Published data indicate that patients with hypothyroidism usually reach scores over + 4. The score between - 29 and + 4 is classified as an unclear result. The authors determine that euthyroid subjects generally are below – 30.

Table 1. Crooks index: thyrotoxicosis clinical diagnosis index

CROOKS INDEX THYROTOXICOSIS CLINICAL DIAGNOSIS INDEX					
Symptoms			Signs		
	Present	Absent		Present	Absent
	Values			Values	
Effort dispnea	1		Palpable Thyroid	3	-3
Rest palpitations	2		Thyroid thrill	2	-2
Astenia	2		Exophthalmos	2	
Preference for heat		-5	Palpebral retraction	2	
Preference for cold	5		Eyelid lag	1	
Temperature indifference	0		Hiperkinetic movements	4	-2
Hyperhydrosis	3		Finger fine tremor	1	
Recent nervousness	2		Warm hands	2	-2
High appetite	3		Wet hands	1	-1
Low appetite		-3	Atrial fibrillation	4	
Weigh gain		-3	Rate <80		-3
Weigh loss	3		Rate 80-90	0	
			Rate >90	3	

Table 2. Billewicz index: hipothyroidsm clinical diagnosis index

BILLEWICZ INDEX HIPOTHYROIDSM CLINICAL DIAGNOSIS INDEX					
Symptoms			Signs		
	Present	Absent		Present	Absent
	Values			Values	
Cold intolerance	4	-5	Slow movements	11	-3
Dry hair	-2	2	Coarse skin	7	-7
Weigh gain	1	-1	Cold skin	3	-2
Constipation	2	-1	Periorbitary edema	4	-6
Hoarseness	5	-6	Heart rate	4	-4
Paresthesia	5	-4	Slow ancle reflex	15	-6
Deafness	2	0			

Table 3. Zulewski index: hipothyroidsm clinical diagnosis index

ZULEWSKI INDEX: HIPOTHYROIDSM CLINICAL DIAGNOSIS INDEX					
Symptoms			Signs		
	Present	Absent		Present	Absent
	Values			Values	
Sweetness reduction	1	0	Slow movements	1	0
Hoarseness	1	0	Slow ankle reflex	1	0
Paresthesia	1	0	Thick skin	1	0
Dry skin	1	0	Periorbitary edema	1	0
Constipation	1	0	Cold skin	1	0
Hearing loss	1	0			
Weigh gain	1	0			

III. Evaluation of Thyroid Hormone Tissue Activity

Almost all human cells express TH receptors, meaning that their action may influence the normal physiological cell function in every tissue (44,45). There are situations, apparently paradoxical, where TH serum concentration does not correlate with tissue activity. Additionally, different organs seem to respond individually to TH, what probably means that there are a variety of particular set of enzymes that metabolize the TH in different tissues. Furthermore, it has been identified several isoforms of TH receptor that are specific of each tissue (46).

The consequences of TH action on different organs can be deduced by the study of clinical manifestations of TD. The evaluation of these factors allows knowing the molecular consequences of TH action and the intensity of their biological function.

1. Peripheral Regulation of Thyroid Hormone Action

A. Deiodinases

Until now only three iodothyronine selenodeiodinases have been described: type I (D1), II (D2) and III (D3) (47). They have both different tissue action and distribution. D1 catalyzes the conversion from T4 to T3. It also can catalyze the T4 inactivation by its conversion to rT3, although this is not their usual activity. Besides this, D1 can inactivate T3 by conversion to T2. The enzyme is expressed mostly in liver, kidney and in less extent in thyroid. Its action contributes to the generation of the circulating T3. D2 catalyzes the conversion from T4 to T3. It can also convert rT3 in T2. D2 is responsible of the intracellular T3 production in the peripheral tissues. The substrate is for its action is circulating T4. D2 is expressed especially in the brain and the pituitary. D3 catalyzes the T4 deiodination by converting it to rT3, and also T3 to T2. Therefore this enzyme has an inhibitory action of the thyroid function. It is expressed mainly in placenta, brain and skin (figure 1). An adult synthesizes about 50 nmol of T3 daily. Around 20% of this quantity (~10 nmol) comes from the thyroid gland whereas the 80% is synthesized in peripheral extrathyroid tissues. Unfortunately, we still do not know the mechanisms that regulate the deiodinases activity in detail.

B. Thyroid Hormone Receptor

The principal TH intracellular action is to regulate the transcription of target genes. TH are liposoluble and enter passively into the cells, although there have been recently identified specific TH transporters. Once in the cytoplasm TH migrate to the nucleus where interact with their specific receptor (TR) (46). The ligand-receptor complex couples with the *thyroid hormone response elements* (TRE) that is located upstream from the promoter area of target genes where exerts a positive or negative regulation (figure 2).

TR belongs to the superfamily of the nuclear hormonal receptors. Its structure presents a central domain (where binds the DNA), a carboxiterminal end (for the union with the ligand) and the aminoterminal end (where interacts with the transcription factors). It has also been described that other nuclear proteins different from the TH can interact with the TRE, and act as regulators. The regulation may be negative (co-repressors) or positive (co-activators). These complexes act through the regulation of the local histone acetylation and interact with the basal transcriptional machinery (48). The T3 affinity for the TR is 10-fold higher than T4 and its efficacy is 10 times higher too. Nevertheless, there is a number of TH actions that are not mediated by the genetic action.

C. Thyroid Hormone Receptor Isoforms and Function

Two principal isoforms of TR has been described: TRα and TRβ. T3 couples to both receptors. Alternative splicing gives an additional heterogeneity to the TRs. The TRα

alternative splicing generates two proteins: TRα-1 and c-erbAα-2. The former does not couple to T3.

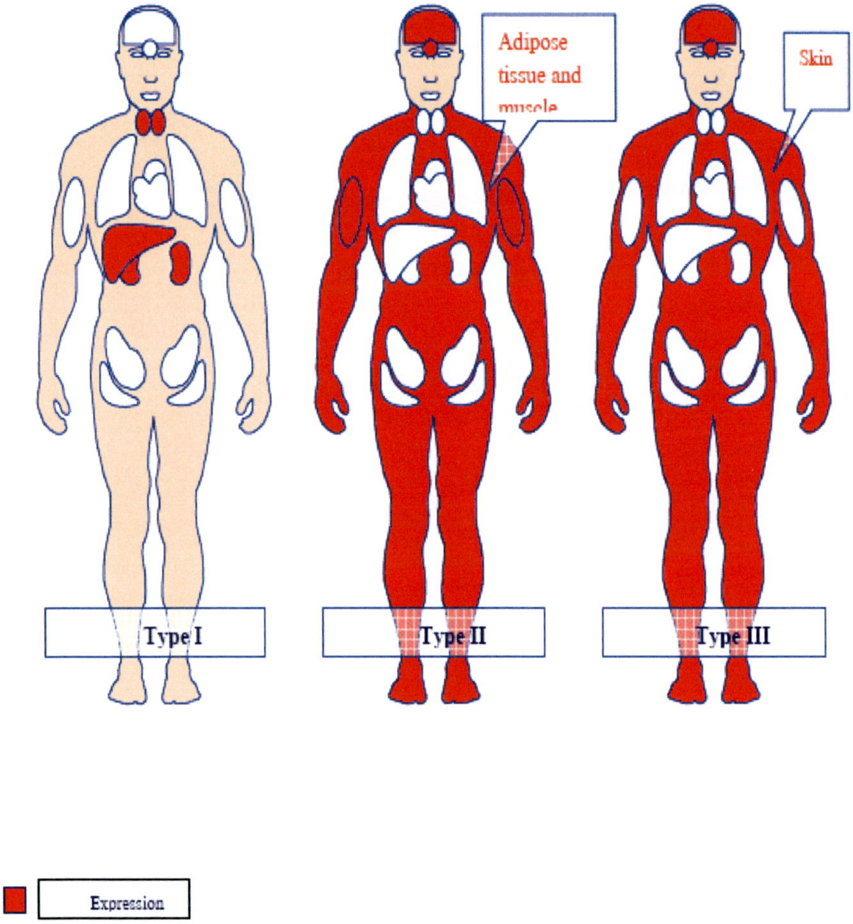

Figure 1.Tissue expression of different deiodinases is specific in each organ. D1, which is the main converter of T3 from circulating T4, is found mainly in thyroid gland, liver and kidney. D2 is responsible of intracellular T3 production from circulating T4 in peripheral tissues, hence its distribution is generalized. However, D3 expression is preponderant in pituitary, brain, muscle and adipose tissue. D3 inactivates T4 generating rT3 and is found mainly in skin and brain.

In addition c-erbAα-2 couples weakly to TREs and consequently cannot transactivate the response to TH. Therefore this TR isoform acts as an inhibitor of the TH action, possibly by competing for the TRE union. Likewise there are two TR derived from the TRβ. The gene has two promoter regions that, alternatively, codify for two different proteins: TRβ-1 and TRβ-2. The expression of both isoforms can be regulated by pituitary transcription factors like Pit-1. The studies that have been done until today have not found new isoforms, although their existence can not be excluded.

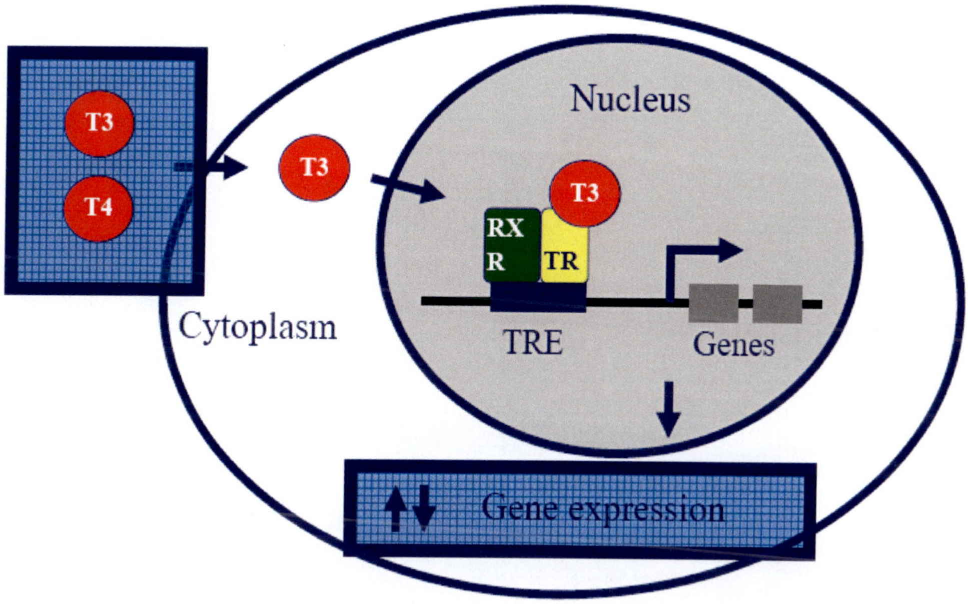

Figure 2.The central activity of thyroid hormones is the transcription regulation of the target genes. This effect is mediated by specific nuclear receptors (TR) with high affinity and specificity for thyroid hormones. T3 migrates to the nucleus after internalization into the cell, where is linked to TR. The complex T3-TR is regulated by Thyroid hormone response elements (TRE) located in the promoting areas of target genes. The formation of complex ligand-LR-TRE is the first critical step to activate the positive or negative regulation of target genes and the subsequent regulation of protein synthesis.

It is plausible that some unknown isoforms may exist and act in a restrict way in some tissues or during some periods of the fetal life. The actual knowledge does not permit to assign a determinate function to each isoform.

It is known that specific receptors interact with several ligands, and moreover T3 can activate its own receptor in an agonist or antagonist direction, depending on the TR isoform subtype with which it interacts (46). This biological activity generates a rise in the expression of a number of proteins and some of them are very well known (6,49). The study of these proteins plasma concentration, as well as other TH activity indicators can be useful to distinguish healthy from unhealthy people, especially those who have borderline hormone serum levels. In the same way it can be also helpful the clinical indexes of thyroid activity (vid supra) (40-43).

D. Distribution

The expression of these receptors varies between the different tissues, what increases the complexity and diversity of TH action between different subjects and even in the same one. TRα-1 and TRβ-1 are expressed in tissues in an ubiquitous way, but TRα-1 is located firstly in muscle and in brown fat (in rodents), and TRβ-1 is expressed mainly in brain, liver and kidney although it is also found in almost all tissues. TRβ-2 is expressed in a specific way in pituitary and in specific hypothalamic areas, as well as in developing brain and internal ear. (Figure 3)

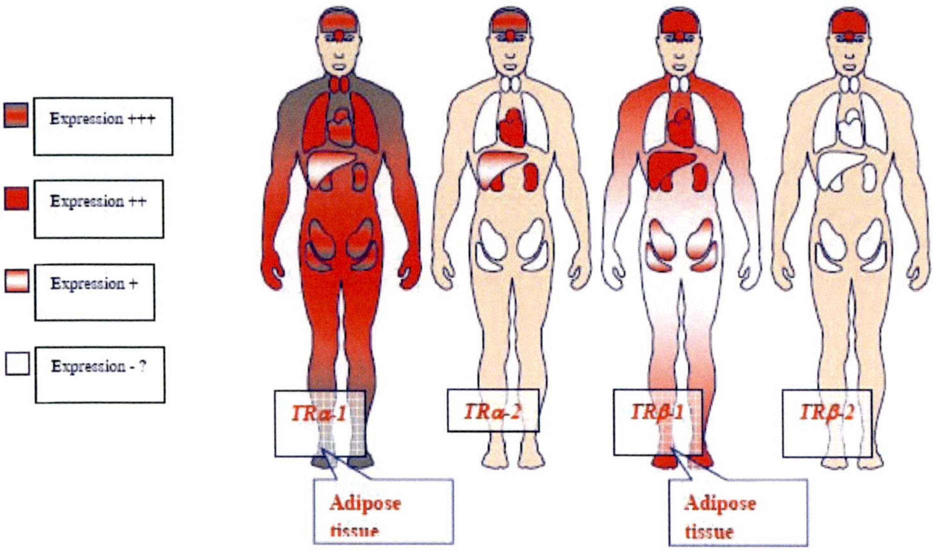

Figure 3. There are two main thyroid hormone receptors (TR): TRα y TRβ. The alternative RNA transcript splicing of TRα generates two proteins: TRα-1 y c-erbAα-2 (TRα-2). There is also two TR derived from TRβ: TRβ-1 y TRβ-2. TRα-1 is expressed principally in heart (is the main receptor in this organ), muscle, bone, and subcutaneous tissue, although is widely distributed in the whole body. TRα-2 is mainly found in brain, pituitary, kidney, heart, and liver. TRβ-1 is predominantly in brain, liver, kidney, and heart. TRβ-2 is specifically expressed in anterior pituitary, certain hypothalamic areas, developing brain and inner ear.

2. Indicators of Tissue Action

As mentioned before, the levels of circulating TH do not directly reflect its action in the cell. This is especially manifest in some situations as pregnancy, low T3 syndrome, alterations in transporter proteins, TH resistance syndromes, subclinical dysfunction, secondary hypothyroidism or iatrogenism by different drugs (amiodarone, lithium, rich iodide compounds, etc) (49). The hypothetical ideal way to measure the hormonal action in the tissues would probably be to study the gene expression modulate by them. This approach is nowadays impossible in clinical practice because its cost and complexity (50).

It is known that the percentage of occupation of the TH receptors by T3 varies notably in different tissues, ranging from 50% to 100% (46, 49).

Likewise it has been studied the origin of intracellular T, comparing the T3 from intracellular conversion (by T4 deiodination, action mediated by D2) with T3 from thyroid origin that enters into the cell from the circulation. This method showed that in liver and kidney the majority of T3 comes from the plasma, whereas in the central nervous system and pituitary T3 comes generally from local conversion, although the plasmatic fraction plays its action in these tissues as well.

3. Indicators of Systemic Action

A. Basal Metabolism

The general systemic action of TH is reproduced by the basal metabolism (45). It is known that T3 increases basal metabolism, promotes thermogenesis and, consequently weight loss. The most important action of T3 is the regulation of cell oxygen consumption by the cell. In fact it is thought that TH regulate around 40% of the consumed oxygen by the body. This function is done trough induction of changes in cellular enzymes, electron transportation and protein synthesis. The facultative thermogenesis occurs as a response to to changes of temperature and depends on the stimulus of the synthesis of mitochondrial uncoupling proteins (UCP). T3 and cathecolamines mediate this effect. The synthesis of UCP stimulates the thermogenesis by uncoupling oxidative phosphorylation, what produces energy loss as heat. It has been seen that cold also activates the D2 activity.

The assessment by indirect calorimetry can be used to calculate the caloric consumption. This investigation has the disadvantage that must be done after resting, fasting and is modified by other diseases or by technical artifacts. All these condition alterate the oxygen consumption. The sensitivity to detect thyroid disease with this test is good (51).

Normal basal metabolism ranges from –15% to +5%. In hyperthyroidism it should be greater than 20%, whereas in hypothyroidism should fall beneath 20%. This test is the only one that measures the consequences of TH in the cellular oxygen consumption by a direct approach. In some circumstances this technique can have clinical utility.

B. Plasma Proteins

Changes in thyroid function induce adjustments in the plasma proteins and several enzyme concentrations. The Sexual Hormone Binding Globulin (SHBG) plasma level is perhaps the best indicator of this group (11,52). SHBG is elevated in patients with hyperthyroidism and is specially sensitive to differentiate patients with real thyroid dysfunction from those with resistance to TH as in the later the SHBG plasma concentration is normal (53). It has also been published that the plasma concentration of Angiotensine-Converter Enzyme (ACE) can help to differentiate between euthyroid sick syndrome and healthy subject (54). The erythrocyte enzymatic activity and the tests on skeletal muscular activity are potentially best indicators of T3 activity in these cells. Likewise, the plasma albumin level is raised in hyperthyroidism and decreased in hypothyroidism.

C. Lipid Metabolism

TH have a number of metabolic actions on target tissues. As a result there is a reduction on plasma total cholesterol concentration, principally because of a fall in low-density lipoproteins. TH stimulate lipogenesis as well as lipolysis. T3 induces the lipogenic enzymes, especially the malic acid dehydrogenase. Therefore the enzyme activity is an excellent marker of T3 action in the liver (55). In addition, T3 accelerates the HMG-CoA reductase and increases the Apoprotein A-1. It is worth to consider that the increase in caloric genesis is principally generated using fat acids as subtract. The decrease in cholesterol plasma level is not only achieved by its hepatic action. TH also contribute to the regulation of lipid receptors expression: the VLDL receptor in brain, muscle, fat tissue and heart, is stimulated by T3.

Similarly TH increase cholesterol biliar excretion that also contributes to reduce blood cholesterol levels.

In hypothyroidism, besides the elevation of total cholesterol, there is a rise in LDL fraction, lipoprotein A and apoprotein A1B and E. The HDL fraction changes are negligible. An increase in triglicerydes plasma level has also been reported and may be related to weight gain and insulinresistance that occur in these patients (56). Some authors defend that subclinic hypothyroidism is an indicator of risk for both arteriosclerosis and myocardial infarction in women older than 64 years old (57,58).

D. Glucose Metabolism

In line with the former findings, it has also been studied which genes are expressed after T3 induction in cultured adipocytes. It was found that 13, out of 1176 studied genes, increase their expression after adding T3 to the medium and 6 genes were infra-regulated. The analysis of these results has shed some light about the possible connection between TH and the development of insulinrresistance (59).

Other authors have related T3 rise with an increase in glucose trapping by cells. It has been also described that the glucose transporter GLUT 4 is regulated by T3. This transporter is expressed predominantly in muscle, adipose tissue and heart. Nevertheless the defects in GLUT 4 are not associated with the development of type 2 diabetes mellitus (60).

4. Indicators of Peripheral Action

As previously indicated, TH act in almost every body system as TR are expressed in virtually all tissues (44). Since each organ have different intensity and isoforms of TR expression and there is also differences in the specific tissue deiodinase activity, it can be assumed that will be important differences in TH response between organs (Figures 1 and 3). The myriad of TH effects is remarkable. They have a fundamental role in important and varied functions like the metabolism of the macronutrients, the regulation of energetic expenditure and oxygen consume, as well as in the regulation of important functions in specific tissues (46).

A. Pituitary

As aforementioned HT, mainly T3, exert a negative effect on TSH secretion by the pituitary thyrotropic cells. T3 also negatively regulates the transcription of both alfa and beta subunits genes. This mechanism is mediated by the intracellular deiodination of T4 into T3. In that way it has been of particularly interest the research on deiodinase expression in TSH producing pituitary tumors. These adenomas overexpress D3 while D2 is underexpressed. This could explain the thyrotropinomas resistance to the TSH negative feedback. The result of increasing D3 action is a reduction of the T3 intracellular concentration in benefit of the inactive rT3. As a consequence the production and secretion of TSH not is not adequately inhibited (61).

Hypothyroidism has been associated to a significantly reduction of IGF-I and IGFBP-3 serum levels, while IGFBP-1 increases in hyperthyroidism as well as in hypothyroidism (62).

B. Gonadal Sphere

Hyperthyroidism is associated with menstrual irregularity and erectile dysfunction. Somehow these alterations are related to variations in the SHBG serum concentrations. As aforementioned, the circulating levels of SHBG are increased in hyperthyroidism. As a result, there are changes in the percentage of circulating free and protein-bound sexual hormones, because testosterone has a greater affinity to SHBG than estradiol. The gonadal steroids metabolism can also be accelerated in these patients. Furthermore, it is also known that the consequence of the stimulus on the estrogenic receptors can perform an antagonic effect in the thyroid function (44).

C. Nervous Tissue and Brain

TH have an essential role in the development of fetal brain in uterus and during the neonatal period. Whatever the cause may be, neonatal hypothyroidism can generate mental retardation and irreversible neurologic defects. The absence of HT produces a decrease in axonal growth and arborization of dendritic cells in cerebral cortex, hippocampus and cerebellum. It has been seen, in rats, that the defects in the cerebral development due to TH deficiency can be reverted when HT are administrated in 2 weeks after birth. Therefore it can be deduced that the prompt administration of T4 in congenital hypothyroidism can prevent the intellectual impairment. T4 deiodination in T3 by D2 in uterus and the maternal transference of T4 can help to maintain the normal T3 concentration in offspring both in normal and in cases of congenital hypothyroidism. The maternal thyroid function status can be important by its effects in the neuropsychological development of children.

The ontogeny of TR isoforms suggests that they have a role in the cerebral development. It is speculated that TRα is especially important for CNS development. TRα is expressed in the whole brain since the beginning of its development; TRβ-1 is expressed minimally, except in the cochlea and in cerebellum; However, just after birth is produced a notable increase (40-fold) in TRβ-1 mRNA expression in the whole brain. This expression reaches its top at 10 days after birth and is maintained until the maturity of adult life. Meanwhile it is seen that in the same organ, TRα-1 and c-erbAα-2 increase their expression twofold at week 2 and decay afterwards until normal concentrations in adult life. This change of receptor expression concurs with a peak of T3 in plasma.

Despite the importance of TH in cerebral development, are known few genes that are regulated directly by these hormones and have been only partially characterized.

D. Liver

TH have multiple effects in liver, including, as already mentioned, the stimulus of the enzymes that regulate lipogenesis and lipolisis (63). TRβ is the isoform that predominates in liver. It has been seen by microarray that there are 55 liver genes specially regulated by TH. Fourteen of those are regulated in a positive way, while 41 in a negatively (46). Malic acid is very sensitive to T3 action in liver, but does not respond in brain, what suggests there are specific tissue factors that modulate the gene transcription mediated by TH. In each blood passage, the liver removes between 5-10% of the plasma T4 concentration. It suggests that there is a mechanism of active hormone (T3 y T4) transport in the cellular membrane to the interior of the hepatocyte.

The triad of reduced biliary excretion, hypocholesterolemia and gall bladder hypotonia that occurs in hypothyroidism can increase the incidence of biliary litiasis in these patients. This alteration is reversible with T4treatment.

Hyperthyroidism is associated with both the necrotic pattern and the cholestasic pattern. The transaminases are increased in around 30% of these patients. The presumed mechanism is related with cellular hypoxia, as a consequence of the increase in oxygen demand without increase in blood flow. Alkaline phosphatase plasma levels increases in 64% of patients with thyrotoxicosis. Although it is not a specific liver alteration, it should be correlated with GGT levels (which increase in 17% of hyperthyroid patients) and bilirrubin (increased in 5%), as indicators of cholestasis.

E. Bone

THs are essential for bone development and growth. Osteoclasts and osteoblasts express TRα (principally TRα-1) and TRβ, and TH stimulate both osteogenesis and osteolysis.

The stimulus for osteogenesis is mediated by proteins involved in the formation of bone matrix, as are Alkaline phosphatase, osteocalcin and collagen. In addition they can have an indirect action, as stimulation of IGF-I synthesis. This suggests that T3 participate in the differentiation and proliferation of osteoblat by regulating the synthesis of growth factors and its actions. Probably the most representative marker of TH in bone formation is osteocalcin. It is increased in situations of accelerated bone loss (thyroid hyperfunction) and decreased in situations of low bone remodelation (hypothyroidism).

The action of TH in osteoclasts is less known. It is thought that THs do not have a direct effect in the bone resorption, although they may have a direct action a paracrine effect by factors secreted by osteoblasts. Several cytokines have been implicated as mediators of this effect. The rise in HT blood levels is usually accompanied by an increase of osteocalcin and alkaline phosphatase (markers of osteoblastic and osteogenic activity), and the balance is favorable to the osteolisys (53). The urinary markers of osteoclastic activity (pyridinolines, telopeptides and beta cross-laps), may be increased in hyperthyroidism (64).

F. Heart

TRα and TRβ are expressed in the heart. The experimental data suggest that TRα-1 has a principal role in the maintenance of cardiac output. THs have ionotropic and cronotropic positive effect and reduce systemic vascular resistance as well. In the same way is also attributed a lusotropic effect (capacity of quick cardiac relaxation) to TH. All these characteristics are related to TH ability in promoting protein synthesis that are critical for cardiac function as the heavy chain of myosin. The increase in contractility is reflected by a greater SERCA synthesis.

According to this data, hyperthyroid patients have an accelerated pre-ejection period (PEP), time of left ventricle (LEVT) ejection and isovolumetric contraction time (ICT). The diastolic function, including the isovolumetric relaxed time is usually supranormal (65). All this alterations are corrected after the administration of beta-blockers. Changes in left ventricular structure and increase in echocardiograph indices of myocardial contractility are observed in thyrotoxic patients, while patients with subclinic hyperthyroidism show an increase in ventricular relaxation velocity (66).

On the contrary, in hypothyroidism all cardiac function is impaired. The ratio PEP/LVET is prolonged. These data are related with improvement of clinic and biochemistry parameters after treatment with L-thyroxin. Subclinic hypothyroidism presents modest prejudice in cardiac function when compare with healthy controls. Substitutive treatment can proportionate an inotropic positive response. Because this reason some authors conclude that the study of cardiac function in the patient with hypothyroidism should be done in a parametric way (comparing each subject with his or her own) and can be justified the use of L-thyroxin because the improvement that produces in cardiac function. This observation is reinforced by the fact that subclinic hypothyroidism is a risk indicator of atherosclerosis and myocardial infarction in older women (37). Endothelial dysfunction has also been associated with hypothyroidism (4).

G. Skeletal Muscle

The patient with hyperthyroidism manifests muscular debility and easy fatigue. This changes have been related with the capacity of T3 to induce the transcription of SERCA1 in the striated muscle and increase in the activity of creatininkinasis. The hyperthyroidism muscular atrophy, when appears, can be related with the increase of urinary 3-metilhistidine. Nevertheless this changes do not permit to distinguish them from euthyroid patients.

Logically, in patients with hypothyroidism, creatininkinase (10 times elevation in severe hypothyroidism) and aldolase are increased. These alterations are corrected in 14 days with hormonal treatment with L-T4. Myoglobin is also elevated, in plasma as well as in urine.

The thyroid function relates well with alquilian reflex. In patients with hypothyroidism it has been observed an alteration in the relaxing phase. It has not been observed an alteration in the relax phase in patients with subclinical disease.

H. Adipose Tissue

TH have an important role in the development and activity of white and brown adipose tissue. TH can induce differentiation of the adipose tissue and stimulate proliferation of adipocytes from preadipocytes. These cells express TRα-1 as well as, in less extent, TRβ-1. The experimental data show that T3 modulate the expression of several genes in the adipose tissue (22). As has been indicated, T3 regulates basal consume of oxygen, the fat storage, lipogenesis and lipolisis.

It has been demonstrated, in humans, that hypothyroidism, chronic hyperthyroidism, as well as the acute administration of T3, do not affect serum leptin levels. Furthermore, it has been also demonstrated that hypothyroid patients have elevated plasma leptin concentrations, although this elevation is correlated with obesity.

IV. Conclusions

The concentration of plasma TSH provides direct information about the thyrotropic cell function and only in an indirect way on the thyroid function, which may involve several limitations. The concentration of TSH is correlated with plasma levels of thyroid hormones but this relationship is imprecise in some circumstances.

The current method of evaluating the thyroid function is clinically useful, but incomplete. In some cases it is not appropriate for a therapeutic adjustment of replacement doses. As a result there are patients who receive treatment that would not require medication and vice versa. Currently, a sensitive diagnostic method able to differentiate between patients with subclinical DT and normal outliers subjects is lacking.

Furthermore, thyroid hormone plasma concentration does not reflect their biological activity in target cells. Tissues have partially autonomous and independent mechanisms that help regulating the particular needs of each organ. Our present knowledge is partial and limited in that regard. The presence, role and expression of different deiodinases and the diverse expression of the different isoforms of thyroid hormone receptors are essential in this particular tissue response to thyroid hormones.

Acknowledgments

We thank Guillermo Garcia del Barrio for his invaluable technical support.

References

[1] Ladenson PW, Singer PA, Ain KB, Bagchi N, Bigos ST, Levy EG, et al. American Thyroid Association guidelines for detection of thyroid dysfunction. *Arch. Intern. Med.* 2000; 160:1573-5.

[2] Dayan CM, Saravanan P, Bayly G. Whose normal thyroid function is better--yours or mine? *Lancet* 2002; 360:353

[3] Cooper DS. Subclinical hypothyroidism. *N. Engl. J. Med.* 2001; 345:260-5.

[4] Duntas LH. Subclinical thyroid disorders: the menace of the Trojan horse. *J. Endocrinol. Invest.* 2003; 26:472-80.

[5] Canaris GJ, Manowitz NR, Mayor G, Ridgway EC. The Colorado thyroid disease prevalence study. *Arch. Intern. Med.* 2000; 160:526-34.

[6] McDermott MT, Ridgway EC. Subclinical hypothyroidism is mild thyroid failure and should be treated. *J. Clin. Endocrinol. Metab.* 2001; 86:4585-90.

[7] Chu JW, Crapo LM. The treatment of subclinical hypothyroidism is seldom necessary. *J. Clin. Endocrinol. Metab.* 2001; 86:4591-9.

[8] Owen PJ, Lazarus JH. Subclinical hypothyroidism: the case for treatment. *Trends Endocrinol. Metab.* 2003; 14:257-61.

[9] Vanderpump MP, Tunbridge WM, French JM, Appleton D, Bates D, Clark F, et al. The incidence of thyroid disorders in the community: a twenty-year follow-up of the Whickham Survey. *Clin. Endocrinol.* 1995; 43:55-68.

[10] Greenspan SL, Klibanski A, Schoenfeld D, Ridgway EC. Pulsatile secretion of thyrotropin in man. *J. Clin. Endocrinol. Metab.* 1986; 63:661-8.

[11] Marqusee E, Haden ST, Utiger RD. Subclinical thyrotoxicosis. *Endocrinol. Metab. Clin. North Am.* 1998; 27:37-49.

[12] Chan V, Jones A, Liendo-Ch P, McNeilly A, Landon J, Besser GM. The relationship between circadian variations in circulating thyrotrophin, thyroid hormones and prolactin. *Clin. Endocrinol.* 1978; 9:337-49.

[13] Salvador J, Wilson DW, Harris PE, Peters JR, Edwards C, Foord SM, et al. Relationships between the circadian rhythms of TSH, prolactin and cortisol in surgically treated microprolactinoma patients. *Clin. Endocrinol.* 1985; 22:265-72.

[14] Mantzoros CS, Ozata M, Negrao AB, Suchard MA, Ziotopoulou M, Caglayan S, et al. Synchronicity of frequently sampled thyrotropin (TSH) and leptin concentrations in healthy adults and leptin-deficient subjects: evidence for possible partial TSH regulation by leptin in humans. *J. Clin. Endocrinol. Metab.* 2001; 86:3284-91.

[15] Fekete C, Sarkar S, Rand WM, Harney JW, Emerson CH, Bianco AC, et al. Agouti-related protein (AGRP) has a central inhibitory action on the hypothalamic-pituitary-thyroid (HPT) axis; comparisons between the effect of AGRP and neuropeptide Y on energy homeostasis and the HPT axis. *Endocrinology* 2002; 143:3846-53.

[16] Stathatos N, Wartofsky L. The euthyroid sick syndrome: is there a physiologic rationale for thyroid hormone treatment? *J. Endocrinol. Invest.* 2003; 26:1174-9.

[17] Beckett GJ, Toft AD. First-line thyroid function tests. TSH alone is not enough. *Clin. Endocrinol.* 2003; 58:20-1.

[18] Meier C, Trittibach P, Guglielmetti M, Staub JJ, Muller B. Serum thyroid stimulating hormone in assessment of severity of tissue hypothyroidism in patients with overt primary thyroid failure: cross sectional survey. *BMJ* 2003; 326:311-2.

[19] Morreale de Escobar G, Obregon MJ, Escobar del Rey F. Is neuropsychological development related to maternal hypothyroidism or to maternal hypothyroxinemia? *J. Clin. Endocrinol. Metab.* 2000; 85:3975-87.

[20] Davies TF, Marians R, Latif R. The TSH receptor reveals itself. *J. Clin. Invest.* 2002; 110:161-4.

[21] Biondi B, Palmieri EA, Lombardi G, Fazio S. Effects of subclinical thyroid dysfunction on the heart. *Ann. Intern. Med.* 2002; 137:904-14.

[22] Adriaanse R, Brabant G, Prank K, Endert E, Wiersinga WM. Circadian changes in pulsatile TSH release in primary hypothyroidism. *Clin. Endocrinol.* 1992; 37:504-10

[23] Wiersinga WM. Functional anatomy, physiology and pathophysiology. In: Pinchera A, editor. Endocrinology and Metabolism, Berkshire: McGraw-Hill, 2001; p. 139-149.

[24] Surks MI, Sievert R. Drugs and thyroid function. *N. Engl. J. Med.* 1995; 333:1688-94.

[25] Galofre JC, Garcia-Mayor RV, Fluiters E, Fernandez-Calvet L, Rego A, Paramo C, et al. Incidence of different forms of thyroid dysfunction and its degrees in an iodine sufficient area. T*hyroidology* 1994; 6:49-54.

[26] Tunbridge WM, Evered DC, Hall R, Appleton D, Brewis M, Clark F, et al. The spectrum of thyroid disease in a community: the Whickham survey. *Clin. Endocrinol.* 1977; 7:481-93.

[27] Huber G, Staub JJ, Meier C, Mitrache C, Guglielmetti M, Huber P, et al. Prospective study of the spontaneous course of subclinical hypothyroidism: prognostic value of thyrotropin, thyroid reserve, and thyroid antibodies. *J. Clin. Endocrinol. Metab.* 2002; 87:3221-6.

[28] Saravanan P, Chau WF, Roberts N, Vedhara K, Greenwood R, Dayan CM. Psychological well-being in patients on 'adequate' doses of l-thyroxine: results of a large, controlled community-based questionnaire study. *Clin. Endocrinol.* 2002; 57:577-85.

[29] Efstathiadou Z, Bitsis S, Milionis HJ, Kukuvitis A, Bairaktari ET, Elisaf MS, et al. Lipid profile in subclinical hypothyroidism: is L-thyroxine substitution beneficial? *Eur. J. Endocrinol.* 2001; 145:705-10.

[30] Caraccio N, Ferrannini E, Monzani F. Lipoprotein profile in subclinical hypothyroidism: response to levothyroxine replacement, a randomized placebo-controlled study. *J. Clin. Endocrinol. Metab.* 2002; 87:1533-8.

[31] Danese MD, Ladenson PW, Meinert CL, Powe NR. Effect of thyroxine therapy on serum lipoproteins in patients with mild thyroid failure: a quantitative review of the literature. *J. Clin. Endocrinol. Metab.* 2000; 85:2993-3001.

[32] Duntas LH. Thyroid disease and lipids. Thyroid 2002; 12:287-93.

[33] Meier C, Staub JJ, Roth CB, Guglielmetti M, Kunz M, Miserez AR, et al. TSH-controlled L-thyroxine therapy reduces cholesterol levels and clinical symptoms in subclinical hypothyroidism: a double blind, placebo-controlled trial (Basel Thyroid Study). *J. Clin. Endocrinol. Metab.* 2001; 86:4860-6.

[34] SoRelle R. Subclinical Hypothyroidism: A Heart Disease Risk? Circulation 2000; 101:E9012-E9012.

[35] Kahaly GJ. Cardiovascular and atherogenic aspects of subclinical hypothyroidism. Thyroid 2000; 10:665-79.

[36] Luboshitzky R, Aviv A, Herer P, Lavie L. Risk factors for cardiovascular disease in women with subclinical hypothyroidism. *Thyroid* 2002; 12:421-5.

[37] Hak AE, Pols HA, Visser TJ, Drexhage HA, Hofman A, Witteman JC. Subclinical hypothyroidism is an independent risk factor for atherosclerosis and myocardial infarction in elderly women: the Rotterdam Study. *Ann. Intern. Med.* 2000; 132:270-8.

[38] Sgarbi JA, Villaca FG, Garbeline B, Villar HE, Romaldini JH. The effects of early antithyroid therapy for endogenous subclinical hyperthyroidism in clinical and heart abnormalities. *J. Clin. Endocrinol. Metab.* 2003; 88:1672-7.

[39] Helfand M, Redfern CC. Screening for thyroid disease: an update. *Ann. Intern. Med.* 1998; 129:144-58.

[40] Crooks J, Murray IP, Wayne EJ. Statistical methods applied to the clinical diagnosis of thyrotoxicosis. *Q J Med.* 1959; 28:211-34.

[41] Billewicz WZ, Chapman RS, Crooks J, Day ME, Gossage J, Wayne E, et al. Statistical methods applied to the diagnosis of hypothyroidism. *Q J Med.* 1969; 38:255-66.

[42] Zulewski H, Muller B, Exer P, Miserez AR, Staub JJ. Estimation of tissue hypothyroidism by a new clinical score: evaluation of patients with various grades of hypothyroidism and controls. *J. Clin. Endocrinol. Metab.* 1997; 82:771-6.

[43] Wayne E. The assessment of thyroid function. Br J Surg 1965; 52:717-21.

[44] Motomura K, Brent GA. Mechanisms of thyroid hormone action. Implications for the clinical manifestation of thyrotoxicosis. *Endocrinol. Metab. Clin. North Am.* 1998; 27:1-23.

[45] Loeb JN. Metabolic changes in thyrotoxicosis. En: Braverman LE and Utiger RD, Eds. The thyroid. 7th ed. Philadelphia: Lippincott-Raven Poblishers, 1996; p. 687-693.

[46] Yen PM. Physiological and molecular basis of thyroid hormone action. *Physiol. Rev.* 2001; 81:1097-142.

[47] Bianco AC, Salvatore D, Gereben B, Berry MJ, Larsen PR. Biochemistry, cellular and molecular biology, and physiological roles of the iodothyronine selenodeiodinases. *Endocr. Rev*. 2002;23:38-89.

[48] McKenna NJ, O'Malley BW. Minireview: nuclear receptor coactivators - an update. *Endocrinology* 2002; 143:2461-5.

[49] Klein I. Clinical, metabolic, and organ-specific indices of thyroid function. Endocrinol *Metab. Clin. North Am.* 2001; 30:415-27.

[50] Burke W. Genetic testing. *N. Engl. J. Med.* 2002; 347:1867-75.

[51] al-Adsani H, Hoffer LJ, Silva JE. Resting energy expenditure is sensitive to small dose changes in patients on chronic thyroid hormone replacement. *J. Clin. Endocrinol. Metab*. 1997; 82:1118-25.

[52] Bunevicius R, Kazanavicius G, Zalinkevicius R, Prange AJ Jr. Effects of thyroxine as compared with thyroxine plus triiodothyronine in patients with hypothyroidism. *N. Engl. J. Med.* 1999; 340:424-9.

[53] Faber J, Perrild H, Johansen JS. Bone Gla protein and sex hormone-binding globulin in nontoxic goiter: parameters for metabolic status at the tissue level. *J. Clin. Endocrinol.* Metab 1990; 70:49-55.

[54] McIver B, Gorman CA. Euthyroid sick syndrome: an overview. *Thyroid* 1997; 7:125-32.

[55] Oppenheimer JH, Silva E, Schwartz HL, Surks MI. Stimulation of hepatic mitochondrial alpha-glycerophosphate dehydrogenase and malic enzyme by L-triiodothyronine. Characteristics of the response with specific nuclear thyroid hormone binding sites fully saturated. *J. Clin. Invest.* 1977; 59:517-27.

[56] Caraccio N, Ferrannini E, Monzani F. Lipoprotein profile in subclinical hypothyroidism: response to levothyroxine replacement, randomized placebo-controlled study. *J. Clin. Endocrinol. Metab.* 2002; 87:1533-8.

[57] Hak AE, Pols HA, Visser TJ, Drexhage HA, Hofman A, Witteman JC. Subclinical hypothyroidism is an independent risk factor for atherosclerosis and myocardial infarction in elderly women: the Rotterdam Study. *Ann. Intern. Med.* 2000; 132:270-8.

[58] Kanaya AM, Harris F, Volpato S, Perez-Stable EJ, Harris T, Baue DC. Association between thyroid dysfunction and total cholesterollevel in an older biracial population: the health, aging and body composition study. *Arch. Intern. Med.* 2002; 162:773-9.

[59] Viguerie N, Millet L, Avizou S, Vidal H, Larrouy D, Langin D. Regulation of human adipocyte gene expression by thyroid hormone. *J. Clin. Endocrinol. Metab.* 2002; 87:630-4.

[60] Torrance CJ, Usala SJ, Pessin JE, Dohm GL. Characterization of a low affinity thyroid hormone receptor binding site within the rat GLUT4 gene promoter. *Endocrinology* 1997; 138:1215-23.

[61] Tannahill LA, Visser TJ, McCabe CJ, Kachilele S, Boelaert K, Sheppard MC, et al. Dysregulation of iodothyronine deiodinase enzyme expression and function in human pituitary tumours. *Clin. Endocrinol.* 2002; 56:735-43.

[62] Iglesias P, Bayon C, Mendez J, Gancedo PG, Grande C, Diez JJ. Serum insulin-like growth factor type 1, insulin-like growth factor binding protein-1, and insulin-like growth factor-binding protein-3 concentrations in patients with thyroid dysfunction. *Thyroid* 2001; 11:1043-8.

[63] Malik R, Hodgson H. The relationship between the thyroid gland and the liver. *QJM* 2002; 95:559-69.

[64] Marcocci C, Golia F, Vignali E, Pinchera A. Skeletal integrity in men chronically treated with suppressive doses of L-thyroxine. *J. Bone Miner. Res.* 1997; 12:72-7.

[65] Dillmann WH. Cellular action of thyroid hormone on the heart. *Thyroid* 2002; 12:447-52.

[66] Petretta M, Bonaduce D, Spinelli L, Vicario ML, Nuzzo V, Marciano F, et al. Cardiovascular haemodynamics and cardiac autonomic control in patients with subclinical and overt hyperthyroidism. *Eur. J. Endocrino* .2001; 145:691-6.

In: Thyroid Hormones: Functions, Related Diseases and Uses ISBN: 978-1-60741-080-5
Editors: F. S. Kuehn, M. P. Lozada

Chapter III

Redox Signaling in Thyroid Hormone Action: A Novel Strategy for Liver Preconditioning

Luis A. Videla and Virginia Fernández
Molecular and Clinical Pharmacology Program, Institute of Biomedical Sciences, Faculty of Medicine, University of Chile, Santiago, Chile

Abstract

Thyroid hormone (L-3, 3',5-triiodothyronine, T_3) exerts important actions on cellular energy metabolism, being mitochondria the major target for its calorigenic effects. Acceleration of O_2 consumption by T_3 is due to transcriptional activation of respiratory genes in target tissues such as liver, leading to increased production of reactive oxygen species (ROS) and the consequent depletion of antioxidant mechanisms. The increase in ROS generation primarily occurs at mitochondrial and other subcellular sites of hepatocytes, concomitantly with a higher respiratory burst activity of Kupffer cells, which act as redox signals regulating important cellular functions such as protein activity and gene expression. Indeed, ROS produced at the Kupffer-cell level activate redox-sensitive transcription factors such as nuclear factor-κB (NF-κB), signal transducer and activator of transcription 3 (STAT3), and activating protein 1 (AP-1), as evidenced by the abolishment of the T_3-induced DNA binding capacity of these proteins by pre-treatment with antioxidants or the Kupffer-cell inactivator $GdCl_3$. Up-regulation of gene expression by T_3 is also accomplished in Kupffer cells, leading to an enhancement in the synthesis and release of the cytokines tumor necrosis factor-α (TNF-α) and interleukin (IL)-1 and IL-6. The TNF-α response elicited by T_3 correlates with the activation of the IκB kinase complex (IKK), which ultimately triggers NF-κB DNA binding with the consequent expression of the NF-κB-responsive genes encoding for inducible nitric oxide synthase, manganese superoxide dismutase, the anti-apoptotic protein Bcl-2, and the type I acute-phase protein haptoglobin. T_3-induced IL-6 signaling T_3 involves the Janus kinase (JAK)-STAT3 pathway up-regulating the expression of both type I (haptoglobin) and type II (β-fibrinogen) acute-phase proteins. In addition to these actions, T_3-dependent TNF-α and IL-6 responses trigger liver cyclin-dependent kinase-2 expression and cellular proliferation, which may be associated with c-jun N-terminal kinase (JNK) and AP-1 activation or with JAK and STAT3 activation, respectively. These data indicate that T_3-induced calorigenesis also triggers non-genomic effects leading to an expression pattern representing adaptive mechanisms to re-establish redox homeostasis and promote cell survival under conditions of ROS toxicity. This redox signaling in T_3 action has been shown to be associated with significant protection against ischemia-reperfusion liver injury. Thus, T_3 administration represents a novel preconditioning strategy with clinical potential. The latter view is of particular importance considering that, with the exception of ischemic preconditioning, all the other protecting strategies studied have not been transferred to clinical application. Noteworthy, T_3 is a widely used and well-tolerated therapeutic agent that has either no important adverse effects or minimal side-effects that can be readily controlled.

Abbreviations

ALT, alanine aminotransferase;
AP-1, activator protein 1;
APP, acute-phase protein;
APR, acute-phase response;
CBP, CREB binding protein;
CDK, cyclin-dependent kinase;
$GdCl_3$, gadolinium chloride;
GSH, reduced (GSSG, oxidized) glutathione;
H_2O_2, hydrogen peroxide;
IKK, inhibitor of κB kinase;
IL, interleukin;
IR, ischemia-reperfusion;
JAK, Janus kinase;
JNK, c-Jun N-terminal kinase;
MnSOD, manganese superoxide dismutase;
NIK, NF-κB-inducing kinase;
NF-κB, nuclear factor-κB;
NOS; nitric oxide synthase;
$O_2^{\bullet-}$, superoxide radical;
PCAF, p300/CBP-associated factor;
QO_2, oxygen consumption;
RNS, reactive nitrogen species;
ROS, reactive oxygen species;
RXR, retinoic acid receptor;
STAT3, signal transducer and activator of transcription 3;
TNF-α, tumor necrosis factor-α;
TNFR, TNF-α receptor; TR, thyroid hormone receptor;
TRADD, TNFR-associated death domain;
TRAF-2, TNFR-associated factor 2;

TRE, thyroid hormone response element;
UCP, uncoupling protein.

Introduction

Thyroid hormones play important roles in cell growth, differentiation, and metabolism, through different and complex mechanisms of action. In mammals, mayor effects are exerted on cellular oxygen consumption (QO_2) and metabolic rate, leading to stimulation and maintenance of basal thermogenesis (Schwartz and Oppenheimer, 1978). The knowledge of these effects of thyroid hormone started with the recognition that 3,3',5-triiodo-L-thyronine (T_3) administration to hypothyroid animals induced a rapid enhancement in liver mitochondrial oxidations (Tata et al., 1963). This action of T_3 is carried out via thyroid hormone receptors (THs) expressed in almost all tissues (Oppenheimer et al., 1974), which are present in multiple isoforms (Pascual et al., 1982) and recognized by specific thyroid hormone response elements (TREs) in DNA, leading to ligand-dependent upregulation of transcription (Larsen et al., 1986). In addition to the above classical genomic model of T_3-dependent calorigenesis, non-genomic mechanisms may also contribute to increase cellular QO_2, with the consequent enhancement in the mitochondrial capacity for oxidative phosphorylation (Soboll, 1993) and generation of reactive oxygen species (ROS)(Fernández and Videla, 1993; Venditti et al., 2003). ROS are known to exert different effects in cells depending on the concentration achieved and time of exposure. These include (i) direct interaction and reaction of ROS with biomolecules leading to their chemical alteration and loss of function or (ii) ROS acting as regulatory mediators, modifying protein function and/or gene expression (Dröge, 2002; Poli et al., 2004). In this article, we (i) review the molecular mechanisms underlying T_3-dependent calorigenesis and ROS generation in the liver, and (ii) discuss the implications of the redox regulation of T_3-induced Kupffer-cell-dependent gene expression in terms of preconditioning against severe liver injury.

Genomic and Non-Genomic Mechanisms in Thyroid Hormone Calorigenesis

T_3 classically regulates gene expression through binding to TRs that recognize TREs in the promoters of T_3-target genes, as heterodimers with retinoic acid receptor (RXR). Upon T_3 binding, co-repressors are released and co-activators such as CREB binding protein/CBP related protein (CBP/p300) and p300/CBP-associated factor are recruited. These co-activators, in turn, recruit several complexes such as histone arginine methyl transferases, histone acetyl-transferase, ATP-dependent chromatin remodelling complexes, and the mediator complex TR-associated protein (Figure 1A), which constitute a bridge between DNA-bound liganded TR/RXR heterodimers and RNA polimerase-II (Yen, 2001; Flamant et al., 2007). Interaction of these complexes with the basal transcription machinery leads to enhanced promoter activity and synthesis of the enzymes involves in energy metabolism and the components of the mitochondrial respiratory chain.

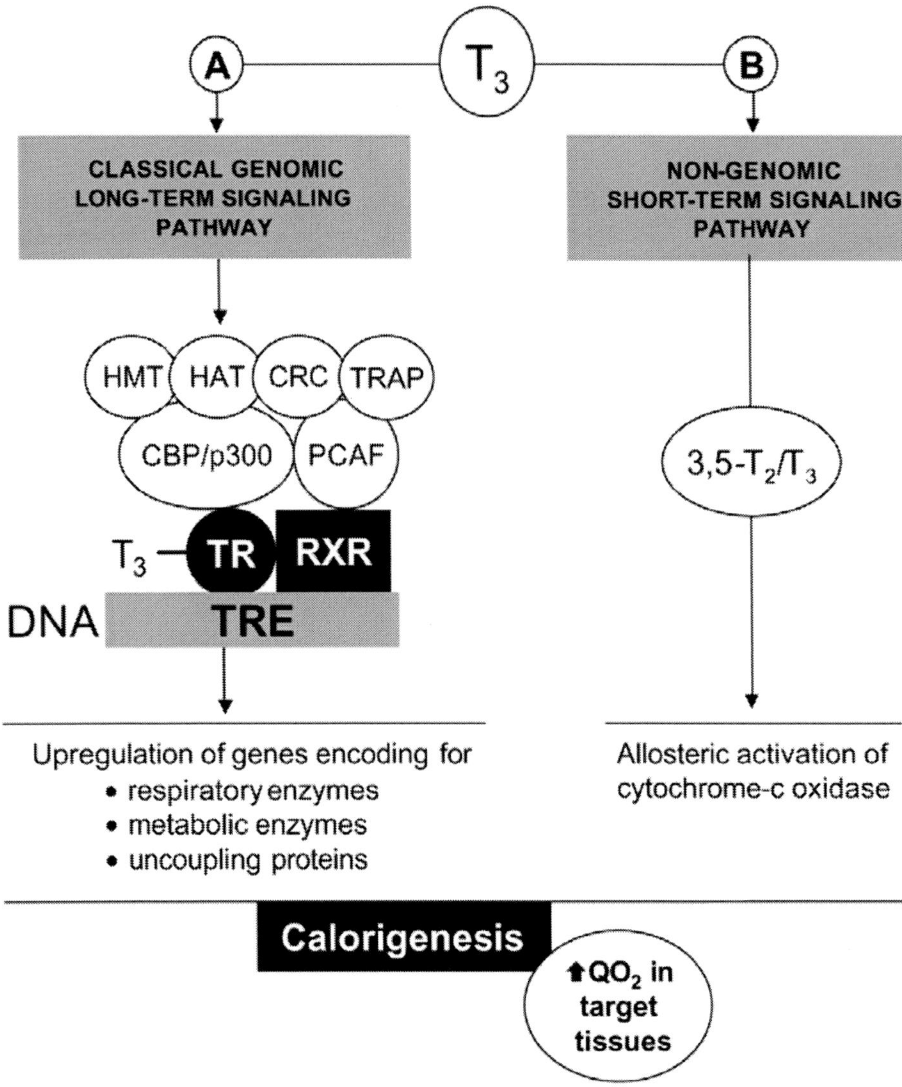

Figure 1. Genomic (A) and non-genomic (B) mechanisms involved in the calorigenic action of thyroid hormones. Abbreviations: CBP, CREB binding protein; CRC, chromatin remodelling complex; HAT, histone acetyltransferase; HMT, histone arginine methyltransferase; 3,5-T2, 3,5-diiodo-L-thyronine; p300, CBP-related protein; PCAF, p300/CBP-associated factor; QO2, rate of oxygen consumption; RXR, retinoic acid receptor; TR, thyroid hormone receptor; TRAP, thyroid hormone receptor-associated protein; TRE, thyroid hormone response element; T_3, 3,3',5-triiodo-L-thyronine.

Consequently, higher rates of oxidative phosphorylation are achieved and the enhancement in ATP production is partially balanced by induction of uncoupling proteins (UCPs), thus determining higher rates of mitochondrial QO_2 (Figure 1A)(Soboll, 1993; Lanni et al., 2003). These calorigenic responses of target cells to T_3 are characterized by being sensitive to inhibitors of transcription and translation and have a latency of hours to days (Yen, 2001), contrary to those elicited by non-genomic mechanisms.

Although most of the effects of T_3 are mediated by TR regulation of target gene transcription in the nucleus and mitochondria, a number of them are independent upon TRs, show rapid onset action (seconds to minutes), and utilize alternate signaling pathways (Yen, 2001; Bassett et al., 2003; Davis et al., 2008). Among them, direct actions of thyroid hormones on oxidative phosphorylation can occur, as shown by the rapid activation of cytochrome-c-oxidase elicited by T_3 and more particularly 3,5-diiodo-L-thyronine (Figure 1B), through binding to its Va subunit that abolishes the allosteric inhibition by ATP (Arnold et al., 1998).

Both genomic long-term and non-genomic short-term signaling pathways of T_3 action are mainly responsible for the enhancement in cellular QO_2 underlying the hyperthyroid state (Figure 1), however, other secondary processes induced by T_3 may also play a role. These include (i) energy expenditure due to futile cycles coupled to increases in catabolic and anabolic pathways of intermediary metabolism; (ii) loss of energy due to higher active cation transport; (iii) higher activity of membrane-bound enzymes of the respiratory chain and metabolite carriers due to changes in lipid composition of mitochondrial membranes (Soboll, 1993); and (iv) O_2 equivalents used in the generation of mitochondrial ROS (Fernández and Videla, 1993).

Relationship Between Thyroid Hormone Calorigenesis And Hepatic ROS Generation

Experimental animals made hyperthyroid by T_3 administration exhibit a thermogenic response that coincides with increases in QO_2 by the liver (Figure 2)(Fernández et al., 1985). Acceleration of hepatic respiration during T_3-induced calorigenesis leads to a marked elevation in the rate of superoxide radical ($O_2^{\bullet-}$) production by liver submitochondrial particles in the presence of NADH or succinate, with higher rates of hydrogen peroxide (H_2O_2) generation, either under basal conditions or in the succinate-supported process, both in the absence and presence of antimycin-A (Figure 2)(Fernández and Videla, 1993). Enhancement in liver mitochondrial H_2O_2 production also occurs in the transition from hypothyroid to hyperthyroid state as a function of the content of autoxidizable electron carriers (Venditti et al., 2003), an effect that is mimicked by cold-induced hyperthyroidism (Venditti et al., 2004).

In addition to T_3-induced liver mitochondrial capacity for ROS generation, the induction of other enzymatic mechanisms also occurs. In fact, development of a hyperthyroid state in rats results in the proliferation of the smooth endoplasmic reticulum, with higher activities of NADPH-cytochrome P450 reductase (Ram and Waxman, 1992) and NADPH oxidase (Fernández et al., 1985). The latter enzymatic activity represents the oxidase activity of cytochrome P450 responsible for $O_2^{\bullet-}$ and H_2O_2 production (Goeptar et al., 1995), which has been related to the induction of the highly pro-oxidant cytochrome P4502E1 isoform by T_3 (Figure 2)(Fernández et al., 2003).

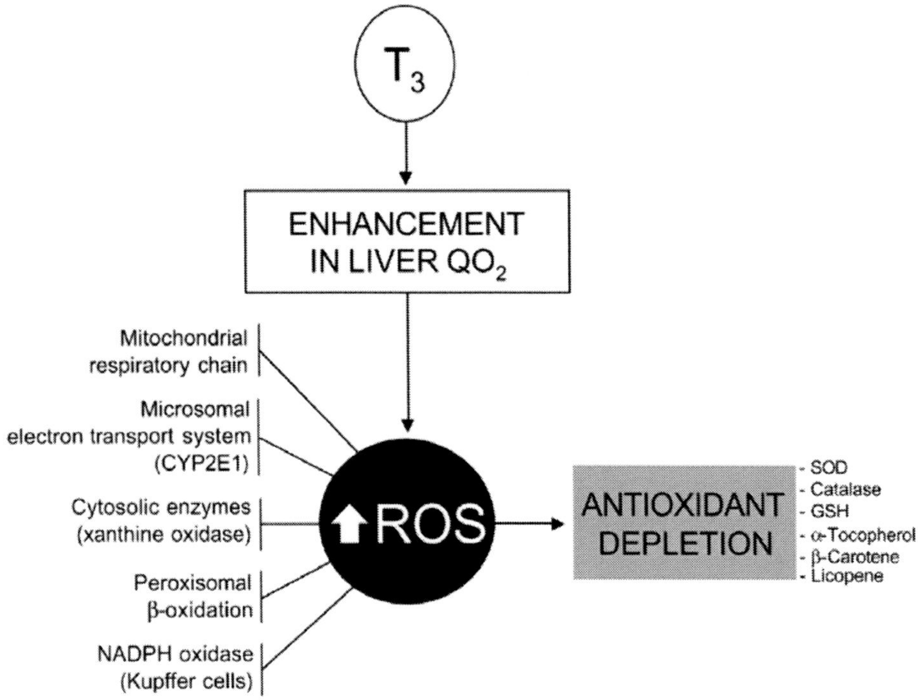

Figure 2. Thyroid hormone calorigenesis and its relationship to reactive oxygen species generation and antioxidant depletion in the liver. Abbreviations: CYP2E1, cytochrome P450 isoform 2E1; GSH, reduced glutathione; QO2, rate of oxygen consumption; ROS, reactive oxygen species; SOD, superoxide dismutase.

These changes, and the increase in the activity of the NADPH-generating system glucose-6-phosphate dehydrogenase (Simon-Giavarotti et al., 1998) are likely to determine high rates of cytochrome P450 reduction in hyperthyroid state, thus explaining the increase in (i) NADPH-dependent antioxidant-sensitive rates of O_2 uptake (Fernández et al., 1988), (ii) NADPH-supported $O_2^{\bullet-}$ generation (Figure 2)(Fernández et al., 1985), and (iii) the biotransformation of a variety of xenobiotics (see Videla, 2000).

T_3-induced liver mitochondrial and microsomal capacity of ROS generation is observed concomitantly with enhancement of cytosolic enzymatic mechanisms such as the $O_2^{\bullet-}/H_2O_2$ generator xanthine oxidase (Huh et al., 1998) and ROS production (Fernández and Videla, 1993) coupled to enhanced fatty acid β-oxidation due to liver peroxisomal proliferation (Figure 2) (Just and Hartl, 1983). Enhancement in hepatic ROS generation is presumed to occur primarily at the parenchymal cell level, with Kupffer cells playing a contributory role, as evidenced by the increase in the respiratory burst activity after T_3 administration (Tapia et al., 1997). The latter process is mainly due to the activity of NADPH oxidase (Figure 2), with a smaller contribution by nitric oxide synthase (NOS)(Wang et al., 1993). Similar to Kupffer cells, T_3-induced liver free-radical generation also occurs in concomitance with enhanced respiratory burst activity and chemiluminescent response in polymorphonuclear leukocytes, both in experimental and human hyperthyroidism (Videla et al., 1993; Fernández and Videla, 1995; Mezosi et al., 2005).

T_3-induced liver free-radical activity is associated with depletion of antioxidant defences (Figure 2)(Asayama et al., 1987; Fernández et al., 1988; Fernández et al., 1991; Simon-Giavarotti et al., 1998; Huh et al., 1998), leading to enhancement in the oxidative stress status of the liver and the consequent elevation in hepatic lipid peroxidation (Fernández et al., 1985; Landriscina et al., 1988; Fernández and Videla, 1996; Venditti et al., 1997; Huh et al., 1998), protein carbonylation (Tapia et al., 1999), and DNA oxidation (Andican et al., 2004). However, this pro-oxidant state achieved in the liver by T_3-induced calorigenesis can be considered as a mild redox alteration, as suggested by the lack of occurrence of morphological changes in liver parenchyma, except for the significant hyperplasia and hypertrophy of Kupffer cells, the resident macrophages of the liver (Tapia et al., 1997). The latter effect of T_3 might be of importance considering that Kupffer cells play a central role in the homeostatic response to liver injury, through the production and release of a wide array of mediators providing physiologically diverse and key paracrine effects on all other liver cells (Tsukamoto, 2002). Thus, transient fluctuation in the levels of ROS and reactive nitrogen species (RNS) may represent regulatory signals controlling protein function or gene expression, either by reversible oxidation and/or nitrosylation of active protein sulfhydryls (Klatt and Lamas, 2000) or via ROS-dependent modulation of the activity of signaling kinases, phosphatases, and redox-sensitive transcription factors, respectively (Dröge, 2002; Poli et al., 2004; Tonks, 2005; Gloire et al., 2006).

Kupffer-Cell Activation and Up-Regulation of Cytokine Expression in Hyperthyroid State

The sinusoidal lining of the liver contains non-parenchymal cells including Kupffer cells, endothelial cells, and stellate cells, which play crucial roles in liver homeostasis and in the pathogenesis of liver disease (Tsukamoto, 2002; Bilzer et al., 2006; Kolios et al., 2006). Kupffer cells account for 80% to 90% of tissue macrophages in the reticuloendothelial system, constitute about 15% of total liver cell population, and are mainly located in periportal areas of the liver lobule (43%; large Kupffer cells), with smaller proportions being found in midzonal (28%) and central (29%) areas (small Kupffer cells)(Bouwens et al., 1986). Large periportal Kupffer cells have higher lysosomal enzyme activities, phagocytic and respiratory burst capacity, and production of tumor necrosis factor-α (TNF-α), interleukin (IL)-1, and prostaglandin E_2 than smaller Kupffer cells from midzonal and central regions (Bilzer et al., 2006). The primary functions of Kupffer cells are phagocytosis and processing of ingested material, antigen presentation, and secretion of biologically active products upon activation, thus representing a key component of innate immunity, the initial, rapid response to potentially dangerous stimuli.

Kupffer cell activation can be triggered by phagocytosable particles and soluble substances through binding to specific receptors on the plasma membrane (Kaisho and Akira, 2006). In the case of T_3, Kupffer cell hyperplasia is a major finding after its *in vivo* administration, an effect that may involve the expansion of Kupffer cell precursors by means of circulating monocyte recruitment, the differentiation of pre-existing local Kupffer cell precursors into mature liver macrophages, or both (Gomes et al., 2004). Under these conditions, Kupffer cell function continuously monitored in the isolated perfused liver from T_3-treated animals by means of colloidal carbon infusion (Cowper et al., 1990), revealed significant increases in the rate of carbon phagocytosis and the associated carbon-induced O_2 uptake (Tapia et al., 1997). The latter parameter is considered to assess the respiratory burst activity of Kupffer cells, a process that is largely dependent on the activity of the ROS-generator NADPH oxidase and abolished by pretreatment with gadolinium chloride ($GdCl_3$)(Tapia et al., 1997), an effective inactivator of large, functional Kupffer cells (Hardonk et al., 1992). The use of $GdCl_3$ to assess Kupffer-cell functioning is further supported by (i) the lack of non-specific actions, as shown by the similar responses in nuclear factor-κB (NF-κB), activator protein 1 (AP-1), and signal transducer and activator of transcription 3 (STAT3) activation (Figure 3A) and in TNF-α release (Fernández et al., 2002) in control animals and euthyroid rats given $GdCl_3$; and (ii) the significant inhibition of hepatic oxidative stress-related parameters induced by T_3 (Tapia et al., 1997; Simon-Giavarotti et al., 2002). In addition to the respiratory burst activity, T_3-induced $GdCl_3$-sensitive liver QO_2 may involve an elevation in the mitochondrial O_2 uptake for energy supply (Cowper et al., 1990) needed for the enhanced carbon phagocytosis observed (Tapia et al., 1997). This contention is supported by the existence of nuclear binding proteins for T_3 in Kupffer cells (Sellitti et al., 1985), which may contribute to trigger the genomic signaling mechanism (Figure 1) determining higher rates of liver macrophage O_2 consumption.

The interdependence between T_3-induced calorigenesis, liver QO_2, and ROS production is associated with significant increases in the hepatic DNA binding of the transcription factors NF-κB (Tapia et al., 2003), STAT3 (Tapia et al., 2006), and AP-1 (Figure 3A)(Fernández et al., 2007a). As shown in Figure 3A, activation of these transcription factors by T_3 administration is suppressed by the *in vivo* pretreatment with $GdCl_3$ prior to hormone treatment. Liver NF-κB and STAT3 activation by T_3 is also abolished by pretreatment with antioxidants (Tapia et al., 2003; 2006). These findings support the view that T_3 induces the redox activation of hepatic NF-κB, STAT3, and AP-1 by actions primarily exerted at the Kupffer cell level, in agreement with the activation of NF-κB by the respiratory burst of colloidal carbon-stimulated Kupffer cells in liver perfusion studies (Romanque et al., 2003). In the liver, Kupffer cells are more sensitive for control of NF-κB activation by ROS than hepatocytes (Tran-Thi et al., 1995; Essani et al., 1997), which is probably due to the highly pro-oxidant state prevailing in Kupffer cells due mainly to NADPH oxidase activity, the active oxidant-driven signaling coupled to NF-κB and AP-1 (Tsukamoto and Lin, 1997), and that most of the antioxidant mechanisms are confined to parenchymal cells (Vrba and Modriansky, 2002). Both NF-κB and AP-1 have prominent transcriptional control over expression of different mediators released by Kupffer cells and other sinusoidal cells, including cytokines, chemokines, and growth factors (Tsukamoto and Lin, 1997). Among them, T_3 administration involving significant NF-κB and AP-1 activation induced mRNA expression of the NF-κB/AP-1-responsive genes for TNF-α, which is correlated with increases in the serum levels of the cytokine (Figure 3B)(Tapia et al., 2003). T_3-induced Kupffer cell-dependent TNF-α response is abolished by pretreatment with the antisense oligonucleotide TJU-2755 (Fernández et al., 2002), a phosphothioate-modified compound targeting the primary RNA transcript of TNF-α (Tu et al., 1998).

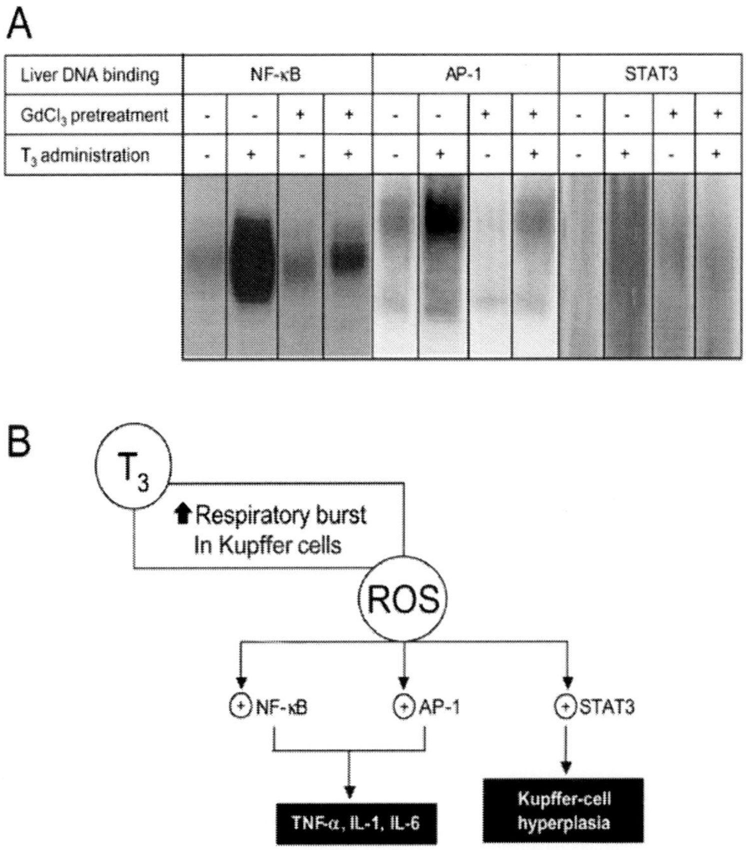

Figure 3. Effects of T_3 administration on rat liver nuclear factor-κB (NF-κB), activating protein 1 (AP-1), and signal transducer and activator of transcription 3 (STAT3) DNA binding in animals with and without gadolinium chloride ($GdCl_3$) pretreatment (A) and T_3-induced Kupffer cell-dependent expression of cytokines and cell proliferation (B). Panel A shows representative autoradiographs of liver NF-κB, AP-1, and STAT3 DNA binding in control rats and T_3-treated animals (0.1 mg/kg, i.p.) and in separate groups of animals subjected to $GdCl_3$ (10 mg/kg, i.v.) 24 h prior to T_3, assessed by electromobility shift assay. Abbreviations: IL-1(6), interleukin 1(6); ROS, reactive oxygen species; TNF-α, tumor necrosis factor-α.

T_3 also elicited (i) an increase in the serum levels of IL-6 (Figure 3B)(Tapia et al., 2006), a cytokine exhibiting NF-κB/AP-1-dependent expression (Tsukamoto and Lin, 1997); and (ii) an elevation in hepatic mRNA expression and serum levels of IL-1 (Figure 3B)(Tapia et al., 2003), a response that may be related to TNF-α induction (Dinarello et al., 1986). In addition to NF-κB and AP-1 activation, the enhancement in STAT3 DNA binding by T_3 administration (Tapia et al., 2006) may be associated with the proliferation of macrophage precursors and their differentiation into Kupffer cells (Figure 3B)(Gomes et al., 2004), considering the central role of STAT3 in gp130-mediated cell growth, differentiation, and survival (Hirano et al., 2000).

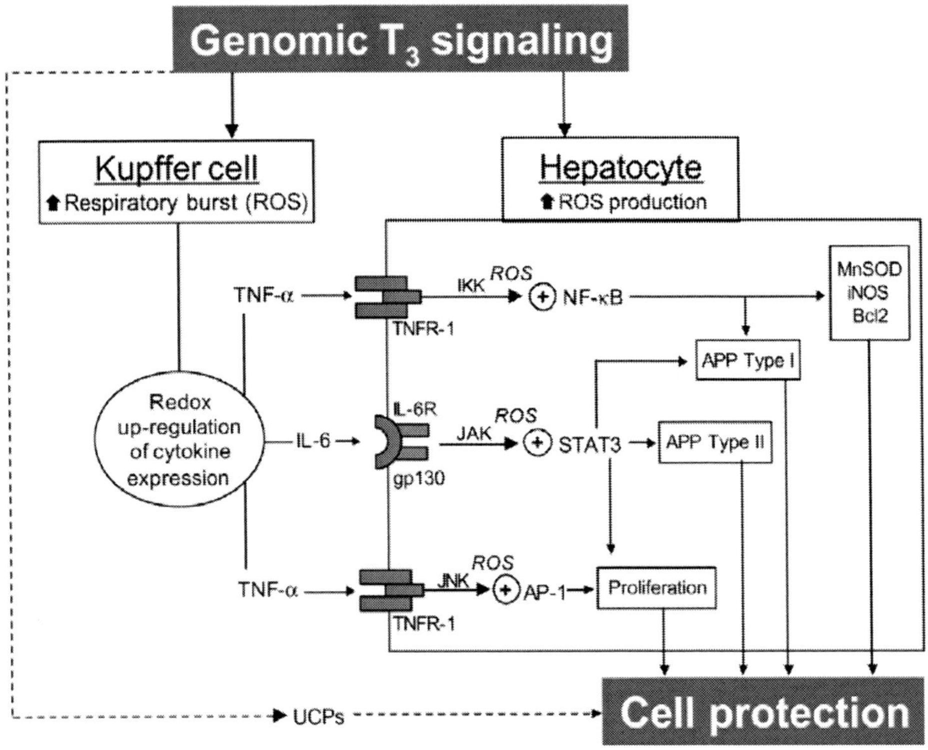

Figure 4. Signaling mechanisms in T_3 calorigenesis leading to reactive oxygen species (ROS) production, redox up-regulation of cytokine expression in Kupffer cells, and hepatocyte activation of genes conferring cytoprotection. Abbreviations: AP-1, activator protein 1; APP, acute phase protein; iNOS, inducible nitric oxide synthase; IKK, inhibitor of κB kinase; IL-6, interleukin 6; IL-6R, IL-6 receptor; JAK, Janus kinase; JNK, c-Jun N-terminal kinase; MnSOD, manganese superoxide dismutase; NF-κB, nuclear factor-κB; STAT3, signal transducer and activator of transcription 3; TNF-α, tumor necrosis factor-α; TNFR-1, TNF-α receptor 1; UCP, uncoupling protein.

T3-Induced Kupffer-Cell-Dependent Up-Regulation of Hepatocyte Antioxidant and Anti-Apoptotic Protein Expression

The effects of cytokines released from Kupffer cells are exerted through their interaction with specific surface receptors in target cells within the liver to mediate signaling from cell membrane to the nucleus (Tsukamoto, 2002; Hayden and Ghosh, 2004). Activated TNF-α receptors (TNFR) mediate the association with different adaptor proteins to regulate kinase or phosphatase activation, lipase stimulation, and protease induction (Hayden and Ghosh, 2004). Thus, coupling of TNF-α with TNFR-1 induces the dissociation of the inhibitor of TNFR activity Silencer of death domain (SODD), allowing binding of the TNFR-associated death domain protein (TRADD), which subsequently recruits downstream adapters resulting in inhibitor of κB (IκB) kinase (IKK), c-Jun N-terminal kinase (JNK), and p38 activation (Hayden and Ghosh, 2004).

In agreement with the above views, the transient TNF-α response elicited by T_3 administration (Figure 3B) correlates with the substantial increase in liver IκB-α phosphorylation (Fernández et al., 2005a; 2005b), evidencing the activation of the IKK complex (Figure 4) (Hyaden and Ghosch, 2004; Gloire et al., 2006). The process requires the recruitment of the adaptor molecules TRADD, TNFR-associated factor-2 (TRAF-2), and receptor-interacting protein (RIP) producing the activation of NF-κB-inducing kinase (NIK), which in turn associates and activates IKK (Garg and Aggarwall, 2002; Gloire et al., 2007). In this signaling cascade, RIP-1 plays a crucial role through direct binding to NF-κB essential modulator (NEMO or IKK-γ), allowing the recruitment of the IKK signalosome upon TNF-α signaling (Zhang et al., 2000), and may involve TNF-α-dependent p65 phosphorylation at serine 529 (Wang and Baldwin, 1998). T_3-induced TNF-α response, liver IKK phosphorylation, and NF-κB activation are abolished by pretreatment with either α-tocopherol or $GdCl_3$, supporting the role of ROS production and Kupffer-cell activation in T_3-dependent signaling leading to up-regulation of hepatic gene expression (Fernández et al., 2005a; 2005b). This is evidenced by the enhanced expression of the NF-κB-responsive genes encoding for inducible NOS (iNOS)(Fernández et al., 2005a), manganese superoxide dismutase (MnSOD), and the anti-apoptotic protein Bcl-2 (Fernández et al., 2005b)(Figure 4). These responses can be interpreted as defense mechanisms against T_3-induced oxidative stress by protecting the liver from ROS toxicity and excessive pro-inflammatory cytokine action.

Up-regulation of hepatic iNOS at hepatocyte and Kupffer-cell levels by T_3 (Fernández et al., 2005a) is expected to achieve large NO generation (Wang et al., 1993), which may (i) scavenge ROS to diminish the pro-oxidant potential oxidizing biomolecules and activating NF-κB; (ii) nitrosylate NF-κB p50 that decreases NF-κB DNA binding; and (iii) induce and/or stabilize IκB to inactivate NF-κB (Janssen-Heininger et al., 2000; Laroux et al., 2000). T_3-induced liver NF-κB DNA binding also up-regulates MnSOD expression, an effect that is abolished by α-tocopherol pretreatment (Fernández et al., 2005b). Induction of MnSOD by T_3 represents an effective protective mechanism against T_3-induced liver $O_2^{\bullet-}$ production occurring at mitochondrial (Fernández and Videla, 1993; Venditti et al., 2003), microsomal (Fernández et al., 1985), and cytosolic (Huh et al., 1998) levels. This response is likely to reduce $O_2^{\bullet-}$ levels by increased $O_2^{\bullet-}$ removal from mitochondria and cytosol, the latter process being due to $O_2^{\bullet-}$ diffusion into the positively changed mitochondrial intermembrane space, $O_2^{\bullet-}$ protonation to form hydroperoxyl radical, and its dismutation in the mitochondrial matrix (Guidot et al., 1995). Coordination in liver T_3-induced expression of iNOS and MnSOD will achieve two goals, an effective $O_2^{\bullet-}$ scavenging and reduction in $O_2^{\bullet-}$ reaction with NO, thus favouring the maintenance of high NO levels that hinder NF-κB signaling. In addition to liver iNOS and MnSOD expression, T_3 administration achieved the redox up-regulation of Bcl-2 in association with IKK/NF-κB activation (Fernández et al., 2005b), a protein reducing apoptosis commitment in disease development and increasing the antioxidation potential of cells (Voehringer and Meyn, 2000). The latter redox aspect of Bcl-2 function is related to a higher intracellular availability of reduced glutathione (GSH), diminishing ROS production (Wiedau-Pazos et al., 1996) and the oxidation of proteins and unsaturated fatty acids (Hockenbery et al., 1993; Virgili et al., 1998). In agreement with this view, repletion of hepatic GSH levels after depletion by T_3 administration is related to the enhancement of either basolateral γ-glutamyl transpeptidase ectoactivity supplying the precursors for intracellular GSH biosynthesis (Carrión et al., 1993), the NADPH-generating enzyme glucose-6-phosphate dehydrogenase supporting oxidized glutathione (GSSG) reduction into GSH (Simon-Giavarotti et al., 1998), or both. Collectively, the analyzed data indicate that T_3 administration elicits the redox up-regulation of iNOS, MnSOD, and Bcl-2 in the liver, in association with the Kupffer cell-dependent release of TNF-α and activation of the IKK/NF-κB cascade, representing antioxidant and anti-apoptotic responses triggered by the underlying oxidative stress status developed (Figure 4).

T3-Induced Kupffer-Cell-Dependent Up-Regulation of Hepatocyte Acute-Phase Response

The acute-phase response (APR) is a major pathophysiologic reaction, in which normal homeostatic mechanisms are replaced by new set points that may contribute to defensive or adaptive capabilities (Ramadori and Christ, 1999). The APR is mainly focused on the liver, being commonly associated with inflammation and a number of states not regarded as inflammatory, including oxidative stress (Samols et al., 2003). This reaction is mediated by both IL-1 like cytokines (IL-1, TNF-α) and IL-6 like cytokines (IL-6, oncostatin M, and others), through the activation of the transcription factors NF-κB, AP-1, STAT3/5, or CCAAT/enhancing-binding protein β (C/EBPβ)(Ramadori and Christ, 1999; Samols et al., 2003; Gruys et al., 2005). These signaling cascades result in the increase in the plasma levels of a number of positive acute phase proteins (APPs) including clotting proteins, transport proteins, anti-proteases, and complement factors, with the parallel decrease of negative APPs such as albumin or transferrin (Gruys et al., 2005).

A major pathway controlling the APR of the liver involves IL-6 signaling through its binding to the gp130 receptor subunit, with the subsequent activation of the gp130-associated JAK/STAT3 system to trigger the expression of APPs (Hirano et al., 2000; Erns and Jenkins, 2004). This cascade was reported to be up-regulated by T_3 administration (Figure 4), as evidenced by the Kupffer-cell-dependent release of IL-6 and activation of hepatic STAT3 (Figure 3) controlling both type I (haptoglobin) and type II (β-fibrinogen) APP genes (Tapia et al., 2006). In addition, this response may be contributed by the T_3-induced TNF-α/IKK/NF-κB pathway (Fernández et al., 2005a; 2005b) controlling type I APP genes (Figure 4), considering that NF-κB activation can synergistically enhance the effects of STAT3 and C/EBPβ upon C-reactive protein induction (Agrawal et al., 2003). In agreement with these data, thyroxine (T_4) administration also increased the hepatic synthesis of the APP α_1-acid glycoprotein, α_2-(acute phase) globulin, haptoglobin (Griffin and Miller, 1973), and ceruloplasmin (Fitch et al., 1999), although the mechanisms underlying these T_4 effects are unknown. Haptoglobin, angiotensinogen, fibrinogen, complement component 4A, and serum amyloid A protein precursor are also upregulated by T_3 in the HepG2 cell line (Lin et al., 2003). Furthermore, T_3 was shown to upregulate the expression of the APP ferritin post-transcriptionally, through enhanced iron-induced displacement of iron regulatory protein from the iron-responsive element present in ferritin mRNA (Leedman et al., 1996).

Upregulation of the hepatic APR by T_3 may represent a defense mechanism against the detrimental effects of oxidative stress occurring both in the liver and in extrahepatic tissues with a calorigenic response (Videla, 2000; Venditti and Di Meo, 2006), considering that the goal of the APR is to restore homeostasis (Ramadori and Christ, 1999; Samols et al., 2003; Gruys et al., 2005). This is achieved by redirecting the gene expression of the liver into a pattern fulfilling immune, transport, coagulation, and antioxidant functions (haptoglobin, ceruloplasmin, and ferritin) that adapt tissues to the metabolic perturbations occurring in inflammatory and oxidative stress conditions (Samols et al., 2003). It is important to note that up-regulation of the hepatic APR (Tapia et al., 2006), iNOS (Fernández et al., 2005a), MnSOD, and Bcl-2 (Fernández et al., 2005b) expression represent nongenomic processes triggered by ROS produced by the calorigenic action of T_3, which are secondary to redox independent genomic pathways (Figure 1A). The latter contention is supported by the lack of effects of α-tocopherol or N-acetylcysteine pretreatment on T_3-induced liver mRNA expression of mitochondrial glycerol-3-phosphate dehydrogenase and the adenine nucleotide translocator 2, two target proteins of thyroid hormone action at the transcriptional level (Videla et al., 2007). Furthermore, T_3-induced liver antioxidant potential through non-genomic mechanisms underlying the APR, iNOS, MnSOD, and Bcl-2 induction may be contributed by up-regulation of UCPs by T_3 (Figure 4) through the classical genomic pathway (Lanni et al., 2003). In fact, upregulation of UCPs may decrease mitochondrial ROS generation due to mild uncoupling by diminishing mitochondrial membrane potential (Lanni et al., 2003) and/or allow the transport of peroxidized unsaturated fatty acid anions to the outer side of the inner mitochondrial membrane, thus decreasing oxidative damage to mitochondrial DNA and proteins (Goglia and Skulachev, 2003).

T3-Induced Kupffer Cell-Dependent Up-Regulation of Hepatocyte Proliferation

Hepatocyte proliferation has been extensively studied after partial hepatectomy (Taub, 1996), a process involving a large number of genes that requires the concurrence of cytokine, growth factor, and metabolic networks (Fausto et al., 2006). Resting hepatocytes in the G0 phase of the cell cycle need to be primed by TNF-α and IL-6 before they can respond to growth factors, with the concomitant activation of NF-κB, STAT3, AP-1, and E/EBPβ, to enter the G1 phase and initiate cell cycle progression. In early GI, hepatocytes respond to growth factors, progress through the cell cycle, overcome the G1 restriction point, and undergo DNA replication (Fausto, 2000). Progression through G1/S phases is regulated by cyclin-dependent kinase 2 (CDK-2)/cyclin E complex with the expression of genes regulating cell progression into late G1/S phases (Jaumot et al., 1999), being cyclin D1 expression in GIIS associated with DNA replication independently of growth factors (Fausto, 2000).

In vivo effects of T_3 as a primary hepatic mitogen leading to hepatocyte proliferation in intact liver are well established (Francavilla et al., 1994; Forbes et al., 2000; Malik et al., 2005), an effect that is also evidenced following hepatocyte transplantation (Oren et al.,

1999). Recently, T_3 administration was found to trigger liver CDK-2 expression and hepatocyte proliferation, as evidenced by the enhancement in Ki-67, a nuclear cell proliferation-associated protein expressed in all active parts of the cell cycle, and in the proliferating cell nuclear antigen (PCNA)(Fernández et al., 2007a). These findings are associated with significant increases in the serum levels of TNF-α and hepatic JNK activation and AP-1 DNA binding (Fernández et al., 2007a), which coincide with the enhancement in the serum IL-6 levels and liver STAT activation (Tapia et al., 2006), being all changes suppressed by $GdCl_3$ treatment prior to T_3. Thus, T_3 triggers hepatocyte proliferation through mechanisms that may involve Kupffer cell-dependent generation of the priming cytokines TNF-α and IL-6, leading to JNK/AP-1 and/or JAK/STAT3 activation (Figure 4), respectively. These findings were observed 52-70 h after the daily administration of T_3 for three consecutive days and may involve earlier increases in cyclin D1, cyclin E, or E2F transcription factor expression and retinoblastoma protein phosphorylation (Pibiri et al., 2001). Collectively, the discussed actions of T_3 may allow transition from G1 to S phase leading to hepatocyte proliferation, the metabolic demands of which could be met by acceleration of energy metabolism through the calorigenic effects of T_3 (Figure 1).

Liver Preconditioning by Thyroid Hormone

Liver functioning implies a variety of aspects of the intermediary metabolism, biotransformation of xenobiotics, excretion, and secretion of different biomolecules, being the high energy demands required to cope with these processes primarily met by fatty acid oxidation. This makes the liver highly dependent on O_2 supply, with consequent generation of ROS and susceptibility to hypoxia or anoxia states. Cellular death in the liver occurs in association with cholestasis, viral hepatitis, drug-induced injury, and ischemia-reperfusion (IR), including liver preservation for transplantation (Malhi et al., 2006). In general terms, IR injury refers to tissue damage produced by blood perfusion to the previously ischemic organ, which in liver is associated with the clinical settings of hepatic resection, transplantation, low-blood pressure states, and abdominal surgery requiring hepatic vascular occlusion (Banga et al., 2005; Massip-Salcedo et al., 2007). IR liver injury underlies Kupffer cell activation, oxidative stress, and production and release of pro-inflammatory mediators playing key roles in inducing critical hepatic failure, which is considered as one of the major causes of primary graft nonfunction in liver transplantation (Lemaster and Thurman, 1995). In this context, liver preconditioning consists in strategies protecting the organ from detrimental effects of subsequent noxious events, such as those underlying chemically-induced injury or IR (Banga et al., 2005; Malhi et al., 2006; Massip-Salcedo et al., 2007). Among them, induction of a mild increase in the oxidative stress status of the liver prior to IR has been studied in experimental animals, as shown for transient ischemia (Peralta et al., 1997), hyperthermia (Terajima et al., 2000), hyperbaric oxygen therapy (Yu et al., 2005), ozone (Ajamieh et al., 2004), and the model oxidants doxorubicin (Ito et al., 2000) and t-butyl hydroperoxide (Rüdiger et al., 2003). This contention is based on the proposal that a moderate enhancement in ROS generation in a defined time interval can elicit an imbalance capable of redox regulation (Dröge, 2002), inducing cytoprotective responses against tissue damage such as those discussed for T_3 administration (Figure 4).

IR liver injury assessed in a model involving 1 hour of partial ischemia induced by vascular clamping followed by reperfusion for 20 h elicited minimal mortality but extensive liver damage (Fernández et al., 2007b). In fact, animals subjected to IR showed substantial distortion of liver architecture, including extensive areas of hepatocyte necrosis in midzone reaching pericentral and periportal areas, neutrophil infiltration, and enlargement of portal and central venules (Fernández et al., 2007b), in agreement with enhancements in the aspartate aminotransferase and TNF-α levels in serum (Table 1). Under these conditions, IR induced a drastic increase in the oxidative stress status of the liver as evidenced by the higher protein oxidation/GSH content ratio observed, which results from both elevated content of protein carbonyls and GSH depletion (Table 1). IR-induced pro-oxidant state in the liver is paralleled by loss in the DNA binding of NF-κB and STAT3 implying loss of cytoprotective potential, as shown by the concomitant diminution in the expression of the APR protein haptoglobin (Table 1) that is controlled by both transcription factors (Agrawal et al., 2003; Erns and Jenkins, 2004; Gruys et al., 2005). Contrary to these responses, the hepatic AP-1 DNA binding activity is increased (Fernández et al., 2008), which may constitute a major determinant of hepatotoxicity under conditions of reduced NF-κB activation and TNF-α response (Tonks, 2005) by inducing a substantial increase in the AP-1/ NF-κB DNA binding ratio (Table 1). Although changes in NF-κB and AP-1 activation are presumed to exhibit a similar pattern after IR, the differential effects found may be due to differences in functional properties of the transcription factors: (i) NF-κB shows a higher sensitivity to activation by ROS than AP-1; and (ii) NF-κB pre-exists in the cells in a latent form while AP-1 requires *de novo* synthesis of its components c-jun and c-fos for full activation of target genes (Meyer et al., 1993). These differences may explain the rapid activation of hepatic NF-κB, compared to AP-1, observed under IR conditions (Takeuchi et al., 2004) or in Kupffer cells exposed to LPS (Tran-Thi et al., 1995), as NF-κB exhibits an early peak (1-3 hours) mainly composed of p50p65 heterodimers and a late peak (12 hours) mainly composed of p50 homodimers that is suppressed by 24-48 hours reperfusion (Takahashi et al., 2001). Diminished DNA binding of hepatic NF-κB after IR injury may involve the induction of several negative-feedback mechanisms, namely, IKK inactivation, binding of newly synthesized IκB proteins to nuclear NF-κB, and/or formation of a modified form of IκBα conjugated with the small ubiquitin-like protein SUMO-1, which is resistant to signal-induced degradation (Karin and Ben-Neriah, 2000). In addition to loss of hepatic NF-κB activation by IR, liver AP-1 DNA binding is significantly enhanced (Table 1)(Fernández et al., 2008). This observation agrees with the view that depression of NF-κB activation increases the susceptibility to TNF-α-induced injury, concurrent with sustained activation of JNK, a major contributor to the death response (Kamata et al., 2005). JNK phosphorylates and activates the c-Jun component of AP-1, being JNK, phosphorylated c-Jun, and AP-1 DNA binding drastically augmented under IR conditions (Takeuchi et al., 2004; Uehara et al., 2005). Sustained JNK activation was reported to depend on TNF-α-induced ROS generation at the mitochondrial level, due to oxidation and inhibition of JNK inactivating phosphatases (Kamata et al., 2005). However, the exact role of these phosphatases in JNK activation and the mechanisms underlying reduction of NF-κB DNA binding remain to be established in liver IR injury.

Table 1. Thyroid hormone (T3) preconditioning against ischemia-reperfusion (IR) liver injury

Parameters		Control-IR / Control-sham	T3-IR / T3-sham
Serum			
	Aspartate aminotransferase	42	12
	TNF-α	2.2	0.9
Liver			
	GSH content	0.6	0.9
	Protein carbonyl content	2.1	1.1
	Protein carbonyl/GSH ratio	3.5	1.2
	NF-κB DNA binding	0.5	1.4
	AP-1 DNA binding	2.5	1.0
	AP-1/NF-κB ratio	5.0	0.7
	STAT3 DNA binding	0.5	0.9
	Haptoglobin expression	0.5	0.9

Values shown correspond to parameters measured in rats subjected to 1 h ischemia followed by 20 h reperfusion (IR) under unpreconditioned (control-IR/control-sham) or T_3-preconditioned (T_3-IR/T_3-sham) conditions. For this purpose, T_3 (0.1 mg/kg, i.p.) was given 48 h prior to the IR protocol, and parameters were measured at the end of the IR period. Abbreviations: AP-1, activator protein 1; GSH, reduced glutathione; NF-κB, nuclear factor-κB; STAT3, signal transducer and activator of transcription 3; TNF-α, tumor necrosis factor-α;

The calorigenic response induced by the administration of a single dose of T_3 to fed rats leads to a transient increase in the oxidative stress status of the liver, which occurs within 24 h after T_3 administration under conditions of higher rates of hepatic O_2 consumption, with significant GSH depletion and protein oxidation enhancement (Fernández et al., 2007b). In addition to these changes that are presumed to occur primarily at the parenchymal cell level, Kupffer cells may play a contributory role, as evidenced by the enhancement in both carbon phagocytosis and the related respiratory burst activity observed at 24 h after T_3 treatment. The latter process returned towards control values 48 h after T_3 treatment, concomitantly with the other oxidative stress-related parameters studied, a treatment that may represent a preconditioning stimulus considering (i) the absence of hepatotoxicity as revealed by the occurrence of normal liver histology and lack of significant changes in the serum levels of aminotransferases; and (ii) the enhancement in the activity of Kupffer cells, macrophages known to play a key role in the homeostatic response to liver injury (Fernández et al., 2007b). In agreement with this contention, T_3 treatment given 48 h before the IR protocol abolished hepatocellular injury associated with IR, with normalization of serum levels of ALT and TNF-α, the oxidative stress status of the liver, the hepatic DNA binding activity of NF-κB, STAT3, and AP-1, and the acute phase response (Table 1)(Fernández et al., 2007b; 2008). Under these conditions, cell protection by T_3 may involve prevention of ROS-dependent oxidative deterioration of biomolecules. In agreement with this view, the administration of the antioxidant N-acetylcysteine prior to the T_3-preconditioning phase increased by more than 3-fold the serum ALT levels after the IR protocol, thus diminishing the hepatoprotection afforded by T_3 (Fernández et al., 2008). In addition, T_3 preconditioning is also related to a gain of liver cell signaling functions represented by recovery of NF-κB and STAT3 DNA binding and APR lost during IR, and normalization of AP-1 activation enhanced by IR (Fernández et al., 2007b; 2008).

Although these responses may protect the liver against IR-induced oxidative stress and TNF-α response, T_3 liver preconditioning may be also related to enhanced cell proliferation (Figure 4) to compensate for liver cells lost due to IR-induced hepatocellular necrosis (Fernández et al., 2007a). These responses may protect the liver against IR-induced oxidative stress by re-establishing redox homeostasis, although actions involving other physiological functions cannot be discarded. In line with these views, recent studies revealed that thyroid hormone activates NF-κB in lymphocytes from rats (Vinayagamoorthi et al., 2005) or human hyperthyroid patients, in association with enhanced oxidative stress status and potentiation of antibody response (Nandakumar et al., 2008). T_3 administration also activates the hepatic JNK/STAT3 pathway in a nutritional model of steatosis, with complete regression of fat accumulation (Perra et al., 2008).

In conclusion, data discussed in this article indicate that redox regulation of gene transcription by T_3 represents an additional non-genomic mechanism to those reported for different cellular processes (Arnold et al., 1998; Yen, 2001; Bassett et al., 2003; Mezosi et al., 2005; Davis et al., 2008), which is dependent upon the genomic pathway triggering energy metabolism with ROS production. The non-genomic actions of thyroid hormones may in turn influence gene transcription by different pathways involving either antioxidant-sensitive NF-κB, AP-1, and STAT3 activation (Tapia et al., 2006; Fernández et al., 2008) or TR and STAT phosphorylation (Bassett et al., 2003; Davis et al., 2008). Furthermore, CREB binding protein (CBP) and the related protein p300 activating liganded TRs in the classical genomic pathway of T_3 action (Figure 1), can function as co-activators of transcription factors such as NF-κB and AP-1 (Yen, 2001). Collectively, these observations suggest the integration of different T_3-signaling inputs to achieve metabolic and redox balance under T_3-induced calorigenic conditions involving oxidative stress. The T_3-induced liver preconditioning (Fernández et al., 2007b) and T_4-dependent heart protection (Pantos et al., 2002) constitute preconditioning strategies that have clinical potential. This is an important issue considering that pharmacological and other liver preconditioning maneuvers have not been transferred to clinical application (Casillas-Ramírez et al., 2006). Furthermore, the usefulness of ischemic preconditioning in human liver resections (Clavien et al., 2003;

Smyrniotis et al., 2006; Heizmann et al., 2008) and in human liver transplantation (Totsuka et al., 2000; Amador et al., 2007), remains controversial (Koneru et al., 2005; Azoulay et al., 2006; Rahbari et al., 2008). T_3 is an endobiotic substance, widely used and well-tolerated therapeutic agent, which at low doses has either no significant adverse effects or minimal side actions than can readily controlled (Brent and Larsen, 1996). However, prevention of IR injury in humans during liver surgery and liver transplantation using reduced-size grafts from living donors await further experimental and clinical studies.

Acknowledgments

This article was supported by grant 1080039 from FONDECYT, Santiago, Chile.

References

Agrawal, A; Cha-Molstad, H; Samols, D; Kushner, I. Overexpressed nuclear factor-kappaB can participate in endogenous C-reactive protein induction, and enhances the effects of C/EBPbeta and signal transducer and activator of transcription-3. *Immunology* 2003; 108: 539-547.

Ajamieh, HH; Menendez, S, Martinez-Sanchez, G; Candelario-Jalil, E; Re, L; Giuliani, A, Fernández, OS. Effects of ozone oxidative preconditioning on nitric oxide generation and cellular redox balance in a rat model of hepatic ischaemia-reperfusion. *Liver International.* 2004; 24: 55-62.

Amador, A; Grande, L; Martí, J; Deulofeu, R; Miquel, R; Solá, A; Rodríguez-Laiz, G; Ferrer, J; Fondevila, C; Charco, R; Fuster, J; Hotter, G; García-Valdecasas, JC. Ischemic preconditioning in deceased donor liver transplantation: a prospective randomized clinical trial. *American Journal of Transplantation* 2007; 7: 2180-2189.

Andican, G; Gelisgen, R; Civelek, S; Seve, A; Seymen, O; Altug, T; Yigit, G; Burcak, G. Oxidative damage to nuclear DNA in hyperthyroid rat liver: inability of vitamin C to prevent the damage. *Journal of Toxicology and Environmental Health* 2004; 67: 413-420.

Arnold, S; Goglia, F; Kadenbach, B. 3,5-Diiodothyronine binds to subunit Va of cytochrome-c oxidase and abolishes the allosteric inhibition of respiration by ATP. *European Journal of Biochemistry* 1998; 252: 325-330.

Asayama, K; Dobashi, K; Hayashibe, H; Megata, Y; Kato, K. Lipid peroxidation and free radical scavengers in thyroid dysfunction in the rat: a possible mechanism of injury to heart and skeletal muscle in hyperthyroidism. *Endocrinology* 1987; 121: 2112-2118.

Azoulay, D; Lucidi, V; Andreani, P; Maggi, U; Sebagh, M; Ichai, P; Lemoine, A; Adam, R; Castaing, D. Ischemic preconditioning for major liver resection under vascular exclusion of the liver preserving the caval flow: a randomized prospective study. *Journal of the American College of Surgeons* 2006; 202: 203-211.

Banga, NR; Homer-Vanniasinkam, S; Graham, A; Al-Mukhtar, A; White, SA; Prasad, KR. Ischaemic preconditioning in transplantation and major resection of the liver. *British Journal of Surgery* 2005; 92: 528-538.

Bassett, JHD, Harvey, CB; Williams, GR. Mechanisms of thyroid hormone receptor-specific nuclear and extra nuclear actions. *Molecular and Cellular Endocrinology* 2003; 213: 1-11.

Bilzer, M; Roggel, F; Gerbes AL. Role of Kupffer cells host defense and liver disease. *Liver International* 2006; 26: 1175-1186.

Bouwens, L; Baekeland, M; De Zanger, R; Wisse, E. Quantitation, tissue distribution, and proliferation kinetics of Kupffer cells in normal rat liver. *Hepatology* 1986; 6: 718-722.

Brent, GA; Larsen, PR. Treatment of hypothyroidism. In: Braverman, LE; Utiger, RD; editors. *Werner and Ingbar's The Thyroid.* Philadelphia: Lippincott-Raven Publishers; 1996, 883-887.

Carrión, Y; Fernández, V; Videla, LA. Influence of thyroid hormone administration on hepatic glutathione content and basolateral γ-glutamyltransferase ectoactivity in the isolated perfused rat liver. *Biochemical Pharmacology* 1993; 45: 2527-2535.

Casillas-Ramírez, A;Mosbah, IB; Ramalho, F; Roselló-Catafau, J; Peralta, C. Past and future approaches to ischemia-reperfusion lesion associated with liver transplantation. *Life Sciences* 2006; 79: 1881-1894.

Clavien, PA; Selzner, M; Rüdiger, HA; Graf, R; Kadry, Z; Rousson, V; Jochum, W. A prospective randomized study in 100 consecutive patients undergoing major liver resection performed with versus without ischemic preconditioning. *Annals of Surgery* 2003; 238: 843-852.

Cowper, KB; Currin, RT; Dawson, TL; Lindert, KA; Lemasters, JJ; Thurman, RG. A new method to monitor Kupffer-cell function continuously in the perfused rat liver. *Biochemical Journal* 1990; 266: 141-147.

Davis, PJ; Leonard, JL; Davis, FB. Mechanisms of nongenomic actions of thyroid hormone. *Frontiers in Neuroendocrinology* 2008; 29: 211-218.

Dinarello, CA; Cannon, JG; Wolff, SM; Bernheim HA; Beutler B; Cerami A; Figari IS; Palladino MA Jr; O'Connor JV. Tumor necrosis factor (cathectin) is an endogenous pyrogen and induced production of interleukin-1. *Journal of Experimental Medicine* 1986; 163: 1433-1450.

Dröge, W. Free radicals in the physiological control of cell function. *Physiological Reviews* 2002; 82: 47-95.

Erns, M; Jenkins, BJ. Acquiring signaling specificity from the cytokine receptor gp130. *Trends in Genetics* 2004; 20: 23-32.

Essani, NA; Fisher, MA; Jaeschke, H. Inhibition of NF-κB activation by dimethyl sulfoxide correlates with suppression of TNF-α formation, reduced ICAM-1 gene expression and protection against endotoxin-induced liver injury. *Shock* 1997; 7: 90-96.

Fausto, N. Liver regeneration. *Journal of Hepatology* 2000; 32: 19-31.

Fausto, N; Campbell, JS; Riehle, KJ. Liver regeneration. *Hepatology* 2006; 43: S45-S53.

Fernández, V; Barrientos, X; Kipreos, K; Valenzuela, A; Videla, LA. Superoxide radical generation, NADPH oxidase activity, and cytochrome P450 content in an experimental hyperthyroid state: relation to lipid peroxidation. *Endocrinology* 1985; 117: 496-501.

Fernández, V; Llesuy, S; Solari, L; Videla, LA, Boveris, A. Chemiluminescence and respiratory responses related to thyroid hormone-induced liver oxidative stress. *Free Radical Research. Communications* 1988; 5: 77-84.

Fernández, V; Simizu, K; Barros, SBM; Azzalis, LA; Pimentel, R; Junqueira, VBC; Videla, LA. Effects of hyperthyroidism on rat liver glutathione metabolism: related enzymes activities, efflux, and turnover. *Endocrinology* 1991: 129:85-91.

Fernández, V; Videla, LA. Influence of hyperthyroidism on superoxide radical and hydrogen peroxide production by rat liver submitochondrial particles. *Free Radical Research Communications* 1993; 18: 329-335.

Fernández, V; Videla, LA. On the mechanism of thyroid hormone-induced respiratory burst activity in rat polymorphonuclear leukocytes. *Free Radical Biology and Medicine* 1995; 19: 359-363.

Fernández, V; Videla, LA. Effect of hyperthyroidism on the biliary release of thiobarbituric acid reactants in the rat. *Toxicology Letters* 1996; 84:149-153.

Fernández, V; Videla, LA; Tapìa, G; Israel, Y. Increases in tumor necrosis factor-α in response to thyroid hormone-induced liver oxidative stress in the rat. *Free Radical Research* 2002; 36: 719-725.

Fernández, V; Massa, L; Quiñones, L; Simon-Giavarotti, KA; Giavarotti, L; D'Almeida, V; Azzalis, LA; Junqueira, VBC; Videla, LA. Effects of γ-hexachlorocyclohexane and L-3,3',5-triiodothyronine on rat liver cytochrome P4502E1-dependent activity and content in relation to microsomal superoxide radical generation. *Biological Research* 2003; 36: 359-365.

Fernández, V; Tapia, G; Varela, P; Videla, LA. Redox regulation of thyroid hormone-induced Kupffer cell-dependent IκB-α phosphorylation in relation to inducible nitric oxide synthase expression. *Free Radical Research* 2005a; 39: 411-418.

Fernández, V; Tapia, G; Varela, P; Castillo, I; Mora, C; Moya, F; Orellana, M; Videla, LA. Redox-up-regulated expression of rat liver manganese superoxide dismutase and Bcl-2 by thyroid hormone is associated with inhibitor of κB-α phosphorylation and nuclear factor-κB activation. *Journal of Endocrinolology* 2005b; 186: 539-547.

Fernández, V; Reyes, S; Bravo, S; Sepúlveda R; Romanque, P; Santander, G; Castillo, I; Varela, P; Tapia, G; Videla, LA. Involvement of Kupffer cell-dependent signaling in T_3-induced hepatocyte proliferation *in vivo*. *Biological Chemistry* 2007a; 388: 831-837.

Fernández, V; Castillo, I; Tapia, G; Romanque, P; Uribe-Echevarría, S; Uribe, M; Cartier-Ugarte, D; Santander, G; Vial, MT; Videla, LA. Thyroid hormone preconditioning: protection against ischemia-reperfusion liver injury in the rat. *Hepatology* 2007b; 45: 170-177.

Fernández, V; Tapia, G; Varela, P; Gaete, L; Vera, G; Mora, C; Vial, MT; Videla, LA. Causal role of oxidative stress in liver preconditioning by thyroid hormone in rats. *Free Radical Biology and Medicine* 2008; 44: 1724-1731.

Fitch, CA; Song, Y; Leverson, CW. Developmental regulation of hepatic ceruplasmin mRNA and serum activity by exogenous thyroxine and dexamethasone. *Proceedings of the Society for Experimental Biology and Medicine* 1999; 221: 27-31.

Flamant, F; Gauthier, K; Samarut, J. Thyroid hormones signaling is getting more complex: STORMs are coming. *Molecular Endocrinology* 2007; 21: 321-333.

Forbes, SJ; Themis, M; Alison, MR; Sarosi, I; Coutelle, C; Hodgson, HJ. Synergistic growth factors enhance rat liver proliferation and enable retroviral gene transfer via a peripheral vein. *Gastroenterology* 2000; 118: 591-598.

Francavilla, A; Carr, BI; Azzarone, A; Polimeno, L; Wang, Z; Van Thiel, DH; Subbotin, V; Prelich, JG; Starzl, TE. Hepatocyte proliferation and gene expression induced by triiodothyronine *in vivo* and *in vitro. Hepatology* 1994; 20: 13237-13241.

Garg, AK; Aggarwal, BB: Reactive oxygen intermediates in TNF signaling. *Molecular Immunology* 2002; 39; 509-517.

Gloire, G; Legrand-Poels, S; Piette, J. NF-κB activation by reactive oxygen species: fifteen years later. *Biochemical Pharmacology* 2006; 72: 1493-1505.

Goeptar, AR; Scheerens, H; Vermeulen, NPE. Oxygen and xenobiotic reductase activities of cytochrome P450. *Critical Reviews in Toxicology* 1995; 25: 25-65.

Goglia, F; Skulachev, VP, A function for novel uncoupling proteins: antioxidant defense of mitochondrial matrix by translocating fatty acid peroxides from the inner to outer membrane leaflet. *FASEB Journal* 2003; 17: 1585-1591.

Gomes, LF; Lorente, S; Simon-Giavarotti, KA; Areco, KN; Araujo-Peres, C; Videla, LA. Tri-iodothyronine differentially induces Kupffer cell ED1/ED2 subpopulations. *Molecular Aspects of Medicine* 2004; 25: 183-190.

Griffin, EE; Miller, LL. Effects of hypothyroidism, hyperthyroidism, and thyroxine on net synthesis of plasma proteins by the isolated perfused rat liver. *Journal of Biological Chemistry* 1973; 248: 4716-4723.

Gruys, E; Toussaint, MJM; Niewold, TA; Koopmans, SJ. Acute phase reaction and acute phase proteins. *Journal of Zhejiant UniversitySCIENCE* 2005; 6B: 1045-1056.

Guidot, DM; Repine, JE; Kitlowski, AD; Flores, SC; Nelson, SK; Wright, RM; McCord, JM. Mitochondrial respiration scavenges extramitochondrial superoxide anion via a nonenzymatic mechanism. *Journal of Clinical Investigation* 1995; 96: 1131-1136.

Hardonk, MJ; Dijkhuis, FWJ; Hultaert, CE; Koudstaal, J. Heterogeneity of rat liver and spleen macrophages in gadolinium chloride elimination and repopulation. *Journal of Leukocyte Biology* 1992; 52: 296-302.

Hayden, MS; Ghosh, S. Signaling to NF-κB. *Genes and Development* 2004; 18: 2195-2224.

Heizmann, O; Loehe, F; Volk, A; Schauer, RJ. Ischemic preconditioning improves postoperative outcome after liver resections: a randomized controlled study. *European Journal of Medical Research* 2008; 13: 79-86.

Hirano, T; Ishihara, K; Hibi, M. Roles of STAT3 in mediating the cell growth, differentiation and survival signals relayed through the IL-6 family of cytokine receptors. *Oncogene* 2000; 19: 2548-2556.

Hochenbery, DM; Oltavi, ZN; Yin, XM; Milliman, CL; Korsmeyer, SJ. Bcl-2 functions in an antioxidant pathway to prevent programmed cell death. *Cell* 1993; 75: 241-251.

Huh, K; Kwon, TH; Kim, JS; Park, JM. Role of the hepatic xanthine oxidase in thyroid dysfunction: effect of thyroid hormones in oxidative stress in rat liver. *Archives of Pharmaceutical Research* 1998; 21: 236-240.

Ito, K; Ozasa, H, Sanada, K; Horikawa, S. Doxorubicin preconditioning: a protection against rat hepatic ischemia-reperfusion injury. *Hepatology* 2000; 31: 416-419.

Janssen-Heininger, YMW; Poynter, M; Baeuerle, PA. Recent advances towards understanding redox mechanisms in the activation of nuclear factor κB. *Free Radical Biology and Medicine* 2000; 28: 1317-1327.

Jaumot, H; Estanyol, JM; Serratosa, J; Agell, M; Bachs, O. Activation of cdk4 and cdk2 during rat liver regeneration is associated with intranuclear rearrangements of cyclin-cdk complexes. *Hepatology* 1999; 29: 385-395.

Just, WW; Hartl, FU. Rat liver peroxisomes, II. Stimulation of peroxisomal fatty-acid beta-oxidation by thyroid hormones.*Hoppe-Seyler's Zeitschrift fur Physiologische Chemie* 1983; 364: 1541-1547

Kaisho, T; Akira, S. Toll-like receptor function and signaling. *Journal of Allergy and Clinical Immunology* 2006; 117: 979-987.

Kamata, H; Honda, S; Maeda, S; Chang, L; Hirata, H; Karin,M. Reactive oxygen species promote TNF-α-induced death and sustained JNK activation by inhibiting MAP kinase phosphatases. *Cell* 2005; 120: 649-661.

Karin, M; Ben-Neriah, Y. Phosphorylation meets ubiquitination: the control of NF-κB activity. *Annual Review of Immunology* 2000; 18: 621-663.

Klatt, P; Lamas, S. Regulation of protein function by S-glutathiolation in response to oxidative stress and nitrosative stress. *European Journal of Biochemistry* 2000; 267: 4928-4944.

Kolios, G; Valatas, V; Kouroumalis, E. Role of Kupffer cells in the pathogenesis of liver disease. *World J. Gastroenterology* 2006; 12: 7413-7420.

Koneru, B; Fisher, A; He, Y; Klein, KM; Skurnick, J; Wilson, DJ; de la Torre, AN; Merchant, A; Arora, R; Samanta, AK. Ischemic preconditioning in deceased donor liver transplantation: a prospective randomized clinical trial of safety and efficacy. *Liver Transplantation* 2005; 11: 196-202.

Landriscina, C; Petragallo, V; Morini, P; Marcotrigiano, GO. Lipid peroxidation in rat liver microsomes: I. Stimulation of the NADPH-cytochrome P450 reductase-dependent process in hyperthyroid state. *Biochemistry International* 1988; 17: 385-393.

Lanni, A; Moreno, M; Lombardi, A; Goglia, F. Thyroid hormone and uncoupling proteins. *FEBS Letters* 2003; 543: 5-10.

Larsen, PR; Herney, JW; Moore, DD. Sequences required for cell-specific thyroid hormone regulation of rat growth hormone promoter activity. *Journal of Biological Chemistry* 1986; 261: 14733-14736.

Laroux, FS; Lefer, DJ; Kawachi, S; Scalia, R; Cockrell, AS; Gray, L; van der Heyde, H; Hoffman, JM; Grisham, MB. Role of nitric oxide in the regulation of acute and chronic inflammation. *Antioxidants and Redox Signaling* 2000; 2: 391-396.

Leedman, PJ; Stein, AR; Chin, WW; Rogers, JT. Thyroid hormone modulates the interaction between iron regulatory proteins and the ferritin mRNA iron-responsive element. *Journal of Biological Chemistry* 1996; 271: 12017-12023.

Lemasters, JJ; Thurman, RG. The many faces of reperfusion injury. *Gastroenterology* 1995; 108:1317-1320.

Lin, KH; Lee, HY; Shih, CH; Yen, CC; Yang, RC; Wang, CS. Plasma protein regulation of thyroid hormone. *Journal of Endocrinology* 2003; 179: 367-377.

Malhi, H; Gores, GJ; Lemasters, JJ. Apoptosis and necrosis in the liver: a tale of two deaths? *Hepatology* 2006; 43: S31-S44.

Malik, R; Habib, M; Tootle, R; Hodgson, H. Exogenous thyroid hormone induces liver enlargement, whilst maintaining regenerative potential, a study relevant to donor preconditioning. *American Journal of Transplantation* 2005; 5: 1801-1807.

Massip-Salcedo, M; Roselló-Catafau, J; Prieto, J; Avíla, MA; Peralta, C. The response of the hepatocyte to ischemia. *Liver International* 2007; 27: 6-16.

Meyer, M; Schreck, R; Baeuerle, PA. H_2O_2 and antioxidants have opposite effects on activation of NF-κB and AP-1in intact cells: AP-1 as secondary antioxidant-responsive factor. *EMBO Journal* 1993; 12: 2005-2915.

Nandakumar, DN; Koner, BC; Vinayagamoorthi, R; Nanda, N; Negri, VS; Goswami, K; Bobby, Z; Hamide, A. Acivation of NF-κB in lymphocytes and increase in serum immunoglobulin in hyperthyroidism: possible role of oxidative stress. *Immunology* 2008; 213: 409-415.

Mezosi, E; Szabo, J; Nagy, EV; Borbely, A; varga, E; Paragh, G; Varga, Z. Nongenomin effect of thyroid hormone on free-radical production in human polymorphonuclear leukocytes. *Journal of Endocrinology* 2005; 185: 121-129.

Oppenheimer, JH; Schwartz, HL; Surks, MI. Tissue differences in the concentration of triiodothyronine nuclear binding sites in the rat: liver, kidney, pituitary, heart, brain, spleen, and testis. *Endocrinology* 1974; 95: 897-903.

Oren, R; Dabeva, MD; Karnezis, AN; Petkov, PM; Rosencrantz, R; Sandhu, JP; Moss, SF; Wang, S; Hurston, E; Laconi, E; Holt, PR; Thung, SN; Zhu, L; Shafritz, DA. Role of thyroid hormone in stimulating liver repopulation on the rat by transplanted hepatocytes. *Hepatology* 1999; 30: 903-913.

Pantos, CI; Malliopoulou, VA; Mourouzis, IS; Karamanoli, EP; Paizis, IA; Steimberg, H; Varonos, DD; Cokkinos, DV. Long-term thyroxine administration protects the heart in a pattern similar to ischemic preconditioning. *Thyroid* 2002; 12: 325-329.

Pascual, AS; Casanova, J; Samuels, HH. Photoaffinity labeling of thyroid hormone receptors in intact cells. *Journal of Biological Chemistry* 1982; 257: 9640-9647.

Peralta, C; Hotter, G; Closa, D; Gelpi, E; Bulbena, O; Roselló-Catafau, J. Protective effect of preconditioning on the injury associated to hepatic ischemia-reperfusion in the rat: role of nitric oxide and adenosine. *Hepatology* 1997; 25: 934-937.

Perra, A; Simbula, G; Simbula, M; Pibiri, M; Kowalik, MA; Sulas, P; Cocco, MT; Ledda-Columbano, GM; Columbano, A. Thyroid hormone (T_3) and TRbeta agonist GC-1 inhibit/reverse nonalcoholic fatty liver in rats. *FASEB J* 2008; 22: 2981-2989.

Pibiri, M; Ledda-Columbano, GM; Cossu, C; Simbula, G; Menegazzi, M; Shinozuka, H; Columbano, A. Cyclin D1 is an early target in hepatocyte proliferation induced by thyroid hormone (T_3). *FASEB Journal* 2001; 15: 1006-10013.

Poli, G; Leonarduzzi, G; Biasi, F; Chiarpotto, E. Oxidative stress and cell signaling. *Current Medicinal Chemistry* 2004; 11: 1163-1182.

Rahbari, NN; Wente, MN; Schemmer, P; Diener, MK; Hoffmann, K; Motschall, E; Schmidt, J; Weitz, J; Büchler, MW. Systematic review and meta-analysis of the effect of portal triad clamping on outcome after hepatic resection. *British Journal of Surgery* 2008; 95: 424-432.

Ram, PA; Waxman, DJ. Thyroid hormone stimulation of NADPH P450 reductase expression in liver and extrahepatic tissues. *Journal of Biological Chemistry* 1992; 267: 3294-3301.

Ramadori, G; Christ, B. Cytokines and the hepatic acute-phase response. *Seminars in Liver Disease* 1999: 19: 141-155.

Romanque, P; Tapia, G; Videla, LA. Kupffer cell stimulation in the isolated perfused rat liver triggers nuclear factor-κB DNA binding activity. *Redox Report* 2003; 8: 341-346.

Rüdiger, HA; Graf, R; Clavien, PA. Sublethal oxidative stress triggers the protective effects of ischemic preconditioning in the mouse liver. *Journal of Hepatology* 2003; 39: 972-977.

Samols, D; Agrawal, A; Krushner, I. Acute phase proteins. In: Oppenheim, JJ; Feldman, M, editors. *Cytokine reference on-line.* London: Academic Press; 2003; 1-16.

Schwartz, HL; Oppenheimer, JH. Physiologic and biochemical actions of thyroid hormone. *Pharmacology and Therapeutics Part B* 1978; 3: 349-376.

Sellitti, DF; Oliver, C; Latham, KR. Antibodies to nuclear thyroid hormone-binding proteins. Antibody characterization and immunofluorescent localization. *Experimental Cell Research* 1985; 158: 223-236.

Simon-Giavarotti, KA; Rodrigues, L; Rodrigues, T; Junqueira, VBC; Videla, LA. Liver microsomal parameters related to oxidative stress and antioxidant systems in hyperthyroid rats subjected to acute lindane treatment. *Free Radical Research* 1998; 29: 35-42.

Simon-Giavarotti, KA; Giavarotti, L; Gomes, LF; Lima, AF; Veridiano, AM; García, EA; Mora OA; Fernández, V; Videla, LA; Junqueira, VBC. Enhancement of lindane-induced liver oxidative stress and hepatotoxicity by thyroid hormone is reduced by gadolinium chloride. *Free Radical Research* 2002; 36: 1033-1039.

Smyrmiotis, V; Theodoraki, K; Arkadopoulos, N; Fragulidis, G; Condi-Pafiti, A; Plemerou-Fragou, M; Vassiliou, J; Dimakakos, P. Ischemic preconditioning versus intermittent vascular occlusion in liver resections performed under selective vascular exclusion: a prospective randomized study. *American Journal of Surgery* 2006; 192: 669-674.

Soboll, S. Thyroid hormone action on mitochondrial energy transfer. *Biochimica et Biophysica Acta*, 1993; 1144: 1-16.

Takahashi, Y; Ganster, RW; Gambotto, A; Shao, L; Kaizu, T; Wu, T; Yagnik, GP; Nakao, A; Tsoulfas, G; Ishikawa, T; Okuda, T; Geller, DA; Murase, N. Role of NF-κB on liver cold ischemia-reperfusion injury. *American Journal of Physiology: Gastrointestinal Liver Physiology* 2001; 283: G1175-G1184.

Takeuchi, D; Yoshidome, H; Kato, A; Ito, H; Kimura, I; Shimizu, M; Morita, Y; Miyazaki, M. Interleukin 18 causes hepatic ischemia/reperfusion injury by suppressing anti-inflammatory cytokine expression in mice. *Hepatology* 2004; 39: 699-710.

Tapia, G; Pepper, I; Smok, G; Videla, LA. Kupffer cell function in thyroid hormone-induced liver oxidative stress in the rat. *Free Radical Research* 1997; 26: 267-279.

Tapia, G; Cornejo, P; Fernández, V; Videla, LA. Protein oxidation in thyroid hormone-induced oxidative stress: relation to lipid peroxidation. *Toxicology Letters* 1999; 106: 209-214.

Tapia, G; Fernández, V; Varela, P; Cornejo, P; Guerrero, J; Videla, LA. Thyroid hormone-induced oxidative stress triggers nuclear factor-κB activation and cytokine gene expression in rat liver. *Free Radical Biology and Medicine* 2003; 35: 257-265.

Tapia, G; Fernández, V; Pino, C; Ardiles, R; Videla, LA. The acute-phase response of the liver in relation to thyroid hormone-induced redox signaling. *Free Radical Biology and Medicine* 2006; 40: 1628-1635.

Tata, JR; Ernster, L; Lindberg, O; Arrhenius ESP; Hedman, R. The action of thyroid hormones at the cell level. *Biochemical Journal* 1963; 86: 408-428.

Taub, R. Transcriptional control of liver regeneration. *FASEB Journal* 1996; 10: 413-427.

Terajima, H; Enders, G; Thiaener, A; Hammer, C; Kondo, T; Thiery, J; Yamamoto, Y; Yamaoka, Y; Messmer, K. Impact of hyperthermic preconditioning on postischemic hepatic microcirculatory disturbances in an isolated perfusion model of the rat liver. *Hepatology* 2000; 31: 407-415.

Tonks, NK. Redox redux: revisiting PTPs and the control of cell signaling. *Cell* 2005; 121: 667-670.

Totsuka, E; Fung, JJ; Urakami, A; Moras, N; Ishii, T; Takahashi, K; Narumi, S; Hakamada, K; Sasaki, M. Influence of donor cardiopulmonary arrest in human liver transplantation: possible role of ischemic preconditioning. *Hepatology* 2000; 31: 577-580.

Tran-Thi, TA; Decker, K; Baeuerle, PA. Differential activation of transcription factors NF-κB and AP-1 in rat liver macrophages. *Hepatology* 1995; 22: 613-619.

Tsukamoto, H; Lin, M. The role of Kupffer cells in liver injury. In: Wisse, E; Knook, DL; Balabaud, C, editors. *Cells of the Hepatic Sinusoid.* Leiden, The Netherlands: Kupffer Cell Foundation; 1997, 244-250.

Tsukamoto, H. Redox regulation of cytokine expression in Kupffer cells. *Antioxidants and Redox Signaling* 2002; 4: 741-748.

Tu, G; Cao, Q; Zhou, F; Israel, Y. Tetranucleoptide GGGA motif in primary RNA transcripts. Novel target site for antisense design. *Journal of Biological Chemistry* 1998; 273: 25125-25131.

Uehara, T; Bennet, B; Sakata, ST; Satoh, Y; Bilter, GK; Westwick, JK; Brenner, DA. JNK mediates hepatic ischemia reperfusion injury. *Journal of Hepatology* 2005; 42: 850-859.

Venditti, P; Balestrieri, M; Di Meo, S; De Leo, T. Effect of thyroid state on lipid peroxidation, antioxidant defenses, and susceptibility to oxidative stress in rat tissues. *Journal of Endocrinology* 1997; 155: 151-157.

Venditti, P; De Rosa, R; Di Meo, S. Effect of thyroid state on H_2O_2 production by rat liver mitochondria. *Molecular and Cellular Endocrinology* 2003; 205: 185-192.

Venditti, P; De Rosa, R; Di Meo, S. Effect of cold-induced hyperthyroidism on H_2O_2 production and susceptibility to stress conditions of rat liver mitochondria. *Free Radical Biology and Medicine* 2004; 36: 348-358.

Venditti, P; Di Meo, S. Thyroid hormone-induced oxidative stress. *Cellular and Molecular Life Sciences* 2006; 63: 414-434.

Videla, LA. Energy metabolism, thyroid calorigenesis, and oxidative stress: functional and cytotoxic consequences. *Redox Report* 2000; 5: 265-275.

Videla, LA; Correa, L; Rivera, M; Sir, T. Zymosan-induced luminol-amplified chemiluminescence of whole blood phagocytes in experimental and human hyperthyroidism. *Free Radical Biology and Medicine* 1993; 14: 669-675.

Videla, LA; Fernández, V; Tapia, G; Varela, P. Thyroid hormone calorigenesis and mitochondrial redox signaling: upregulation of gene expression. *Frontiers in Bioscience* 2007; 12: 1220-1228.

Vinayagamoorthi, R; Koner, BC; Kavitha, S; Nandakumar, DN; Priya, PP; Goswami, K. Potentiation of humural immune response and activation of NF-κB pathway in lymphocytes in experimentally induced hyperthyroid rats. *Cellular Immunology* 2005; 238: 56-60.

Virgili, F; Santini, MP; Canali, R; Polakowska, RR; Heads, A; Perozzi, G. Bcl-2 overexpression in the HaCat cell line is associated with a different fatty acid composition and sensitivity to oxidative stress. *Free Radical Biology and Medicine* 1998, 24: 93-101.

Voehringer, DW; Meyn, RE. Redox aspects of Bcl-2 function. *Antioxidants and Redox Signaling* 2000; 2: 537-550.

Vrba, J; Modriansky, M. Oxidative burst of Kupffer cells: target for liver injury treatment. *Biomedical Papers* 2002; 146: 15-20.

Wang, JF; Komarov, P; de Groot, H. Luminol chemiluminescence in rat macrophages and granulocytes: the role of NO, O_2^-/H_2O_2, and HOCl. *Archives of Biochemistry and Biophysics* 1993; 304: 189-196.

Wang, D; Baldwin, AS, Jr. Activation of nuclear factor κB-dependent transcription by tumor necrosis factor α is mediated through phosphorylation of RelA/p65 on serine 529. *Journal of Biological Chemistry* 1998; 273: 29411-29416.

Wiedau-Pazos, M; Trudell, JR; Altenbach, C; Kane, DJ; Hubbell, WL; Bredesen, DE. Expression of bcl-2 inhibits cellular radical generation. *Free Radical Research* 1996; 24: 205-212.

Yen, PM. Physiological and molecular basis of thyroid hormone action. *Physiological Reviews* 2001; 81: 1097-1142.

Yu, SY; Chiu, JH; Yang, SD; Yu, HY; Hsied, CC; Chen, PJ; Lui, WY; Wu, CW. Preconditioned hyperbaric oxygenation protects the liver against ischemia-reperfusion injury in rats. *Journal of Surgical Research* 2005; 128: 28-36.

Zhang, SQ; Kovalenko, A; Cantarella, G; Wallach, D. Recruitment of the IKK signalosome to the p55 TNF receptor: Rip and A20 bind to NEMO (IKKgamma) upon receptor stimulation. *Immunity* 2000; 12: 301-311.

Reviewed by: Professor Yedy Israel, Ph.D., Laboratory of Gene Therapy, Department of Pharmacological and Toxicological Chemistry, Faculty of Chemical and Pharmaceutical Sciences, University of Chile, Olivos 1007, Independencia, Santiago, RM, Chile (yisrael@uchile.cl).

In: Thyroid Hormones: Functions, Related Diseases and Uses ISBN: 978-1-60741-080-5
Editors: F. S. Kuehn, M. P. Lozada

Chapter IV

Different Effect of Thyroxine on Behavior and the Brain Serotonin Receptors of Catalepsy-Prone and Catalepsy-Resistant Mouse Strains

Alexander V.Kulikov*[*1], Eugene A. Zubkov*[*]
***and Vladimir S. Naumenko*[1]**
[1]Laboratory of Behavioral Neurogenomics, Institute of Cytology and Genetics, Siberian Branch of Russian Academy of Sciences, Novosibirsk, Russia
[2]Novosibirsk State University, Novosibirsk, Russia

Abstract

Thyroid hormones are used for treatment of patients with depressive disorders. In order to find genetic and molecular factors defining the sensitivity to thyroid hormones, the effects of chronic thyroxine (T4) treatment (2 mg/l, 60 days, in drinking water) on locomotor activity, anxiety-related, depressive-like behavior and freezing reaction (catalepsy) as well as on the 5-HT_{1A} and 5-HT_{2A} serotonin receptors in the brain were investigated in catalepsy-resistant AKR/J and catalepsy-prone ASC/Icg (Antidepressant Sensitive Catalepsy) strains. The latter was selectively bred for the high predisposition to catalepsy from intercross between CBA/Lac and AKR/J parental strains. In AKR mice T4 increased predisposition to catalepsy and locomotion in the open field test compared with the respective controls, but did not affect forced swim immobility. In contrast, in ASC mice T4 significantly decreased predisposition to catalepsy and immobility time in the forced swim test without any effect on locomotion in the open field. No influence of T4 on anxiety-related behavior in mice of these strains was shown. T4 treatment significantly increased head-twitch response to 5-HT_{2A} receptor agonist, DOI (1 mg/kg, ip) and the receptor mRNA level in the cortex in AKR, but not in ASC mice. Although

[*] Address for correspondence: Kulikov Alexander V., SD Laboratory of Behavioral Neurogenomics Institute of Cytology and Genetics 10 Lavrentyev Avenue Novosibirsk, 630090, Russia. Fax: 7-383-3331278 Phone: 7-383-3323101 e-mail: akulikov@ngs.ru.

the hormone did not affect 5-HT$_{1A}$ receptor mRNA level in the hippocampus and midbrain of ASC mice, a marked attenuation of hypothermic effect of 5-HT$_{1A}$ receptor agonist, 8-OH-DPAT (1 mg/kg, ip) in the T4-treated ASC was found. It was suggested that the cortical 5-HT$_{2A}$ receptor mediated the T4-induced activation of locomotion, while the 5-HT$_{1A}$ receptor was involved in the anticataleptic and antidepressant effects of the hormone. The results indicate that hereditary predisposition to catalepsy can predict behavioral effect of chronic T4 treatment in mice.

Introduction

Thyroid hormones are used for treatment of patients with depressive disorders. Chronic administration of high doses of thyroxine (T4) are effective in therapy of some depressive illness [4-9,16,56,60]. Small doses of triiodothyronine accelerate and augment clinical effect of tricyclic antidepressant [24,25,44,51]. At the same time, the mechanisms of sensitivity of the brain to thyroid hormones are still unknown and the clinical effects of chronic treatment with exogenous thyroid hormones are hardly predictable.

Data of few experimental studies of effect of chronic thyroid hormones administration on animal behavior are contradictory. Increase of locomotion in the open field test in T4-treated Wistar rats [55] was not confirmed [62]. Chronic T4 treatment did not affect anxiety-related behavior [62], but decreased sexual motivation [62] and produced antidepressant effect in the forced swim test [55] in Wistar rats.

It was supposed that the variability in sensitivity to hormone could be dependent on genotype and inherited brain neurotransmitter specificity [6]. The brain serotonin system was proposed as a target for thyroid hormones [4,26]. Thyroidectomy decreased density [39] and mRNA level [38] of the 5-HT$_{2A}$ receptor in the cortex of Wistar rats. Chronic T3 treatment decreased 5-HT$_{2A}$ receptor density in the cortex of mice [22] and rats [58]. At the same time, high doses of T4 and T3 increased the 5-HT$_{2A}$ receptor density in the cortex of rats [43]. Long-term treatment with T4 increased the 5-HT$_{2A}$ receptor sensitivity to the agonist DOI in Wistar rats [62].

Catalepsy (tonic immobility, immobility reflex, animal hypnosis) is a state of pronounced motor inhibition characterized by a failure to correct externally imposed, awkward posture. The phenomenon is a kind of passive defensive (cryptic) behavior and it is found in all vertebrates [18,27]. In birds and mammals, catalepsy is usually associated with fear and manifested as freezing in response to appearance of a predator or other threatening stimuli as an alternative to flight [18,20,27]. This reaction has also been suggested to be an element of female courtship behavior [28], male submissive behavior [19], and the behavior of pups when transported by their mothers [13]. At the same time, an exaggerated form of catalepsy is a syndrome of such severe disease as schizophrenia [1,21,57,59]). In rats genetic catalepsy was associated with depressive-like features [35].

A close link between thyroid hormones and catalepsy was shown [42]. Thyroidectomy predisposed Wistar rats to catalepsy, while selective breeding rats for catalepsy resulted in the decrease of blood T4 level [3]. On the other hand, chronic treatment of thyroidectomized Wistar and catalepsy-prone GC (Genetic Catalepsy) rats with T4 significantly reduced the immobility time [31]. At the same time, hormone did not alter immobility in catalepsy-resistant Wistar rats [62]. Moreover, hereditary catalepsy is linked to brain serotonergic system [49]. Catalepsy-prone GC rats have a decreased 5-HT_{2A} receptor density in the striatum compared with catalepsy-resistant Wistar animals [30].

Cataleptic-like immobility can be produced by repeated pinching of mouse at the scruff of the neck ("pinch-induced" catalepsy) [2,47]. Significant genetic variability in the predisposition to catalepsy in inbred mouse strains was shown [36]. Among 10 inbred mouse strains studied catalepsy was found only in mice of CBA strain – 54% of males and females in this strain displayed immobility time more than 60 s, while immobility was never observed in mice of AKR strain. Hereditary catalepsy in mice was demonstrated to be associated with 5-HT_{1A} and 5-HT_{2A} receptors [30,49,50]. Moreover, hereditary catalepsy in mice was shown to be linked to the 5-HT_{1A} receptor gene [29,32]. Recently at the Institute of Cytology and Genetics (Novosibirsk, Russia) ASC/Icg (Antidepressant Sensitive Catalepsy) mouse line highly predisposed to catalepsy was selectively bred from an initial backcross population between catalepsy-prone CBA and catalepsy-resistant AKR mouse strains [10,29,33]. ASC mice displayed numerous depressive-like behavioral features [10] and were sensitive to long-term treatment of a classical antidepressant, imipramine [63]. Mice of ASC were distinguished from animals of parental AKR strain by sensitivity to hypothermic effect of 5-HT_{1A} receptor agonist, 8-OH-DPAT. The drug produced significant decrease in body temperature in ASC mice, but failed to alter body temperature in AKR animals [29].

The main aim of the article was comparative study the effects of chronic T4 treatment on behavior and the serotonin receptors in catalepsy-prone ASC and catalepsy-resistant AKR mice. It was planned to compare the effects of T4 on: (1) catalepsy, (2) locomotion in the open-field, (3) anxiety related behavior in the light/dark box, (4) immobility in the forced swim test, (5) DOI-induced head-twitch, (6) 8-OH-DPAT-induced hypothermia and (7) the level of mRNA of 5-HT_{2A} and 5-HT_{1A} receptors in the brain.

Experimental Procedures

Animals. Experiments were performed on adult males of ASC/Icg (n=50) and AKR/J (n=53) strains. The AKR strain was maintained in the Institute of Cytology and Genetic during 40 years using brother-sister inbreeding and, therefore, was highly inbred. The ASC/Icg mouse line was selectively bred for high predisposition to catalepsy from a backcross generation BC(CBA x F_1(CBA x AKR)) between catalepsy-prone CBA/LacJ and catalepsy-resistant AKR/J mouse strains. Thirty-four couples with pronounced catalepsy were selected from the backcrosses to produce the S_1 mice. The S_2 mice were obtained by crossing 37 cataleptic couples from different families of the S_1. The S_3 and S_4 mice were produced by mating cataleptic mice from different 34 and 18 families of the S_2 and S_3, respectively. This scheme of crossing decreases the effect of founder. Starting with the S_5 breeding was accompanied by inbreeding – only cataleptic brothers and sisters were crossed [10,29]. Pups were isolated from their mothers at the age of one month, separated by sex and kept under the standard conditions in groups of 10 per cage (40 x 25 x 12 cm). The ASC mice were the 12th generation of selection for catalepsy and the 8th generation of brother-sister inbreeding. At the experiment beginning all animals were 2 months of age and weighting 22.3 ± 0.5 g. The mice of each strain were divided into two groups, control (18 ASC and 20 AKR) and T4-treated (18 ASC and 20 AKR). During the experiment mice of the four groups were housed 4-6 per cage of 50 x 25 x 15 cm at temperature of 22°C with 12:12 light/dark cycle. T4-treated mice of both strains were given L-thyroxine (Berlin-Chemie, Germany) in drinking water (2 mg/l) for 60 days. Control animals were given water for the same period. On the 61th day T4 was replaced by water and mice were isolated in individual cages of the same size. Behavioral test were started on the 63th day (two days after isolation). All experimental procedures were in compliance with the European Communities Council Directive of November 24, 1986 (86/309/EEC).

In order to evaluate the effect of T4 on serum thyroxine concentration other 7 ASC and 7 AKR mice were treated with the same dose of hormone for 14 days. Control 7 ASC and 6 AKR males received water for the same period. These 14 ASC and 13 AKR mice were decapitated after 14 days (on the 15th day) of treatment their blood serum was collected and kept at -20°C until T4 assay.

The catalepsy test. Immobility reaction was assayed according to the early described procedure [36]. Animals were firmly pinched between two fingers for 5 s at the scruff of the neck, placed on parallel bars, with the forepaws at 5 cm above the hind legs and then were released gently. The catalepsy duration (s) was recorded from the instant the animals were released to the instant when the animals shifted their front paws from their initial position on the upper bar or made gross body or head movements. The trial ended either when the animal started to move or after 120 s of immobility. Every animal was submitted to 10 successive trials with 2-min intervals. Mice were kept in the home cages between the trials. A mouse was considered as cataleptic if its immobility time was above 20 s in no less than 3 of 10 trials. Catalepsy was evaluated by percentage of cataleptics. This kind of scoring was highly reliable and the cataleptic score was replicated in 85% mice one week later.

In the open-field, light/dark and forced swim tests mouse movements were automatically registered by special tracking system consisting of arena, digital video camera, computer and EthoStudio tracking software [37], which frame-by-frame analyses captured video and detects animal in each frame using a threshold algorithm [46]. The center of animal was calculated as the means of the coordinates of all dark pixels on the animal back. White mice (AKR) were marked with a black permanent dye (a single black mark about 3 cm in diameter was put on animal's back) 3 days before the open field test.

The open field test. Two days after the catalepsy assay mice were tested in the open-field apparatus made of perplex 80 x 80 x 25 cm and colored white. The arena was brightly illuminated with a white lamp of 300 W set at a height of 180 cm. A mouse was placed by the wall at equal distances from two corners. The number of rears and distance (cm) run by the center of animal for 5 min was used as indexes of vertical and horizontal activities, respectively. The apparatus was careful cleared after each test.

The light/dark test. A day after the open field mice were tested for anxiety-related behavior in the light/dark box made of perplex and consisting of the light (30 x 30 x 25 cm) and dark (30 x 30 x 25 cm) compartments. The light compartment was open, colored white and brightly illuminated with a white lamp of 300 W set at a height of 180 cm, while the dark compartment was closed and colored black. The compartments were connected with the open (7 x 7 cm). A mouse was placed on the center of the light compartment faced to the dark compartment. The time (%) spent in the light compartment were registered for 5 min and served as an index of anxiety. The apparatus was careful cleared after each test.

The forced swim test. A day after the light/dark box mice were tested for depressive-like behavior in the forced swim test. Mouse was placed in square reservoir of 18 x 18 x 22 cm filled 3/4 with water at 25°C and after 40 s period of adaptation its movements was registered during 3 min. Immobility time (s) was evaluated by the time when the velocity of the mouse center shift was below 2 cm/s [17]. Water was changed after each test.

A half of mice in each group were used for measurement of functional activity of the 5-HT_{1A} and 5-HT_{2A} serotonin receptors.

The 8-OH-DPAT-induced hypothermy. The hypothermic effect of 5-HT_{1A} receptor agonist, 8-hydroxy-2-di-N-propylaminotetralin (8-OH-DPAT, Sigma Inc, 1 mg/kg in saline, i.p.) was evaluated by the difference in body temperature before and 30 min after the drug administration. Body temperature was measured by means of KJT thermocouple (Hanna Instruments, Singapore) with copper-constantan rectal probes for mice (Physitemp Instruments).

The head twitch test. Two days after the number of head twitches was visually counted for 20 min after single administration of 5-HT_{2A} receptor agonist (DOI, R.B.I., 1 mg/kg in saline, i.p.). The head twitch score used as an index of functional activity of 5-HT_{2A} receptors.

RT-PCR assay of 5-HT_{1A} and 5-HT_{2A} receptor mRNA. Another half of mice in the groups was decapitated, their brains were removed and the frontal cortex, hippocampus and midbrain were dissected, frozen with liquid nitrogen and kept at -66°C. For RT-PCR of 5-HT_{1A} and 5-HT_{2A} receptor mRNA expression, the method describe in detail earlier was used [41]. Total RNA was extracted with guanidinium thiocyanate-phenol-chloroform method according to Chomczynski and Sacchi [15] with modifications [41]. The RNA samples were treated with RNase free DNase for 10 min at 37°C to remove genomic DNA contamination [45]. The concentration of total RNA was determined by absorbance at 260 nm and its purity was estimated by 260/280 ratio. The RNA integrity was evaluated by electrophoresis in 0.8% agarose gel. Only RNA samples with clear visible 28S and 18S rRNA bands were used. The absence of DNA contamination in RNA preparations was checked by PCR analysis using primers for β-actin and 1 μl of total RNA diluted five times [40,45]. No sign of genomic β-actin fragment was detected by 32 cycles of amplification.

Total RNA, 8 μl (1 μg) was mixed with 180 ng of random hexamer primer and 2.25 μmol of sterile KCl in the volume of 16 μl, denatured at 94°C for 5 min, annealed at 41°C for 15 min, and then 15 μl of mixture containing reverse transcriptase M-MLV (200U) (Biosan, Russia), Tris HCl (pH 8.3, 0.225 μmol), dNTP mixture (0.015 μmol of each) (SibEnzyme, Russia), dithiothreitol (0.225 μmol) and $MnCl_2$ (0.03 μmol) were added. The mixture (at the final volume of 31 μl) was incubated at 41°C for 60 min. The synthesized cDNA was stored at -20°C.

An aliquot of 1 μl of cDNA was mixed with 2 μl of PCRx10 buffer, 1 μl of dNTP mixture, 0.03 μmol of $MgCl_2$, 5 μl of mixture of appropriate sense and antisense primers (250 pmol of each; 5-HT_{2A} primers: 5'-agaagccaccttgtgtgtga-3' and 5'-ttgctcattgctgatggact-3', 5-HT_{1A} primers: 5'-ccccccaagaagagcctgaa-3' and 5'-ggcagccagcagaggatgaa-3', β-actin primers: 5'-cggaaccgctcattgcc-3' and 5'-acccacactgtgcccatcta-3'), 1U of Taq-polymerase (SibEnzyme,

Russia) and sterile water to the final volume of 20 μl. PCR was carried out at the following protocol: (i) 5 min at 94°C; (ii) 40 s at 94°C, 40 s at 58°C ($5\text{-}HT_{2A}$) or 64°C ($5\text{-}HT_{1A}$) or 61°C (β-actin), 40 s at 72°C, 32 ($5\text{-}HT_{2A}$ and $5\text{-}HT_{1A}$) or 20 (β-actin) cycles; (iii) 4 min at 72°C.

The control tubes containing 1 μl of external standard DNA (100 ng/μl for β-actin or 10 ng/μl for the receptors) instead of cDNA and the same reagent mixture were amplified together with the corresponding sample tubes. We used genomic DNA extracted from the liver of C57BL/6J mice as the external standard containing 200 copies of the target genes per 1 ng [40,41]. Negative controls included the same reagent mixture except that cDNA and DNA were omitted.

The sample PCR products with the corresponding standards and the negative controls were then resolved by electrophoresis in the same 2% agarose gel, stained with ethidium bromide and scanned with Biometra™ system. The band intensities for samples and standards were analyzed using Scion Image software (Scion Corporation, http://www.scioncorp.com). The band intensities for the samples were calibrated by corresponding standard DNA, and the number of copies of $5\text{-}HT_{1A}$, $5\text{-}HT_{2A}$ and β-actin per 1 μl of cDNA was calculated. Expression of receptor mRNA was evaluated by the number of copies per 100 copies of respective β-actin mRNA.

Blood serum T4 concentration assay. Total T4 concentration in serum was assayed with immunoenzymatic method as described earlier [3].

Statistical analysis. Effect of T4 on catalepsy was evaluated by 2x2 table χ^2 statistics. Other behavioral traits were presented as means ± SEM and analyzed with two-way ANOVA followed by Newman-Keuls post-hoc comparison.

Results

No difference in the total serum T4 level in control AKR (45.0 ± 6.6 nM) and ASC (46.1 ± 5.6 nM, $p>0.05$) mice was found. Chronic T4 treatment (2 mg/l for 14 days) produced similar significant increase of serum thyroxine concentration (305.8 ± 29.7 nM in AKR and 255.2 ± 11.4 nM in ASC, $F_{1,23} = 190.6$, $p<0.001$). No effect of strain x treatment interaction was shown ($F_{1,23} = 2.3$, $p>0.05$). The result indicated that the T4 treatment was effective to maintain high hormone concentration in mouse blood.

None of 20 control AKR mice showed catalepsy, while 7 of 20 T4-treated AKR displayed pronounce immobility reaction (35%, $\chi^2 = 8.48$, $p<0.01$). On the contrary, chronic T4 administration significantly decreased the percentage of cataleptics in catalepsy-prone ASC mice: 13 of 18 (72%) in control and 7 of 18 (38%) in T4-treated ($\chi^2 = 4.05$, $p<0.05$, Figure 1).

Significant effects of strain ($F_{1,72} = 39.4$, $p<0.001$), T4 ($F_{1,72} = 11.3$, $p<0.01$), but not strain x T4 interaction ($F_{1,72} = 1.3$, $p>0.05$) on locomotion in the open field were revealed (Table 1). The control AKR mice showed about two-fold higher locomotion than the control ASC mice ($p<0.001$). However, chronic T4 treatment significantly increased locomotion in mice of AKR ($p<0.01$), but not in ASC ($p>0.05$) strains. A marked influence of genotype ($F_{1,72} = 14.3$, $p<0.001$) on the number of rears was shown. At the same time, this trait was not affected with T4 treatment ($F_{1,72} = 1.7$, $p>0.05$) (Table 1).

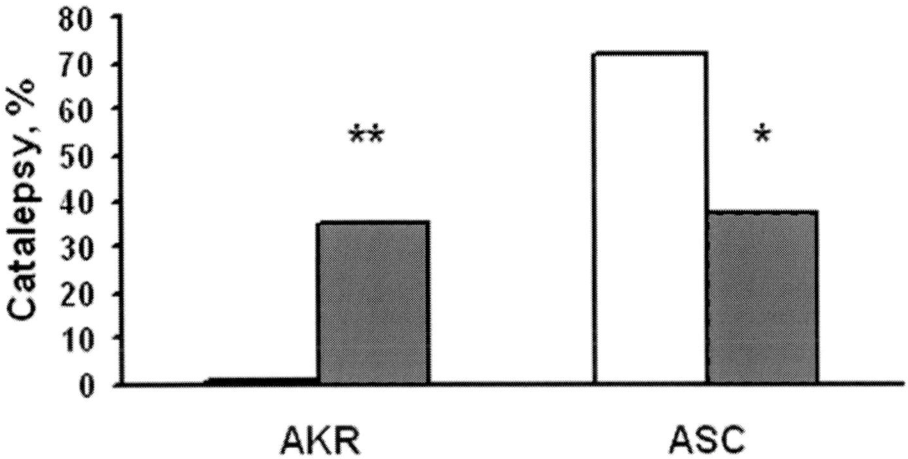

*p<0.05, **p<0.01 vs respective control.

Figure 1. Percentage of cataleptics in the control (open bars) and T4-treated (gray bars) AKR and ASC mice. Hormone was administered for 60 days in drinking water (2 mg/l) to male mice kept in groups of 4-6 animals.

Table 1. Vertical (rear numbers) and horizontal (distance run, cm) activities of the control and T4-treated AKR and ASC mice

Trait	Strain			
	AKR		ASC	
	Control (n=20)	T4 (n=20)	Control (n=18)	T4 (n=18)
Rear number	18.9±2.2	26.0±6.4	7.0±1.4	9.6±1.7
Distance run (cm)	1520.0±147.6	2170.0±183.9**	776.1±87.1***	1097.2±129.2

**p<0.01, p<0.001 vs AKR control.

No effect of strain ($F_{1,72}$ <1), T4 ($F_{1,72}$ = 3.5, p>0.05) or their interaction ($F_{1,72}$ <1) on the time spent in the light compartment was detected (Figure 2).

Untreated AKR mice were more immobile compared to untreated ASC mice in the forced swim test ($F_{1,72}$ = 192.2, p<0.001). Significant effect of the strain x T4 interaction on immobility time was found ($F_{1,72}$ = 13.8, p<0.001). T4-tratment did not alter immobility time in the forced swim test in AKR (p>0.05), but significantly decreased the trait value in ASC mice (p<0.001, Figure 3).

Control mice of AKR and ASC strains did not differ neither in the number of DOI-induced head twitches ($F_{1,37}$ = 4.5, p>0.05) nor in the 5-HT_{2A} receptor mRNA level in the frontal cortex (31.9 ± 3.6 in AKR and 36.9 ± 2.6 in ASC, $F_{1,24}$ = 4.2, p>0.05).. At the same time, a considerable interstrain difference in the thyroxine effect was found. T4 treatment significantly increased the number of DOI-induced head twitches (60.0 ± 7.6 vs. 40.0 ± 2.2, p<0.01) and the 5-HT_{2A} receptor mRNA expression in the cortex of AKR mice (up to 58.7 ± 4.0, p<0.001), but not in ASC (69.1 ± 5.5 vs. 53.2 ± 3.8, p>0.05) (Figure 4). Highly significant effect of T4 treatment ($F_{1,24}$ = 18.4, p<0.001) and genotype x T4 interaction ($F_{1,24}$ = 14.2, p<0.001) on the receptor mRNA was shown.

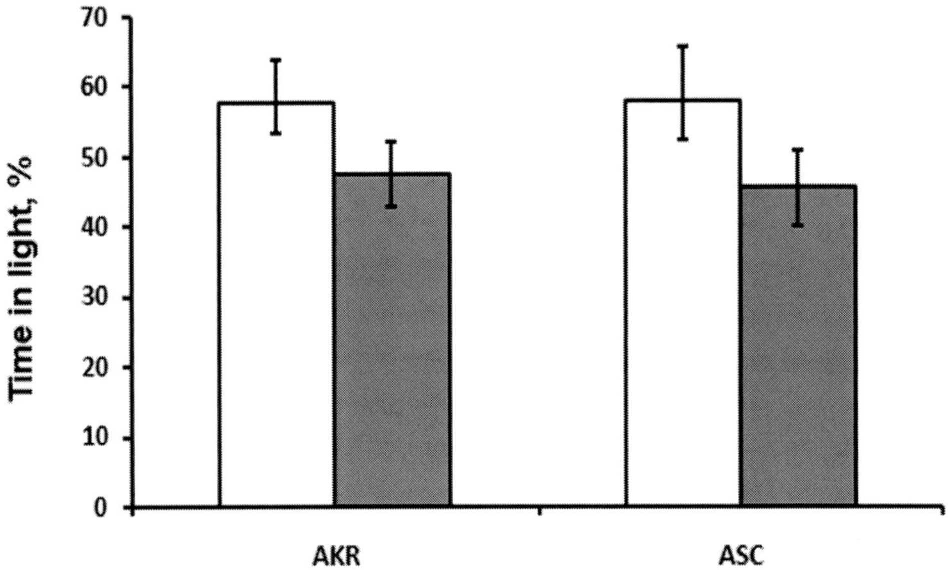

Figure 2. Effect of chronic T4 treatment (2 mg/l, 60 days) on the time spent in the light compartment (%) in AKR and ASC mice. Open bars represent control, while gray bars – T4-treated animals.

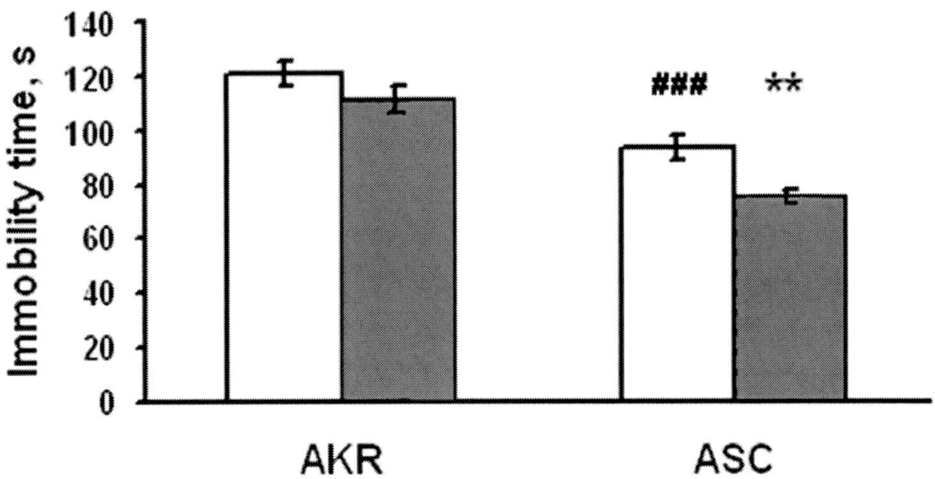

**p<0.01 vs respective control, ###p<0.001 vs AKR control.

Figure 3. Immobility time (s) in the forced swim test in the control (open bars) and T4-treated (gray bars) AKR and ASC mice.

Significant interstrain difference in 8-OH-DPAT – induced hypothermia was revealed ($F_{1,38} = 38.7$, $p<0.001$). 5-HT_{1A} receptor agonist 8-OH-DPAT induced hypothermia in ASC (-3.5 ± 0.4°C), but not in AKR mice (-0.4 ± 0.4°C). A marked effect of strain x treatment interaction was found ($F_{1,38} = 5.7$, $p<0.05$).

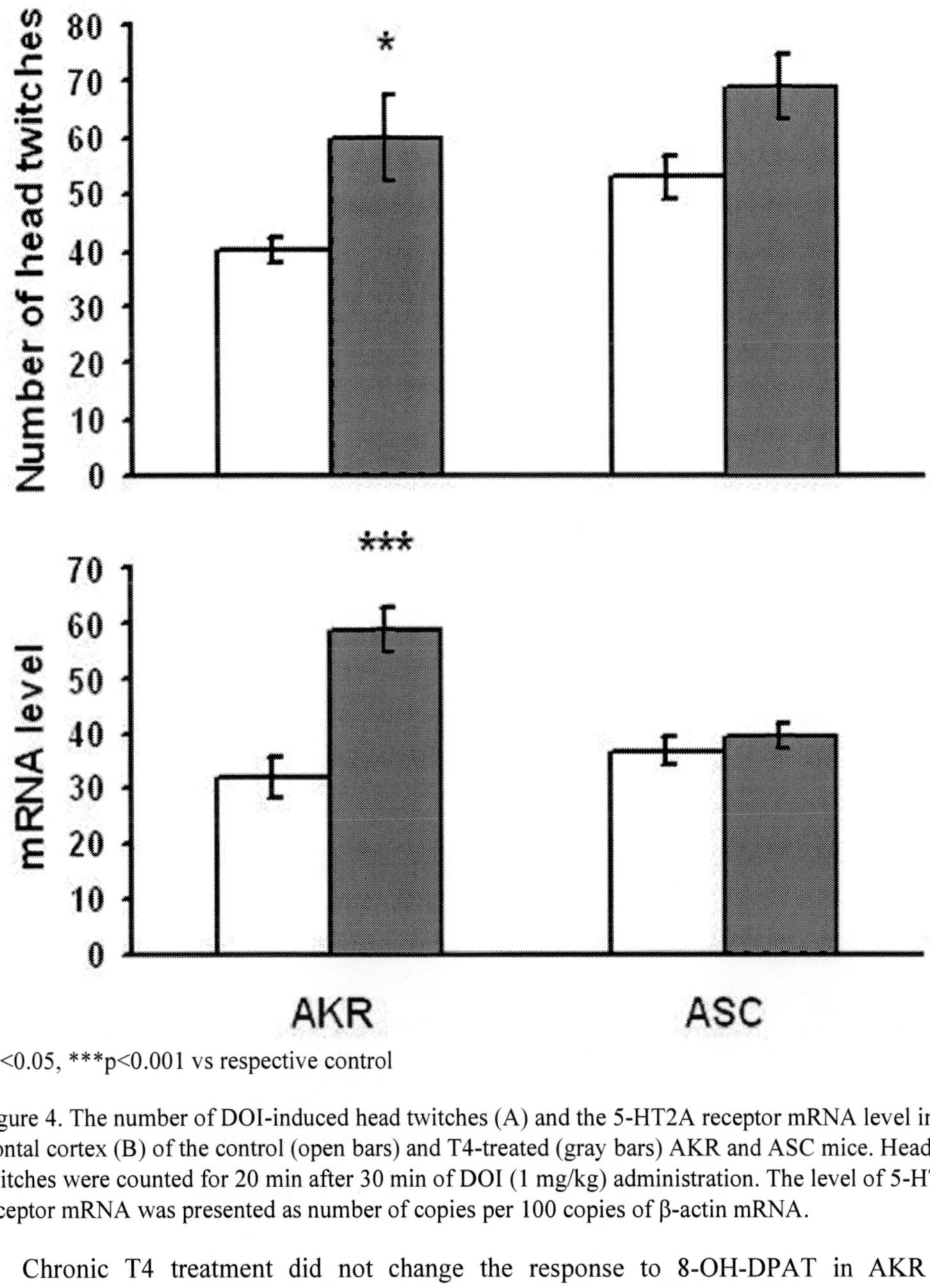

*p<0.05, ***p<0.001 vs respective control

Figure 4. The number of DOI-induced head twitches (A) and the 5-HT2A receptor mRNA level in the frontal cortex (B) of the control (open bars) and T4-treated (gray bars) AKR and ASC mice. Head twitches were counted for 20 min after 30 min of DOI (1 mg/kg) administration. The level of 5-HT_{2A} receptor mRNA was presented as number of copies per 100 copies of β-actin mRNA.

Chronic T4 treatment did not change the response to 8-OH-DPAT in AKR mice ($p>0.05$), but significantly decreased hypothermic effect in ASC mice (down to -2.0 ± 0.3°C, $p<0.01$, Figure5). Concentrations of the 5-HT_{1A} receptor mRNA in the hippocampus and midbrain of the control ASC mice were significantly higher than in these structures in the untreated AKR animals ($F_{1,25} = 17.0$, $p<0.001$ in hippocampus, and $F_{1,28} = 15.1$, $p<0.001$ in midbrain). Chronic T4 treatment did not affect the receptor mRNA level in the hippocampus and in the midbrain in AKR and ASC mice (Figure 5).

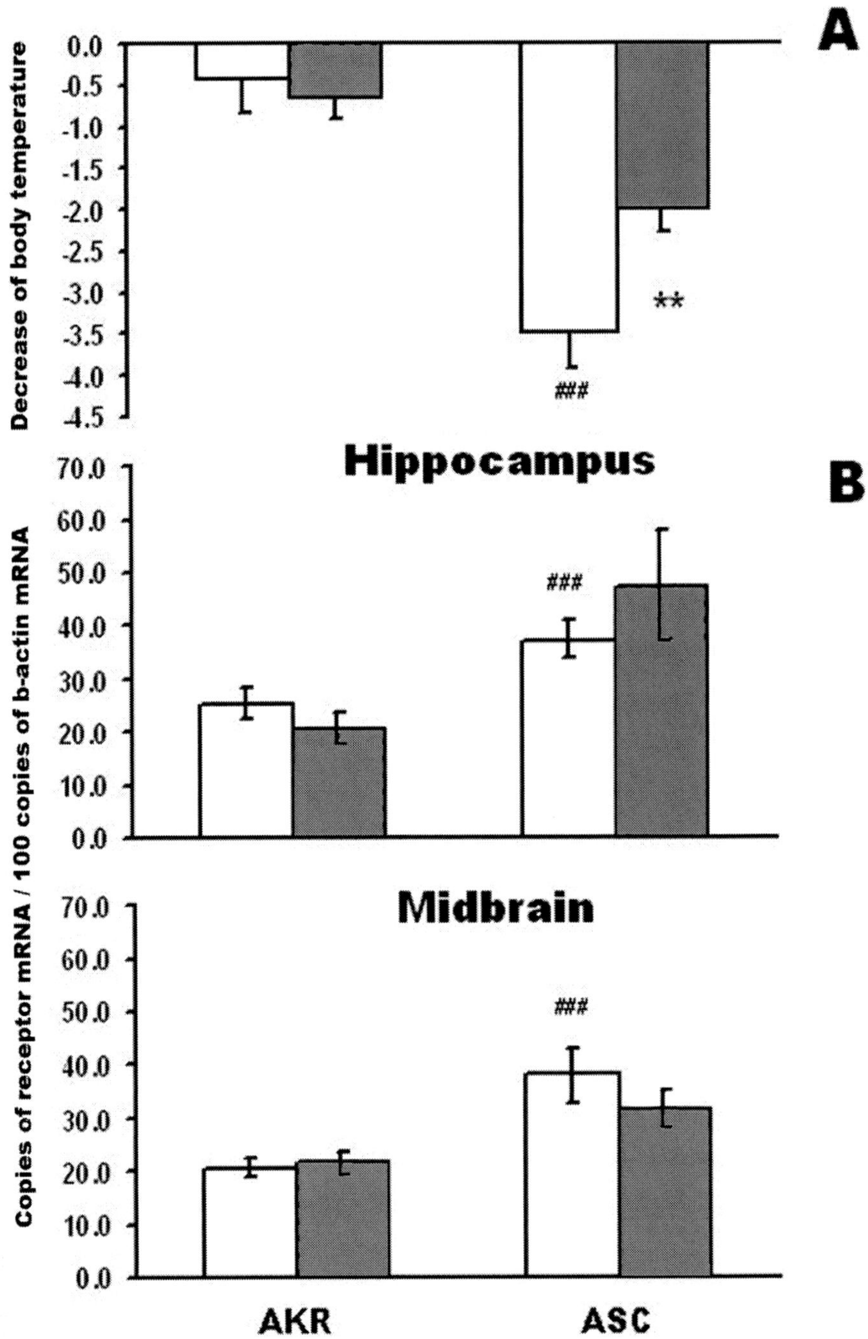

***p<0.001 vs respective control, ###p<0.001 vs AKR control.

Figure 5. The hypothermic effect of 8-OH-DPAT (A) and the 5-HT_{1A} receptor mRNA level in the hippocampus and midbrain (B) of the control (open bars) and T4-treated (gray bars) AKR and ASC mice. The hypothermic effect was evaluated by body temperature decrease 30 min after administration of 8-OH-DPAT (1 mg/kg). The level of 5-HT1A receptor mRNA was presented as number of copies per 100 copies of β-actin mRNA.

Discussion

The main result of the study was that effects of chronic T4 treatment on behavior were dependent on the genetically defined predisposition to catalepsy. The ASC line were created by the long-term selective breeding backcrosses between catalepsy-prone CBA and catalepsy-resistant AKR mice for high predisposition to catalepsy [10,29] and they carried out about 25% of the AKR genome [33]. Despite of the considerable shared part of the AKR and ASC genomes, mice of these strains show significant differences in the behavioral characteristics. The control AKR mice did not demonstrate catalepsy, while 72% of the control ASC mice were cataleptics. The untreated AKR mice showed increased locomotion in the open field and immobility in the forced swim compared with the control ASC mice. The data was consistent with early data obtained on mice of the S_8 generation of selection and was considered as an evidence of genetic association between catalepsy and these traits [10].

Chronic T4 treatment did not affect the time spent in the light compartment of the light/dark box in mice of both strains studies. Since the time in light is a valuable index of anxiety [54] it seems that chronic T4 fails to alter anxiety-related behavior in mice. This conclusion is consistent with our earlier observations that rat's anxiety-related behavior is resistant to thyroid hormone alterations [3,62].

At the same time, chronic T4 administration produced different effect on locomotion in the open field, immobility in the forced swim and catalepsy in AKR and ASC mice. Hormone significantly increased the open-field locomotion in AKR mice, but failed to alter the trait in ASC mice. At the same time, chronic T4 administration decreased the immobility time only in catalepsy-prone ASC mice but not in catalepsy-resistant AKR mice. Since chronic T4 treatment did not significantly affect locomotion in ASC mice, the observed decrease of immobility in the T4 treated ASC mice did not seem to result from an increase of locomotion, but it was caused by a specific antidepressant-like effect of the hormone. The opposite effect of T4 on catalepsy in the AKR and ASC mice was shown. T4 significantly decreased freezing in the catalepsy-prone ASC, but produced a marked cataleptogenic effect on catalepsy-resistant AKR mice. The anticataleptic effect of T4 in ASC mice is consistent with that found in catalepsy-prone GC rats [31]. At the same time, the cataleptogenic effect of T4 in catalepsy-resistant AKR mice was demonstrated for the first time. The result unambiguously indicated an association the effects of T4 on catalepsy, locomotion and immobility in the forced swim with genetically defined predisposition to catalepsy.

Numerous experimental observations demonstrated the involvement of 5-HT_{2A} and 5-HT_{1A} serotonin receptors in the regulation of immobility in the forced swim test [12]. The key role of 5-HT_{1A} receptors in the control of catalepsy was also well demonstrated: (i) activation of 5-HT_{1A} receptors decreased neuroleptic-induced catalepsy [14,23,52,53,64,65]; (ii) 5-HT_{1A} receptor agonists 8-OH-DPAT and flesinoxan attenuated expression of hereditary catalepsy in GC rats and CBA mice [34,50] and (iii) a linkage of genetic catalepsy in mice to the 5-HT_{1A} receptor gene was shown [29,32]. At the same time, hereditary predisposition to catalepsy in rats and mice was accompanied with a decrease of 5-HT_{2A} receptors density in striatum [30,49] and an increase of the receptor density in the cortex of catalepsy-prone CBA mice [30]. Thyroid hormones are also able to regulate both density and mRNA level of the 5-

HT_{2A} receptor in rat brain: their deficit produced by thyroidectomy significantly decreased the number of the receptor sites [39] and 5-HT_{2A} mRNA level [38] in the frontal cortex of Wistar rats. Therefore, an involvement of the 5-HT_{1A} and 5-HT_{2A} receptors in the determination of the genetically defined variability of the effects of T4 on behavior could be expected.

An intrigue result of the present article was demonstration that chronic T4 treatment increased the mRNA level in the cortex and activated 5-HT_{2A} receptor in AKR mice. This result is in concordance with increase of DOI-induced head-shakes in T4 treated Wistar rats [62] and decrease of the density [39] and the mRNA concentration [38] in thyroidectomized Wistar rats. Therefore, thyroid hormones seem to perform a consistent tonic control on the cortical 5-HT_{2A} receptors: hormone deficit suppresses while their excess activates the receptors. Since no thyroid response element was found in 5-HT_{2A} receptor gene promoter, it is unlikely that thyroid hormones affect directly the receptor gene expression. At the same time, the sensitivity of the 5-HT_{2A} receptors to T4 is dependent on genotype and T4 fails to affect the mRNA level and functional activity of the receptor in ASC mice.

Untreated AKR and ASC mice significantly differed in functional activity and the level of the 5-HT_{1A} receptor mRNA in the brain structures. The receptor functional activity evaluated by hypothermic effect of 8-OH-DPAT was higher in ASC compared with AKR mice. This result is in good concordance with earlier data [29]. The 5-HT_{1A} receptor mRNA level in the hippocampus and midbrain was higher in ASC compared with AKR mice.

The role of thyroid hormones in the regulation of 5-HT_{1A} receptors is less clear. An increase of the receptor density in the hippocampus of thyroidectomized rats [61] was not confirmed [39]. In the present study we found no effect of T4 treatment on the 5-HT_{1A} receptor mRNA in the hippocampus and midbrain of AKR and ASC mice. At the same time, a significant decrease of 8-OH-DPAT hypothermic effect of chronic T4 treatment in ASC mice indicated a possible involvement of thyroid hormone in the regulation of 5-HT_{1A} receptor function at posttranslational level.

What do these finding speak about possible association between thyroid hormones, the serotonin receptors and behavior? A positive correlation between effects of T4 on locomotion in the open field and 5-HT_{2A} receptor was shown. In AKR mice, chronic T4 treatment increased locomotion, the mRNA level and functional activity of the 5-HT_{2A} receptor, while hormone produced no significant effects on locomotion and 5-HT_{2A} receptor of ASC mice. At the same time, the 5-HT_{2A} receptor did not seem to mediate the effects of T4 on catalepsy and immobility in the forced swim. Despite of the positive association between T4 and 5-HT_{2A} receptor in mice, the hormone produced the opposite effects on catalepsy in AKR and ASC mice. Moreover, catalepsy in rats was shown to be associated with decreased thyroid hormone level [3,31,62]. Although the 5-HT_{2A} receptor of ASC mice was resistant to the chronic T4 treatment, hormone significantly decreased immobility time in the forced swim in animal of this strain. The chronic T4 treatment did not affect immobility in AKR mice which 5-HT_{2A} receptor was sensitive to hormone.

At the same time, the anticataleptic and antidepressant effects of T4 in ASC mice were accompanied with the decrease of the 5-HT_{1A} receptor functional activity. So, a possible involvement of the receptor function regulation in the anticataleptic and antidepressant effects of chronic T4 treatment can be hypothesized. This hypothesis is consistent with the commonly accepted hypothesis on the key role of the 5-HT_{1A} receptor desensitization in the mechanism of antidepressant drug action [11,48] and in the mechanism of catalepsy [14,23,64,65].

High doses of thyroid hormones ameliorate mood in some depressive patients but are ineffective in others [6]. The present data explain and provide some biological predictors of the clinically observed variability in sensitivity to T4. Chronic T4 treatment produced anticataleptic and antidepressant effect on catalepsy-prone GC rats and ASC mice. On the contrary, in catalepsy-resistant Wistar rats or AKR mice the hormone treatment was not effective or even produced a pronounced cataleptogenic effect. So, the neurobiological and molecular alterations associated with the genetically defined predisposition to catalepsy are biological predictors for the antidepressant and anticataleptic effects of thyroid hormones. The present findings build a bridge between the experimental and clinical observations: it can be hypothesized that T4 ameliorates behavior in some depressive patients, but produces an opposite effect on relatively healthy individuals.

Acknowledgments

The work was supported by the Siberian Division of Russian Academy of Sciences "Integration" (grant № 18) and the Russian Program "Molecular and Cell Biology" (grant № 20.9).

References

[1] Abrams, R., Taylor, M.A. and Coleman-Stolurow, K. (1979) Catatonia and mania: patterns of cerebral dysfunction. *Biol Psychiatry*, 14, 111-117.

[2] Amir, S., Brown, Z.V., Amir, Z. and Ornstein, K. (1981) Body-pinches induced long lasting cataleptic-like immobility in mice: Behavioral characterization and the effects of naloxone. *Life Sci*., 10, 1189–1194.

[3] Barykina, N.N., Chuguy, V.F., Alekhina, T.A., Kolpakov, V.G., Maksiutova, A.V. and Kulikov, A.V. (2002) Effects of thyroid hormone deficiency on behavior in rat strains with different predisposition to catalepsy. *Physiol Behav*., 75, 733–737.

[4] Bauer, M., Heinz, A. and Whybrow, P.C. (2002) Thyroid hormones, serotonin and mood: of synergy and significance in adult brain. *Molecular Psychiatry*, 7, 140–156.

[5] Bauer, M., Hellweg, R., Graft, K.J. and Baumgathner, A. (1998) Treatment of refractory depression with high-doze thyroxine. *Neuropsychopharmacology*, 18, 444–455.

[6] Bauer, M., London, E.D., Silverman, D.H.S., Rasgon, N., Kirchheiner, J. and Whybrow, P.C. (2003) Thyroid and mood modulation in affective disorders: insights from molecular research and functional brain imaging. *Pharmacopsychiatry*, 36, 215–221.

[7] Bauer, M,. Priebe, S., Berghofer, A., Bschor, T., Kiesslinger, K. and Whybrow, P.C. (2001) Subjective response to and tolerability of long-term supraphysiological doses of levothyroxine in refractory mood disorders. *J Affect Disord.*, 64, 35–42.

[8] Bauer, M.S. and Whybrow, P.C. (1990) Rapid cyclic bipolar affective disorder. Treatment of refractory rapid cycling with high-dose levothyroxine: a preliminary study. *Arch Gen Psychiatry*, 47, 435–440.

[9] Baumgartner, A., Bauer, M. and Hellweg, R. (1994) Treatment intractable non-rapid cycling bipolar affective disorder with high-doze thyroxine: an open clinical trial. *Neuropsychopharmacology*, 10, 183–189.

[10] Bazovkina, D.V., Kulikov, A.V., Kondaurova, E.M. and Popova, N.K. (2005) Selection for the predisposition to catalepsy enhances depressive-like traits in mice. *Russ J Genet.*, 41, 1222–1228.

[11] Blier, P. and de Montigny, C. (1994) Current advances in and trends in the treatment of depression. *Trends Pharmac Sci.*, 15, 220–226.

[12] Borsini, F. and Meli, A. (1988) Is the forced swimming test suitable model for revealing antidepressant activity? *Psychopharmacology*, 94, 147–160.

[13] Brewstrer, J. and Leon, M. (1980) Facilitation of maternal transport by Norway rat pups. *J Com Physiol Psychol.*, 94, 80-88.

[14] Broekkamp, C.L., Oosterloo, S.K., Berendsen, H.H. and van Delft, A.M. (1988) Effect of metergoline, fenfluramine, and 8-OHDPAT on catalepsy induced by haloperidol or morphine. *Naunyn-Schmiedebergs Arch Pharmacol.*, 338, 191–195.

[15] Chomczynski, P. and Sacchi, N. (1987) Single-step method of RNA isolation by guanidinium thiocyanate – phenole – chloroform extraction. *Anal Biochem.*, 162, 156-159.

[16] Cleare, A.J., McGregor, A. and O'Kean, V. (1996) Thyroxine replacement increases central 5-HT activity and reduces depressive symptoms in hypothyroidism. *Neuroendocrinology*, 64, 65–69.

[17] Crowley, J.J., Jones, M.D., O'Leary, O.F. and Lucki, I. (2004) Automated tests for measuring the effects of antidepressants in mice. *Pharmacol Biochem Behav.*, 78, 269–274.

[18] Dixon, A.K. (1998). Ethological strategies for defense in animals and humans: Their role in some psychiatric disorders. *Br J Med Psychol.*, 71, 417-445.

[19] Erskine, M.S., Barfield, R.J. and Coldan, B.D. (1980) Postpartum aggression in rats. II Dependence on maternal sensitivity to young and effects of experience with pregnancy and parturition. *J Comp Physiol Psychol.*, 94, 495-505.

[20] Gallup, G.G. (1977) Tonic immobility: The role of fear and predation. *Psychol Res.*, 27, 41-61

[21] Garver, G.L. (1984) Disease of the nervous system: Psychiatric disorders. In Kaplan, L.A., Pesce, A.J. (eds), *Clinical chemistry: theory analysis and correlations.* Sent Louis, C.V. Mosby, pp. 864-881.

[22] Heal, D.J. and Smith, S.L. (1988) The effects of acute and repeated administration of T3 to mice on 5-HT1 and 5-HT2 function in the brain and its influence on the actions of repeated electroconvulsive shock. *Neuropharmacol.*, 27, 1239–1248.

[23] Invernizzi, R.W., Cervo, L. and Samanin, R. (1988) 8-Hydroxy-2-(di-n-propylamino) tetralin, a selective serotonin1A receptor agonist, blocks haloperidol-induced catalepsy by an action on raphe nuclei medianus and dorsalis. *Neuropharmacology*, 27, 515–518.

[24] Joffe, R.T. and Levitt, A.J. (1993) The thyroid and depression. In Joffe, R.T. and Levitt, A.J. (eds), *The thyroid axis and psychiatric illness*. Washington, American Psychiatric Press Inc., pp. 195-253.

[25] Joffe, R.T., Sokolov, T.H. and Singer, W. (1995) Thyroid hormone treatment of depression. *Thyroid*, 5, 235–239.

[26] Kirkegaard, C. and Faber, J. (1998) The role of thyroid hormones in depression. *Eur J Endocrinol.*, 138, 1 – 9.

[27] Klemm, W.R. (1990) Behavioral inhibition, brainstem mechanisms of behavior. In Klemm, W.R., and Vertes, R.P. (eds), *Brainstem Mechanisms of Behavior*. New York, Willey, pp. 497-533.

[28] Komisaruk, B.R. (1974) Reproductive Behavior. In Motagna, W. and Sadler, W. (eds.), *Neural and hormonal interaction in the reproductive behavior of female rats*. New York, Plenum Press, pp. 97-129.

[29] Kondaurova, E.M., Bazovkina, D.V., Kulikov, A.V. and Popova, N.K. (2006) Selective breeding for catalepsy changes the distribution of microsatellite D13Mit76 alleles linked to the 5-HT_{1A} serotonin receptor gene in mice. *Genes Brain Behav.*, 5, 596-601

[30] Kulikov, A.V., Avgustinovich, D.F., Kolpakov, V.G., Maslova, G.B. and Popova, N.K. (1995) 5-HT_{2A} serotonin receptors in the brain of rats and mice hereditarily predisposed to catalepsy. *Pharmacol Biochem Behav.*, 50, 383–387.

[31] Kulikov, A.V., Barykina, N.N., Tikhonova, M.A., Chuguy, V.F., Kolpakov, V.G. and Popova, N.K. (2002) Effect of chronic thyroxine treatment on catalepsy in rats. *Neurosci Lett.*, 330, 207–209.

[32] Kulikov, A.V., Bazovkina, D.V., Moisan, M.P. and Mormede, P. (2003) The mapping of the gene of susceptibility to catalepsy in mice using polymorphic microsatellite markers. *Dokl Biol Sci.*, 393, 531–534.

[33] Kulikov, A.V., Bazovkina, D.V., Kondaurova, E.M. and Popova, N.K. (2008) Genetic structure of hereditary catalepsy in mice. *Genes Brain Behav.*, 7, 506-512.

[34] Kulikov, A.V., Kolpakov, V.G., Maslova, G.B., Kozintsev, I. and Popova, N.K. (1994) Effect of selective 5-HT_{1A} agonists and 5-HT_2 antagonists on inherited catalepsy in rats. *Psychopharmacology*, 114, 172–174.

[35] Kulikov, A.V., Kolpakov, V.G. and Popova, N.K. (2006) The genetic cataleptic (GC) rat strain as a model of depression disorders. In Kaluev, A. (ed) *Animal models in biological psychiatry*. Nova Science Publishers, New York, pp 59-73.

[36] Kulikov, A.V., Kozlachkova, E.Y., Maslova, G.B. and Popova, N.K. (1993) Inheritance of predisposition to catalepsy in mice. *Behavior Genetics*, 23, 378–384.

[37] Kulikov, A.V., Kulikov, V.A. and Bazovkina, D.V. (2005) Digital registration and analysis of visual information in behavioral experiment. *Zh Vyssh Nerv Deiat.*, 55, 126–132 [In Russian].

[38] Kulikov, A.V., Maksyutova, A.V., Ivanova, E.A., Khvorostov, I.B. and Popova, N.K. (2002) The effect of thyroidectomy on the expression of the mRNA of 5-HT_{2A}

serotonin receptors in the rat frontal cortex. Dokl. Akad. Nauk, 383, 417–419 [In Russian].

[39] Kulikov, A.V., Moreaux, X. and Jeanningros, R. (1999) Effects of experimental hypothyroidism on 5-HT_{1A}, 5-HT_{2A} uptake sites and tryptophan hydroxilase activity in mature rat brain. Neuroendocrinology, 69, 453–459.

[40] Kulikov, A.V. and Naumenko, V.S. (2007) Problems of mRNA quantification in the brain using RT-PCR. In Kwang, L.B. (ed) New Messenger RNA Research Communications. Nova Science Publishers, New York, pp. 53-68.

[41] Kulikov, A.V., Naumenko, V.S., Voronova, I.P., Tikhonova, M.A. and Popova, N.K. (2005) Quantitative RT-PCR assay of 5-HT_{1A} and 5-HT_{2A} serotonin receptor mRNAs using genomic DNA as an external standard. *J Neurosci Methods*, 141, 97–101.

[42] Kulikov, A.V. and Popova, N.K. (2007) Thyroid hormones, serotonin and behavior. The role of genotype. In Czerbska, M.T. (ed.) *Psychoendocrinology Research Trends*. Nova Science Publishers, New York, pp. 321-341.

[43] Mason, G.A., Bondy, S.C., Nemeroff, C.B., Walker, C.H. and Prange, A.J. (1987) The effects of thyroid state on beta-adrenergic and serotonergic receptors in rat brain. *Psychoneuroendocrinol.*, 12, 261-270.

[44] Musselman, D.L. and Nemeroff, C.B. (1996) Depression and endocrine disorders: focus on the thyroid and adrenal system. *Br J Psychiatry*, Suppl 168, 123–128.

[45] Naumenko, V.S. and Kulikov, A.V. (2006) Quantitative assay of 5-HT_{1A} serotonin receptor gene expression in the brain. *Mol Biol.*, 40, 37–44.

[46] Noldus, L.P., Spink, A.J. and Tegelenbosch, R.A. (2001) EthoVision: a versatile video tracking system for automation of behavioral experiments. *Behav Res Methods Instrum Comput.*, 33, 398–414.

[47] Ornstein, K. and Amir, S. (1981) Pinch-induced catalepsy in mice. *J Comp Phychol.*, 95, 827–835.

[48] Pineyro, G. and Blier, P. (1999) Autoregulation of serotonin neurons: role in antidepressant drug action. *Pharmacol Rev.*, 51, 533–591.

[49] Popova, N.K. and Kulikov, A.V. (1995) On the role of brain serotonin in expression of genetic predisposition to catalepsy in animal models. *Am J Med Genet.*, 60, 214–220.

[50] Popova, N.K., Kulikov, A.V., Avgustinovich, D.F., Vishnevetskaia, G.B. and Kolpakov, V.G. (1994) Participation of brain 5-HT_{1A} serotonin receptors in regulating hereditary catalepsy. *Bull Eksp Biol Med.*, 118. 633–635 [In Russian].

[51] Prange, A.J. (1996) Novel uses of thyroid hormones in patients with affective disorders. *Thyroid*, 6, 537–543.

[52] Prinssen, E.P., Colpaert, F.C. and Koek, W. (2002) 5-HT_{1A} receptor activation and anti-cataleptic effects: high-efficacy agonists maximally inhibit haloperidol-induced catalepsy. *Eur J Pharmacol.*, 453, 217–221.

[53] Prinssen, E.P., Koek, W. and Kleven, M.S. (2000) Effects of WAY 100635 on antipsychotic-induced catalepsy in 5-HT depleted animals: a role for tonic activation of 5-HT(1A) receptors. *Eur J Pharmacol.*, 395, 143–147.

[54] Ramos, A., Berton, O., Mormede, P. and Chaouloff, F. (1997) A multiple-test study of anxiety-related behaviours in six inbred rat strains. *Behav Brain Res.*, 85, 57-69.

[55] Redei, E.E., Solberg, L.C., Kluczynski, J.M. and Pare, W.P. (2001) Paradoxical hormonal and behavioral responses to hypothyroid and hyperthyroid states in the Wistar-Kyoto rat. *Neuropsychopharmacology*, 24, 632–639.

[56] Rudas, S., Schmitz, M., Pichler, P. and Baumgathner, A. (1999) Treatment of refractory chronic depression and dysthymia with high-doze thyroxine. *Biol Psychiatry*, 45,229–233.

[57] Sanberg, P.R., Bunsey, M.D., Giordano, M. and Norman, A.B. (1988) The catalepsy test: Its ups and downs. *Behav Neurosci.*, 102, 748-759.

[58] Sandrini, M., Vitale, G., Vergoni, A.V., Ottani, A. and Bertolini, A. (1996) Effect of acute and chronic treatement with triiodothyronine on serotonin levels and serotonergic receptor subtypes in the rat brain. *Life Sci.*, 58, 1551–1559.

[59] ingerman, B. and Raheja, R. (1994) Malignant catatonia--a continuing reality. *Ann Clin Psychiatry*, 6, 259-266.

[60] Stancer, H.C. and Persad, E. (1982) Treatment of intractable rapid-cycling manic-depressive disorder with levothyroxine. Clinical observations. *Arch Gen Psychiatry*, 39, 311–312.

[61] Tejani-Butt, S.M., Yang, J. and Kaviani, A. (1993) Time course of altered thyroid states on 5-HT_{1A} receptors and 5-HT uptake sites in rat brain: an autoradiographic analysis. *Neuroendocrinology*, 57, 1011–1018.

[62] Tikhonova, M.A., Kulikov, A.V., Lebedeva, E.I., Barykina, N.N., Amstislavskaya, T.G. and Popova, N.K.. (2005) On association between cortical 5-HT_{2A} receptors and behavior in rats with experimental thyroid disturbances. *Pharmacol Biochem Behav.*, 82, 506–514.

[63] Tikhonova, M.A., Lebedeva, V.V., Kulikov, A.V., Bazovkina, D.V. and Popova, N.K. (2006) Effect of imipramine on the behavior and cerebral 5-HT_{1A} serotonin receptors in mice genetically predisposed to catalepsy. *Bull Exp Biol Med.*, 141, 48–50.

[64] Wadenberg, M.L. (1996) Serotonergic mechanisms in neuroleptic-induced catalepsy in the rat. *Neurosci. Biobehav. Rev.*, 20, 325– 339.

[65] Wadenberg, M.L., Cortizo, L. and Ahlenius, S. (1994) Evidence for specific interaction between 5-HT1A and dopamine D2 receptor mechanisms in the mediation of extrapiramidal motor function in the rat. *Pharmacol Biochem Behav.*, 47, 509–513.

In: Thyroid Hormones: Functions, Related Diseases and Uses ISBN: 978-1-60741-080-5
Editors: F. S. Kuehn, M. P. Lozada

Chapter V

Involvement of Thyroid Hormones in the Regulation of Mitochondrial Oxidations in Mammals and Birds

A. Collin[*1], *R. Joubert*[1], *Q. Swennen*[2,3], *M. Damon*[4], *S. Métayer Coustard*[1], *S. Skiba-Cassy*[5], *N. Everaert*[2], *J. Buyse*[2] *and S. Tesseraud*[1]

[1]INRA, UR83 Recherches Avicoles, F-37380 Nouzilly, France
[2]Department of Biosystems. Laboratory for Livestock Physiology, Immunology and Genetics of Domestic Animals, K.U. Leuven, Kasteelpark Arenberg, 30, 3001 Leuven, Belgium
[3]Centre for Environmental Sciences, Hasselt University, 3590 Diepenbeek, Belgium
[4]INRA, UMR1079 Systèmes d'Elevage Nutrition Animale et Humaine, F-35590 Saint-Gilles, France and
Agrocampus Ouest, UMR1079 Systèmes d'Elevage Nutrition Animale et Humaine, F-35000 Rennes, France
[5]INRA, UMR1067 Nutrition Aquaculture et Génomique, F-64310 Saint-Pée-sur-Nivelle, France;
IFREMER, UMR1067 Nutrition Aquaculture et Génomique, F-29280 Plouzané, France and
Université Bordeaux 1, UMR 1067 Nutrition Aquaculture et Génomique, F-33405 Talence, France.

Abstract

Thyroid hormones are major hormones regulating development and energy expenditure in mammals and avian species. They modulate the transcription of target genes by interacting with intracellular thyroid receptors that bind to thyroid hormone

[*] Correspondence : collin@tours.inra.fr.

response elements (TRE) located on DNA. Mitochondria are also reported to be targets of thyroid hormones, with early or delayed effects occurring through several pathways. In mammals, a direct short-term activation of enzymes involved in the respiratory chain results in higher rates of mitochondrial oxidative phosphorylation and the generation of reactive oxygen species (ROS). Additional long-term effects are mediated through changes in the mitochondrial coupling of oxidative phosphorylation, partly via a mechanism involving uncoupling proteins (UCP) and increasing proton leak. Moreover, triiodothyronine is reported to regulate fatty acid utilization, through the activation of enzymes involved in β-oxidation. Part of the mechanisms regulated by these hormones is dependent on the coordinated stimulations of the transcription of the nuclear and mitochondrial genomes. The present review focuses on the central role of thyroid hormones in the regulation of mitochondrial oxidations in light of the recent data obtained in mammals and birds.

Keywords: triiodothyronine, thyroxine, mitochondria, reactive oxygen species, O_2 consumption

Introduction

Thyroid hormones (TH) are reported to be major regulators of energy metabolism and mitochondrial functioning in both mammalian and avian species (Decuypere *et al.*, 1981; Silva, 1995). The two main thyroid hormones produced by the thyroid gland, common to all vertebrates, are L-thyroxine (3,5,3',5'-tetraiodothyronine T4) and, in lower amounts, L-triiodothyronine (3,5,3'-triiodo-L-thyronine or T3). These hormones are the result of the iodination and condensation of the tyrosine residues from thyroglobulin (Silvestri *et al.*, 2005b). Besides T4 and T3, small amounts of other iodothyronine, reverse triiodothyronine (r-T3) and 3,5-diiodo-L-thyronine (3,5-T2) are also reported to exert a significant physiological effect (Lanni *et al.*, 2001).

The production of thyroid hormones is controlled through a hypothalamic-pituitary-thyroid axis (figure 1). The T4 and T3 released by thyroid gland exert a negative feedback on the generation of both the hypothalamic thyroid-releasing-hormone (TRH) and the pituitary thyroid-stimulating-hormone (TSH). It is noteworthy that the main source of T3, r-T3 and 3,5-T2 is not the thyroid gland but peripheral tissues (mainly liver and kidneys) in which T4 and T3 are altered by deiodinating enzymes called deiodinases (Darras *et al.*, 2006). Three types of deiodinase have been described until now: type I (or D1) catalyzing the outer ring deiodination of T4 producing T3 and the inner-ring deiodination of T4 producing r-T3, mainly in liver and kidney but also in brain, thyroid gland, intestine and placenta (St Germain and Galton, 1997; Bianco *et al.*, 2002). Type II deiodinase (D2) converts T4 in T3 by a outer ring deiodination mainly in brain, brown adipose tissue of young mammals, but also in skeletal muscle (Bianco *et al.*, 2002; Darras *et al.*, 2006). Finally, the inner-ring deiodination of T3 and T4 is also catalyzed by type 3 deiodinase (D3) mainly in the central nervous system, fetal tissues, skin and placenta (St Germain and Galton, 1997; Darras *et al.*, 2006). As thyroid hormone receptors (TR) preferentially bind T3, the activity of thyroid hormones will depend on the control of peripheral T3 availability by the spatial and temporal regulations of TH synthesis and degradation (Decuypere *et al.*, 2005).

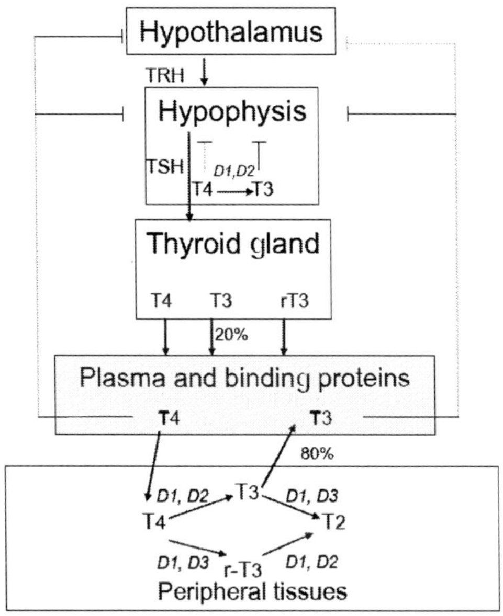

Figure 1. Schematic representation of thyroid axis in mammal and avian species. TRH: thyroid-releasing-hormone; TSH: thyroid-stimulating-hormone; T4: thyroxine (3,5,3',5'-tetraiodothyronine); T3: triiodothyronine (3,5,3'-triiodo-L-thyronine); r-T3: reverse triiodothyronine and T2: diiodo-L-thyronines. D1: type I deiodinase; D2: type II deiodinase; D3: type III deiodinase (from Decuypere and Kühn, 1988 and Mouillet, 2000).

The pathways involved in thyroid-mediated oxidations may correspond to short-term pathways such as the activation of cytoplasmic or mitochondrial enzymes and proteins, and long-term pathways including the transcription of nuclear and mitochondrial genes. Mitochondrial oxidations include O_2 consumption (and hence heat production or thermogenesis) and ATP production, re-oxidation of the reduced components of the respiratory chain and fatty acid oxidation, these pathways being associated to mechanisms producing reactive oxygen species (ROS). The present review focuses on the central role of thyroid hormones in the regulation of these mitochondrial oxidations in light of the recent data obtained in mammals and in avian species.

The Stimulation of Mitochondrial Activity by Short-Term Mechanisms

An increasing number of studies highlight a short-term increase in mitochondrial O_2 consumption and oxidations after a TH treatment. Part of the mechanisms regulated by these hormones is directly the result of biochemical interactions with mitochondrial enzymes and proteins, and they are likely to be interdependent (Silvestri *et al.*, 2005b). These pathways act either directly or indirectly (through an increase in ATP turnover) on mitochondrial activity.

Maintenance of Transmembrane Ionic Gradients

A small portion of the increase in O_2 consumption and hence metabolic rate under thyroid stimulation is indirect and due to the maintenance of transmembrane ionic gradients (Na^+/K^+ and Ca^{2+} gradients) in the cell, which consumes ATP and hence triggers mitochondrial activity (Silva, 2003). Indeed, the maintenance of the Ca^{2+} gradient between the sarcoplasmic reticulum and cytosol is of significant energy cost and regulates cell health. Hyperthyroidism will tend to reduce this gradient and increase the demand for ATP to maintain it.

Substrate Cycles

In addition to the stimulation of ion cycling, several substrate cycles are triggered by thyroid hormones. The metabolism of all three macronutrients (lipids, proteins and carbohydrates) is susceptible to be accelerated after T3 treatment. Two striking examples will be developed below: the regulation of lipogenesis/lipolysis turnover and the glycerol-3-phosphate/NADH shuttle.

It is well known that the effect of T3 on energy expenditure partly involves lipogenesis/lipolysis cycling (Freake and Oppenheimer, 1995). This cycling is mediated by transcriptional pathways but also by a direct effect on activities of proteins, which is detailed here. On the one hand, the lipogenic effect of thyroid hormones is evidenced in warm-blooded species (Weirich *et al.*, 1987; Silva, 2003), where malic enzyme activity, playing a key role in fatty acid synthesis, is strongly stimulated by T3. On the other hand, thyroid hormones are shown to trigger muscular fatty acid oxidations. The injection of T3 rapidly increases carnitine-palmitoyl-transferase activity in rat skeletal muscle, which stimulates the entry of fatty acids into mitochondria and thus triggers mitochondrial fatty acid oxidation (de Lange *et al.*, 2008).

Thyroid hormones could also decrease the efficiency of ATP synthesis through the glycerol-3-phosphate/NADH shuttle. Briefly, to re-enter into mitochondria after its reduction in the cytoplasm, nicotinamide adenine dinucleotide (NADH) has to be oxidized to NAD through the NADH shuttles. One of these shuttles is the glycerol-3-phosphate/NADH shuttle that regenerates NAD by transferring H^+ and e^- into mitochondria. The pathway using this shuttle produces 2 molecules of ATP per atom of oxygen reduced to H_2O, while the alternative malate-aspartate pathway results in 3 molecules of ATP/atom O reduced. The glycerol-3-phosphate (G3P)/NADH shuttle is under the control of the mitochondrial G3P dehydrogenase (or mGPD), the activity of this enzyme being stimulated by thyroid hormones (Silva, 2003).

Thyroid Hormones Modify Signaling Pathways Involved in the Regulation of Cellular Energy Metabolism

Thyroid hormones also affect rapidly and directly cellular signaling pathways, including the phosphorylation of protein kinase C, cAMP-dependent protein kinase and pyruvate kinase M2, and hence stimulate their activity and the downstream pathways (Davis and Davis,

1996). Several studies have recently focused on the involvement of AMP-activated protein Kinase (AMPK) in thyroid regulation of energy metabolism. This cellular energy sensor regulates the uptake and oxidation of both glucose and long chain fatty acids (Hardie, 2007). In chicken muscle, the phosphorylation of AMPK subunit α was also recently shown to be increased in hyperthyroid as compared to hypothyroid chickens (Collin *et al.*, 2007). Two laboratories demonstrated that an injection of T3 increased AMPK activation as soon as 6 hours (de Lange *et al.*, 2008) and even 2 hours (Irrcher *et al.*, 2008) post-injection in rat muscle. This activation is susceptible to activate fatty acid oxidation at the mitochondrial level, through both the direct phosphorylation of peroxisome proliferator-activated receptor gamma coactivator-1α (PGC1-α; Jäger *et al.*, 2007) and a longer-term transcriptional pathway. It is however noteworthy that AMPK activation by T3 is tissue-dependent, being increased in muscle but decreased in liver of rats. Finally, the p38 mitogen-activated protein kinase (P38 MAPK) pathway may also be recruited following T3-stimulation, and could be with AMPK activation a nongenomic pathway of T3-induction of mitochondrial biogenesis in skeletal muscles (Irrcher *et al.*, 2008).

Thyroid Hormones Modulate the Efficiency of Energy Transduction System

Besides the mechanisms described above, most of the short-term effects of thyroid hormones on mitochondrial oxidations are mediated through the modulation of the mitochondrial energy-transduction system efficiency (Silvestri *et al.*, 2005b). It is for example well recognized that the effect of thyroid hormones on O_2 consumption in liver and skeletal muscle occurs within the first hour post-treatment in mammals (Nelson, 1990; Soboll *et al.*, 1992). These changes are unaffected by inhibitors of protein synthesis, suggesting that they do not occur through transcriptional or translational pathways (O'Reilly and Murphy, 1992). They may rather involve both interactions with enzymes of the respiratory chain and mitochondrial uncoupling (Goglia *et al.*, 1999; Lombardi *et al.*, 2007).

A direct non-nuclear diiodothyronine-mediated stimulation of mitochondrial respiration rate and cytochrome oxidase (COX) activity is reported in rat liver and bovine heart (Horst *et al.*, 1989; Goglia *et al.*, 1994, Lombardi *et al.*, 1998). Cytochrome oxidase is a key multimeric enzyme controlling mitochondrial O_2 consumption and hence the intensity of energy metabolism and thermogenesis. The short-term stimulation of this enzyme activity by 3,5-T2 might occur via a specific binding of 3,5-T2 on the COX subunit Va, which abolishes ATP inhibition of COX activity (Arnold *et al.*, 1998).

Lombardi *et al.* (2007) recently evidenced another direct effect of 3,5-T2 on the mitochondrial respiration of hypothyroid rats. Mitochondrial oxidation of reduced substrates at the level of the inner membrane enables the phosphorylation of ADP and hence ATP production. This reaction is possible through the coupling of the respiratory chain with the H^+-pumping across the mitochondrial inner membrane that generates an electrochemical potential, which drives the transport of protons back to the mitochondrial matrix and stimulates ATP synthesis (Maloney *et al.*, 1974). However, this coupling is imperfect and two mechanisms were suggested to explain mitochondrial uncoupling (Luvisetto, 1997): (1) the existence of a proton leak through the inner membrane independently from ATP synthase, (2) a slippage of electron transfer into the respiratory chain decreasing the yield of H^+-extraction when O_2 is consumed.

One hour after 3,5-T2 injection, both coupled (+27%) and uncoupled (+42%) respiration rates are increased in the hypothyroid rat (Lombardi *et al.*, 2007). The rapid effect of 3,5-T2 on proton leak of hypothyroid rats could be of significant physiological effect since proton leak may account for 52% of resting O_2 consumption of skeletal muscle in rat (Rolfe *et al.*, 1994). The underlying mechanism might be an increase in the spontaneous mitochondrial proton leak caused by a change in the composition and permeability of the phospholipidic bilayer (Harper *et al.*, 1993). Indeed, thyroid hormones increase membrane cardiolipin content through the stimulation of cardiolipin synthase activity, and thus enhance the activity of several mitochondrial carriers (Paradies *et al.*, 1997; Cao *et al.*, 1995).

Among mitochondrial proteins also affecting membrane proton conductance, adenine nucleotide translocase (ANT) and uncoupling proteins (UCP) could mediate part of the short-term uncoupling effect of thyroid hormones (Collin *et al.*, 2005). For instance, in skeletal muscle, non-esterified fatty acids (NEFA) seem to be cofactors essential for the uncoupling activity of UCP3, the uncoupling protein specific to muscle and adipose tissue in mammals. Lombardi *et al.* (2002) report that hypothyroidism-hyperthyroidism transition is accompanied by an increase in the endogenous levels of mitochondrial NEFA. It also enhances the sensitivity of mitochondrial respiration rate and of membrane potential to NEFA, in good correlation with the level of UCP3 protein. The ANT contribution to NEFA-induced changes in mitochondrial uncoupling is low in both the hypothyroid and euthyroid states but becomes more relevant in the hyperthyroid state associated to high NEFA concentrations.

Thyroid Hormones Trigger Mitochondrial Reactive Oxygen Species (ROS) Generation

The redox reactions occurring within the mitochondrial respiratory electron transport chain are associated to the reduction of O_2 in $O_2^{\cdot-}$ (superoxide anion). This highly reactive free radical will oxidize various biomolecules, hence generating ROS (Turrens, 2003). Generation of these species and of reactive nitrogen species (RNS) occurs at low levels under normal conditions and may regulate protein function through reversible oxidation and/or nitrosation of protein sulfhydryls (Klatt and Lamas, 2000). However, persistent production of large amounts of ROS are reported to cause several damages through the induction of significant oxidation of biomolecules, changes in gene expression and signal transduction, that may even lead to cell death (Droge, 2002). In many tissues including liver, a pro-oxidant activity is developed as the result of the interdependent mechanisms of thyroid thermogenesis, cellular O_2 consumption, and ROS generation (Videla, 2000; Venditti and Di Meo, 2006). Oxidative stress is reported in hyperthyroid animals of several species (Videla *et al.*, 1988; Tapia *et al.*, 1997), and recent results of our laboratory indicate higher levels of thiobarbituric acid reactive substances (TBARS) in the skeletal muscle of chickens chronically treated with T3 as compared to euthyroid chickens (Collin *et al.*, 2007). In mammals, it is noteworthy that T3-induced oxidative stress depends on the muscle metabolic type. Indeed, increases in TBARS upon T3 stimulation were reported in slow oxidative muscles with type I fibers but not in muscles mainly containing type IIb glycolytic fibers (for a review, see Venditti and Di Meo, 2006).

Part of this T3-induced oxidative stress is attributed to mitochondrial mechanisms. Indeed, in isolated mitochondria, both complex I and III of the respiratory chain are identified as sites of $O_2^{\cdot-}$ production (Anderson and Neufer, 2006). Hepatic mitochondrial fraction from hyperthyroid rats releases hydrogen peroxide at higher rates than those of euthyroid animals, either under basal conditions or when complex I and III of the respiratory chain are specifically stimulated (Fernandez and Videla, 1993).

Nevertheless, thyroid hormones also seem to trigger concomitant anti-oxidant pathways that may attenuate thyroid-induced oxidative stress. In rat skeletal muscle, the release of NEFA, superoxide and coenzyme Q occurring under T3 stimulation is reported to increase the UCP3 specific activation, which could be a physiological anti-oxidant response when mitochondrial oxidations are triggered by thyroid hormones (Silvestri *et al.*, 2005a). Indeed, the contribution of UCP3 to proton leak is debated and this protein is suggested to be rather involved in limiting ROS generation and/or lipotoxicity in cells (Mozo *et al.*, 2005; Costford *et al.*, 2007). Additional thyroid hormone-activated mitochondrial mechanisms, including increased expressions of uncoupling proteins and enzymes re-establishing redox homeostasis in cells (Varela *et al.*, 2006; Videla *et al.* 2007), may also contribute to provide protection against excessive ROS accumulation.

Triiodothyronine can also affect both cytoplasmic and mitochondrial functions, thereby modulating the metabolism of several tissues, through long-term pathways controlling transcription of target genes and mitochondriogenesis.

The Mitochondrial Target of Thyroid Hormones: Long-Term Pathways

A large part of oxidative pathways mediated by thyroid hormones is dependent on the coordinated stimulations of the transcription of the nuclear and mitochondrial genomes. The long-term oxidative effect of thyroid hormones is also exerted through the stimulation of mitochondrial biogenesis. Mitochondriogenesis, including the assembly of the phospholipid membrane, DNA replication and coordinated expression of nuclear and mitochondrial genes, is stimulated by T3 after a period longer than 24h (Pillar and Seitz, 1997; Mutvei *et al.*, 1989). This pathway is mediated through the binding of T3 to thyroid receptors and/or coactivators.

Thyroid receptors and thyroid response elements

Thyroid receptors (TR) belong to the superfamily of nuclear receptors. They present a central DNA-binding domain (DBD) containing two "zinc-fingers", a ligand-binding domain, a hinge region and an amino-terminal (A/B) domain (Lazar, 1993; Yen *et al.*, 2001). They are encoded by two separate genes, and translated into multiple TR isoforms by alternated splicing (TRα and TRβ, also named NR1A1 and NR1A2, respectively, according to the nomenclature of nuclear hormone receptors) and are reported to be the cellular homologs of the viral oncogene product v-erb (Sap *et al.*, 1986; Weinberger *et al.*, 1986).

These nuclear receptors directly act as transcription factors in binding as monomers, homodimers or heterodimers to the thyroid hormone response elements (TRE) as demonstrated by in vitro studies (Forman *et al.*, 1988; Nelson *et al.*, 1994). Unliganded TR can also bind to TRE and hence modulate the transcription of target genes. These TRE are usually located upstream from the minimal promoter, but can also be found in 3'-flanking sequences downstream from the coding region (Bigler and Eisenman, 1995; Zhang *et al.*, 1992). Although a putative consensus hexamer half-site sequence of (G/A)GGT(C/G)A has been suggested (Cheng, 2000), TRE sequences may present a high heterogeneity in the number, spacing and orientation of their half-sites (for an extended review, see Yen, 2001).

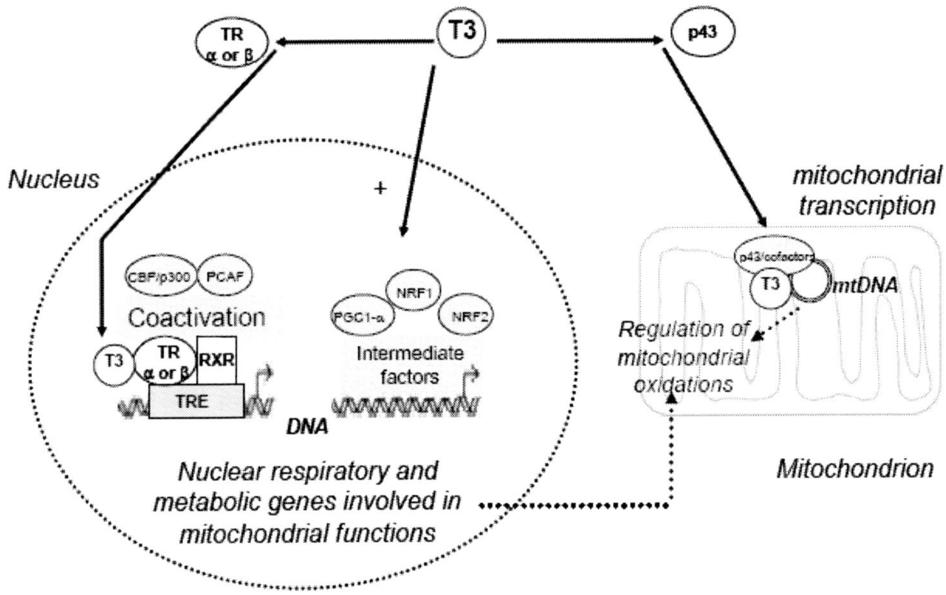

Figure 2. Nuclear and mitochondrial triiodothyronine (T3)-mediated activation of the transcription of genes involved in mitochondrial oxidations. The nuclear pathway involves nuclear thyroid receptors (TR) that may bind DNA on thyroid hormone response elements (TRE) when liganded with other receptors such as retinoic acid receptor (RXR). These dimeres can form complexes with specific co-activators such as CREB binding protein (CBP), CBP related protein p300 and p300/CBP-associated factor (PCAF). T3 may also stimulate nuclear transcription by indirect activation of intermediate factors such as nuclear respiratory factor-1 (NRF-1) and NRF-2 or the peroxisome proliferator-activated receptor gamma coactivator 1α (PGC-lα). Induction of mitochondrial transcription is also stimulated through a binding with truncated TR such as p43 and interactions with truncated TR and cofactors.

Briefly, thyroid receptors can bind TRE sites with half-sites characterized by palindromes (TREpal), direct repeats (DRs), and inverted palindromes (IPs), with optimal spacing for these half-site positions being zero, four, and six nucleotides, respectively (TREpal0, DR4, and IP6).

Casas *et al.* (1999) have also identified in rat mitochondria two truncated forms of the nuclear receptor TRα1 (p43 and p28, with molecular weight of 43 and 28 kDa, respectively). These isoforms are translated in the cytosol before being imported into the mitochondria, where they regulate the transcription of mitochondrial genes (Wrutniak *et al.*, 1995; Wrutniak-Cabello *et al.*, 2001). In vitro, p43 overexpression stimulates mitochondrial biogenesis and respiratory chain activity (Wrutniak *et al.*, 1995), while mice overexpressing p43 were recently shown to present altered muscular metabolic types with for example a more oxidative gastrocnemius muscle (Casas *et al.*, 2008).

Transcription Factors Involved in T3-Activated Gene Expression

Thyroid receptors can bind to TRE in the form of heterodimers such as TR/retinoic acid receptor (RXR) heterodimers, forming complexes with specific co-activators, thus regulating histone acetylation and gene transcription (Figure 2; Varela *et al.*, 2006). Some T3-responsive genes do not require TR binding but may be indirectly stimulated via the activation of intermediate factors, such as nuclear respiratory factor-1 and -2 (NRF-1 and NRF-2) or PGC-lα (Yen, 2001; Weitzel *et al.*, 2001), although this latter hypothesis was recently debated by Wulf *et al.* (2007). Branvold *et al.* (2008) recently demonstrated that cAMP response element binding protein (CREB) is also phosphorylated following T3 administration, and may regulate the expression of several genes presenting a CREB response element on their promoter sequence, including PGC1-α and cytochrome c. In line of this finding, Casas *et al.* (2008) recently evidenced that PGC-1α and peroxisome proliferator-activated receptor delta (PPARδ), two major regulators of muscle phenotype (Lin *et al.*, 2002; Wang *et al.*, 2004), were upregulated in p43 transgenic mice, suggesting that these proteins could also be downstream targets of mitochondrial activity and in turn may regulate mitochondrial oxidations.

Upregulation of Genes Involved in Mitochondrial O2 Consumption

A large number of genes involved in mitochondrial respiration are regulated following T3-binding with thyroid receptors and/or direct or indirect transcriptional activation. Among them can be cited several nuclear-encoded respiratory genes such as cytochrome c or ATP synthase subunits in rats (Pillar and Seitz, 1997) or cytochrome oxidase in chickens (Collin *et al.*, 2007).

The proton leak across the inner mitochondrial membrane also accounts for a part of the mechanisms of energy dissipation and hence O_2 consumption in liver and muscles (Rolfe and Brown, 1997). Attention has currently been focused on uncoupling proteins, among which UCP1 is known to play a calorigenic role in the brown adipose tissue (BAT) of young mammals (Enerback *et al.*, 1997). Expression of UCP1 gene is strongly stimulated by thyroid hormones (Silva, 1988), acting in synergy with the sympathetic nervous system to stimulate BAT cold-induced thermogenesis. Indeed, T3 content is modulated in BAT by a type II deiodinase, which is strongly activated by adrenergic stimulation. The upregulation by T3 of the expression of other uncoupling proteins, UCP2 and UCP3 in mammals, and of avian UCP (avUCP) in birds is also well documented (Gong *et al.*, 1997; Masaki *et al.*, 2000; Damon *et al.*, 2002, De Lange *et al.*, 2001; Collin *et al.*, 2003). However, the contribution of these UCPs to proton leak and thermogenesis is still controversial (Talbot *et al.*, 2004; Collin *et al.*, 2005; Mozo *et al.*, 2005; Costford *et al.*, 2007)

Upregulation of Genes Involved in Mitochondrial Fatty Acid Oxidations

Besides the upregulation of the respiratory machinery, the mitochondrial utilization of fatty acids is also activated by thyroid hormones through the transcription of several genes involved in fatty acid oxidation. For example, Silvestri *et al.* (2005a) report in muscles of T3-treated rats an increase in the expression of carnitine palmitoyl transferases CPT1 and CPT2, involved in the long-chain fatty acid transfers into mitochondria. This is associated with higher rates of mitochondrial acyl-coenzyme A (CoA) thioesterase I (MTE-I) involved in fatty acid utilization. An increase in the messenger RNA of one isoform of CPT1 and in β-hydroxyacyl dehydrogenase mRNA was also observed in chronically T3-treated chickens compared to euthyroid ones (Collin *et al.*, 2007), suggesting the T3-mediated induction of both the entry and the oxidation of fatty acids in muscle mitochondria. Altogether these data suggest that transcriptional pathways are associated with the direct stimulation of enzyme activities to trigger lipid handling after T3 stimulation.

Conclusion

An increasing amount of studies have shown that TH play a key role in the regulation of mitochondrial activity through the control of O_2 consumption and thermogenesis, fatty acid utilization and oxidative stress/antioxidant pathways. The mechanisms involved are dependent on the coordinated stimulations of the transcription of the nuclear and mitochondrial genomes, but also on direct effects on target enzymes. A lot of information on these pathways has been gathered in comparing hyper- or hypothyroid states. A major objective of studies dealing with TH-mediated mitochondrial oxidations is now to better understand their integration in physiological regulations, according to nutritional status and environmental factors. This implies to consider other hormonal pathways such as the adrenergic system or insulin signaling that can interact with TH action.

Aknowledgments

R. Joubert is a PhD student supported by a grant from INRA and Région Centre, France, Q. Swennen is supported by the Research Foundation – Flanders, and N. Everaert is supported by IWT-grant number 040510.

References

Anderson EJ, Neufer PD. Type II skeletal myofibers possess unique properties that potentiate mitochondrial H(2)O(2) generation. *Am J Physiol Cell Physiol.* 2006 290(3):C844-C851.

Arnold S, Goglia F, Kadenbach B. 3,5-Diiodothyronine binds to subunit Va of cytochrome-c oxidase and abolishes the allosteric inhibition of respiration by ATP. *Eur J Biochem* 1998 252:325-330.

Bianco AC, Salvatore D, Gereben B, Berry MJ, Larsen PR. Biochemistry, cellular and molecular biology, and physiological roles of the iodothyronine selenodeiodinases. *Endocr Rev*. 2002 23(1):38-89.

Bigler J, and Eisenman RN. Novel location and function of a thyroid hormone response element. *EMBO J*. 1995 14: 5710-5723.

Branvold DJ, Allred DR, Beckstead DJ, Kim HJ, Fillmore N, Condon BM, Brown JD, Sudweeks SN, Thomson DM, Winder WW. Thyroid Hormone effects on LKB1, MO25, phospho-AMPK, phospho-CREB, and PGC-1{alpha} in Rat Muscle. *J Appl Physiol*. 2008 Jul 31. [Epub ahead of print].

Cao SG, Cheng P, Angel A, Hatch GM. Thyroxine stimulates phosphatidylglycerolphosphate synthase activity in rat heart mitochondria. *Biochim Biophys Acta*. 1995 1256(2):241-244. Erratum in: Biochim Biophys Acta 1995 Oct 26;1259(1):123.

Casas F, Daury L, Grandemange S, Busson M, Seyer P, Hatier R, Carazo A, Cabello G, Wrutniak-Cabello C. Endocrine regulation of mitochondrial activity: involvement of truncated RXRalpha and c-Erb Aalpha1 proteins. *FASEB J*. 2003 17(3): 426-436.

Casas F, Pessemesse L, Grandemange S, Seyer P, Gueguen N, Baris O, Lepourry L, Cabello G, Wrutniak-Cabello C. Overexpression of the mitochondrial T3 receptor p43 induces a shift in skeletal muscle fiber types. *PLoS ONE*. 2008 Jun 25;3(6):e2501.

Casas F, Rochard P, Rodier A, Cassar-Malek I, Marchal-Victorion S, *et al*. A variant form of the nuclear triiodothyronine receptor c-ErbAalpha1 plays a direct role in regulation of mitochondrial RNA synthesis. *Mol Cell Biol*. 1999 19: 7913–7924.

Cheng SY. Multiple mechanisms for regulation of the transcriptional activity of tyroid hormone receptors. *Rev Endocr Metabolic Disorders* 2000 1/2: 9-18.

Collin A, Cassy S, Buyse J, Decuypere E, Damon M. Potential involvement of mammalian and avian uncoupling proteins in the thermogenic effect of thyroid hormones. *Domest Anim Endocrinol*. 2005 29(1):78-87.

Collin A., Swennen Q., Métayer-Coustard S., Skiba-Cassy S., Joubert R., Briclot G., Crochet S., Decuypere E., Buyse J., Tesseraud S. Regulation of mitochondrial and tissue oxidations by thyroid hormones in chicken muscle. 2nd International Symposium on Energy and Protein metabolism and nutrition (ISEP); 2007/09/09-13; Vichy (FRA). Ortigues-Marty, I. (Ed.) Energy and protein metabolism and nutrition. *EAAP Publication* n° 124. Wageningen Academic Publishers, Wageningen (NLD); 2007. 65-66.

Collin A, Taouis M, Buyse J, Ifuta NB, Darras VM, Van As P, Malheiros RD, Moraes VM, Decuypere E. Thyroid status, but not insulin status, affects expression of avian uncoupling protein mRNA in chicken. *Am J Physiol Endocrinol Metab* 2003 284:E771-777.

Costford SR, Seifert EL, Bézaire V, F Gerrits M, Bevilacqua L, Gowing A, Harper ME. The energetic implications of uncoupling protein-3 in skeletal muscle. *Appl Physiol Nutr Metab*. 2007 32(5):884-894.

Damon M, Lombardi T, Vincent A, Herpin P. Differential effect of triiodothyronine on mitochondrial energy coupling in piglet glycolytic and oxidative muscle. *Biochim Biophys Acta* 2002 1555 suppl 1:K8.

Darras VM, Verhoelst CH, Reyns GE, Kühn ER, Van der Geyten S. Thyroid hormone deiodination in birds. *Thyroid*. 2006 16(1):25-35.

Davis PJ, Davis FB. Nongenomic actions of thyroid hormone. *Thyroid* 1996;6:497-504.

Decuypere E, Hermans SC, Michels H, Kühn ER, Verheyen J. Thermoregulatory response and thyroid hormone concentrations after cold exposure in young chicks treated with iopanoic acid and saline. *Adv Physiol Sci* 1981 33:291-298.

Decuypere E, Kühn ER. Thyroid hormone physiology in galliformes: age and strain related changes in physiological control. *Am Zool.* 1988 28:401-415.

Decuypere E, Van As P, Van der Geyten S, Darras VM. Thyroid hormone availability and activity in avian species: a review. *Domest Anim Endocrinol.* 2005 29(1):63-77.

De Lange P, Lanni A, Beneduce L, Moreno M, Lombardi A, Silvestri E, Goglia F. Uncoupling protein-3 is a molecular determinant for the regulation of resting metabolic rate by thyroid hormone. *Endocrinol* 2001 142:3414-3420.

De Lange P, Senese R, Cioffi F, Moreno M, Lombardi A, Silvestri E, Goglia F, Lanni A. Rapid activation by 3,5,3'-L-triiodothyronine of AMPK/ACC and Akt/PKB signaling pathways: relation to changes in fuel metabolism and myosin heavy chain protein content in rat gastrocnemius muscle in vivo. *Endocrinology.* 2008 Aug 14. [Epub ahead of print].

Droge W. Free radicals in the physiological control of cell function. *Physiol Rev* 2002 82: 47-95.

Enerback S, Jacobsson A, Simpson EM, Guerra C, Yamashita H, Harper ME, Kozak LP. Mice lacking mitochondrial uncoupling protein are cold-sensitive but not obese. *Nature* 1997 387:90-94.

Fernández V, Videla LA. Influence of hyperthyroidism on superoxide radical and hydrogen peroxide production by rat liver submitochondrial particles. *Free Radic Res Commun.* 1993 18(6):329-335.

Forman BM, Yang CR, Stanley F, Casanova J, Samuels HH. c-erbA protooncogenes mediate thyroid hormone-dependent and independent regulation of the rat growth hormone and prolactin genes. Mol Endocrinol. 1988 2(10):902-911.

Freake HC, Oppenheimer JH. Thermogenesis and thyroid function. *Annu Rev Nutr.* 1995 15:263-291.

Goglia F, Lanni A, Barth J, Kadenbach B. Interaction of diiodothyronines with isolated cytochrome c oxidase. *FEBS Lett* 1994 346:295-298.

Goglia F, Moreno M, Lanni A. Action of thyroid hormones at the cellular level: the mitochondrial target. *FEBS Lett.* 1999 452(3):115-120.

Gong DW, He Y, Karas M, Reitman M. Uncoupling protein-3 is a mediator of thermogenesis regulated by thyroid hormone, beta 3-adrenergic agonists, and leptin. *J Biol Chem* 1997 272:24129-24132.

Hardie DG. AMP-activated/SNF1 protein kinases: conserved guardians of cellular energy.
Nat Rev Mol Cell Biol. 2007 8(10):774-785.

Harper ME, Ballantyne JS, Leach M, Brand MD. Effects of thyroid hormones on oxidative phosphorylation. *Biochem Soc Trans* 1993 21:785-1792.

Horst C, Rokos H, Seitz HJ. Rapid stimulation of hepatic oxygen consumption by 3,5-di-iodo-L-thyronine. *Biochem J* 1989 261:945-950.

Irrcher I, Walkinshaw DR, Sheehan TE, Hood DA. Thyroid hormone (T3) rapidly activates p38 and AMPK in skeletal muscle in vivo. *J Appl Physiol.* 2008 104(1):178-185.

Jäger S, Handschin C, St-Pierre J, Spiegelman BM. AMP-activated protein kinase (AMPK) action in skeletal muscle via direct phosphorylation of PGC-1alpha. *Proc Natl Acad Sci U S A*. 2007 104(29):12017-12022.

Klatt P, Lamas S. Regulation of protein function by S-glutathiolation in response to oxidative and nitrosative stress. *Eur J Biochem*. 2000 267(16):4928-4944.

Lanni A, Moreno M, Lombardi A, de Lange P, Goglia F. Control of energy metabolism by iodothyronines. *J Endocrinol Invest*. 2001 24(11):897-913.

Lazar MA. Thyroid hormone receptors: multiple forms, multiple possibilities. *Endocr Rev*. 1993 14(2):184-193.

Lin J, Wu H, Tarr PT, Zhang CY, Wu Z, Boss O, Michael LF, Puigserver P, Isotani E, Olson EN, Lowell BB, Bassel-Duby R, Spiegelman BM. Transcriptional co-activator PGC-1 alpha drives the formation of slow-twitch muscle fibres. Nature. 2002 418(6899):797-801.

Lombardi A, Lanni A, de Lange P, Silvestri E, Grasso P, Senese R, Goglia F, Moreno M. Acute administration of 3,5-diiodo-L-thyronine to hypothyroid rats affects bioenergetic parameters in rat skeletal muscle mitochondria. *FEBS Lett*. 2007 581(30):5911-6.

Lombardi A, Lanni A, Moreno M, Brand MD, Goglia F. Effect of 3,5-di-iodo-L-thyronine on the mitochondrial energy-transduction apparatus. *Biochem J* 1998 330:521-526.

Lombardi A, Silvestri E, Moreno M, De Lange P, Farina P, Goglia F, Lanni A. Skeletal muscle mitochondrial free-fatty-acid content and membrane potential sensitivity in different thyroid states: involvement of uncoupling protein-3 and adenine nucleotide translocase. *FEBS Lett*. 2002 532(1-2):12-16.

Luvisetto S. Hyperthyroidism and mitochondrial uncoupling. *Biosci Rep* 1997 17:17-21.

Maloney PC, Kashket ER, Wilson TH. A protonmotive force drives ATP synthesis in bacteria. *Proc Natl Acad Sci U S A* 1974 71:3896-3900.

Masaki T, Yoshomatsu H, Kakuma T, Hidaka S, Kurokawa M., Sakata T. Enhanced expression of uncoupling protein 2 gene in rat white adipose tissue and skeletal muscle following chronic treatment with thyroid hormone. *FEBS Lett* 2000 418:323-326.

Mouillet L. 2000. Iodothyronines et métabolisme énergétique chez le caneton en croissance au froid. Thèse de Doctorat de l'Université Claude Bernard Lyon I. 137pp.

Mozo J, Emre Y, Bouillaud F, Ricquier D, Criscuolo F. Thermoregulation: what role for UCPs in mammals and birds? *Biosci Rep*. 2005 25(3-4):227-49.

Mutvei A, Husman B, Andersson G, Nelson BD. Thyroid hormone and not growth hormone is the principle regulator of mammalian mitochondrial biogenesis. *Acta Endocrinol (Copenh)* 1989; 121: 223-228.

Nelson BD. Thyroid hormone regulation of mitochondrial function. Comments on the mechanism of signal transduction. *Biochim Biophys Acta*. 1990 1018(2-3):275-277.

Nelson CC, Hendy SC, Faris JS, Romaniuk PJ. The effects of P-box substitutions in thyroid hormone receptor on DNA binding specificity. Mol Endocrinol. 1994 8(7):829-840.

O'Reilly I, Murphy MP. Studies on the rapid stimulation of mitochondrial respiration by thyroid hormones. *Acta Endocrinol (Copenh)*. 1992 127(6):542-546.

Paradies G, Petrosillo G, Ruggiero FM. Cardiolipin-dependent decrease of cytochrome c oxidase activity in heart mitochondria from hypothyroid rats. *Biochim Biophys Acta*. 1997 1319(1):5-8.

Pillar TM, Seitz HJ. Thyroid hormone and gene expression in the regulation of mitochondrial respiratory function. *Eur J Endocrinol* 1997; 136: 231-239.

Rolfe DF, Hulbert AJ, Brand MD. Characteristics of mitochondrial proton leak and control of oxidative phosphorylation in the major oxygen-consuming tissues of the rat. *Biochim Biophys Acta.* 1994 1188(3):405-416.

Rolfe DFS, Brown GC. Cellular energy utilization and molecular origin of standard metabolic rate in mammals. *Physiol Rev* 1997 77:731-758.

Sap J, Muñoz A, Damm K, Goldberg Y, Ghysdael J, Leutz A, Beug H, Vennström B. The c-erb-A protein is a high-affinity receptor for thyroid hormone. *Nature.* 1986 324(6098):635-640.

Silva JE. Full expression of uncoupling protein gene requires the concurrence of norepinephrine and triiodothyronine. *Mol Endocrinol* 1988 2:706-713.

Silva JE. Thyroid hormone control of thermogenesis and energy balance. *Thyroid* 1995 5:481-492.

Silva JE. The Thermogenic Effect of Thyroid Hormone and Its Clinical Implications. *Ann Intern Med* 2003 139: 205-213.

Silvestri E, Moreno M, Lombardi A, Ragni M, de Lange P, Alexson SE, Lanni A, Goglia F. Thyroid-hormone effects on putative biochemical pathways involved in UCP3 activation in rat skeletal muscle mitochondria. *FEBS Lett.* 2005a 579(7):1639-1645.

Silvestri E, Schiavo L, Lombardi A, Goglia F. Thyroid hormones as molecular determinants of thermogenesis. *Acta Physiol Scand.* 2005b 184(4):265-283.

Soboll S, Horst C, Hummerich H, Schumacher JP, Seitz HJ. Mitochondrial metabolism in different thyroid states. *Biochem J.* 1992 281 (Pt 1):171-173.

St Germain DL, Galton VA. The deiodinase family of selenoproteins. *Thyroid.* 1997 7(4):655-668.

Talbot DA, Duchamp C, Rey B, Hanuise N, Rouanet JL, Sibille B, Brand MD. Uncoupling protein and ATP/ADP carrier increase mitochondrial proton conductance after cold adaptation of king penguins. J Physiol. 2004 558(Pt 1):123-135.

Tapia G, Pepper I, Smok G, Videla LA. Kupffer cell function in thyroid hormone-induced liver oxidative stress in the rat. *Free Radic Res.* 1997 26(3):267-279.

Turrens JF. Mitochondrial formation of reactive oxygen species. *J Physiol.* 2003 552(Pt 2):335-344.

Varela P, Tapia G, Fernández V, Videla LA. The role of thyroid hormone calorigenesis in the redox regulation of gene expression. *Biol Res.* 2006 39(4):611-617.

Venditti P, Di Meo S. Thyroid hormone-induced oxidative stress. *Cell Mol Life Sci.* 2006 63(4):414-434.

Videla LA. Energy metabolism, thyroid calorigenesis, and oxidative stress: functional and cytotoxic consequences. *Redox Rep* 2000 5: 265-275.

Videla LA, Fernández V, Tapia G, Varela P. Thyroid hormone calorigenesis and mitochondrial redox signaling: upregulation of gene expression. *Front Biosci.* 2007 12:1220-1228.

Videla LA, Sir T, Wolff C. Increased lipid peroxidation in hyperthyroid patients: suppression by propylthiouracil treatment. *Free Radic Res Commun.* 1988 5(1):1-10.

Wang YX, Zhang CL, Yu RT, Cho HK, Nelson MC, Bayuga-Ocampo CR, Ham J, Kang H, Evans RM. Regulation of muscle fiber type and running endurance by PPARdelta. PLoS Biol. 2004 Oct;2(10):e294. Erratum in: PLoS Biol. 2005 Jan;3(1):e61.

Weinberger C, Thompson CC, Ong ES, Lebo R, Gruol DJ, Evans RM. The c-erb-A gene encodes a thyroid hormone receptor. *Nature*. 1986 324(6098):641-646.

Weirich RT, Schwartz HL, Oppenheimer JH. An analysis of the interrelationship of nuclear and plasma triiodothyronine in the sea lamprey, lake trout, and rat: evolutionary considerations. *Endocrinology*. 1987 120(2):664-677.

Weitzel JM, Radtke C, Seitz HJ. Two thyroid hormone-mediated gene expression patterns in vivo identified by cDNA expression arrays in rat. *Nucleic Acids Res*. 2001 29(24): 5148-5155.

Wrutniak C, Cassar-Malek I, Marchal S, Rascle A, Heusser S, Keller JM, Fléchon J, Daua M, Samarut J, Ghysdael J, Cabello G. A 43-kDa protein related to c-Erb A alpha 1 is located in the mitochondrial matrix of rat liver. *J Biol Chem*. 1995 270: 16347–16354.

Wrutniak-Cabello C, Casas F, Cabello G. Thyroid hormone action in mitochondria. *J Mol Endocrinol*. 2001;26:67–77.

Wulf A, Harneit A, Weitzel JM. T3-mediated gene expression is independent of PGC-1alpha. *Mol Cell Endocrinol*. 2007 270(1-2):57-63.

Yen PM. Physiological and molecular basis of thyroid hormone action. *Physiol Rev*. 2001 81(3): 1097-1142.

Zhang W, Brooks RL, Silversides DW, West BL, Leidig F, Baxter JD, and Eberhardt ML. Negative thyroid hormone control of human growth hormone gene expression is mediated by 3'-untranslated/3'flanking DNA. *J Biol Chem* 1992 267: 15056-15063.

In: Thyroid Hormones: Functions, Related Diseases and Uses ISBN: 978-1-60741-080-5
Editors: F. S. Kuehn, M. P. Lozada

Chapter VI

Immuno-Pathogenesis of Thyroid Associated Ophthalmopathy (TAO). The Effect of Novel Treatment of TAO with Anti-TNFα and Anti-CD 20 Monoclonal Antibodies

***Jan Komorowski*[*,1] *and Henryk Stępień*[2]**
[1]Department of Clinical Endocrinology
[2]Department of Immunoendocrinology, the Medical University of Łódź, Poland

Abstract

The etiology of Graves' ophthalmopathy (TAO), representing the most common extrathyroidal manifestation of Graves'disease (GD), is multifactorial. In spite of majority of GD patients having some evidence of ocular involvement, only a minority (3-5%) develops severe TAO. Graves' ophthalmopathy is an autoimmune disease of the orbit involving both the retroorbital connective tissue and the extraocular muscles, but its pathogenesis is still incompletely understood. Multiple genetic (class II HLA genes and cytotoxic T lymphocyte associated-4 regions), environmental (smoking, stress, and iodine uptake), and endogenous factors are involved in the pathogenesis of GD (the thyroid cell itself appears to play a major role in the disease progression through the expression of a number of immunologically active peptides such as adhesion molecules, cytokines, CD40, and complementary regulatory proteins). Examination of retroorbital tissues in the initial inflammatory phase of TAO reveals an accumulation of hydrophilic glycosaminoglycans, increased fat volume, marked T and B lymphocytic infiltration, and presence of many pro-inflammatory cytokines and growth factors. Peripheral blood levels of pro-inflammatory cytokines released from T and B lymphocytes or by the thyroid follicular cells (IFNγ, IL-1β, IL-2, sIL-2R TNFα, IL-6, IL-6R) and antibodies of

* Professor Jan Komorowski M.D., Ph.D., Chair of Endocrinology, Department od Clinical Endocrinology, Medical University of Łódź,, ul. Sterlinga 3, 91-425 Łódź, Poland. Tel.: + (48 42) 633-19-31; Fax: + (48 42) 636 54 27, E-mail: komorowski.j@wp.pl.

TSH receptor (TRAb) secreted from B lymphocytes are markers of the immune system activity. Updated the efficacy of the new anti-cytokine and anti-lymphocyte treatment of the Graves' ophthalmopathy has been revived. In this reviewed study the positive results of anti-B lymphocyte (anti-CD20; rituximab] and anti-TNFα monoclonal antibodies (infliximab; etanercept) administration as new therapeutic options in the treatment of patients with active TAO were described.

Keywords: cytokines, lymphocytes T, B, TNFα, anti-TNFα, CD20, anti-CD20, thyroid associated ophthalmopathy, Graves' disease

I. Introduction

Thyroid orbitopathy (TAO) occurring in 25-20% of patients with Graves' disease (Cawood et al., 2004) is one of autoimmunological diseases. Its pathomechanism has not been fully explained so far (Heufelder et al., 2000). Clinical symptoms such as exopthalmus, oedema of a soft tissue around orbits, eyelids retraction, oculomotor muscle disfunction, pain, diplopia, optical nerve neuropathy and vision disorders result from enlargement of the external eye muscles and increased volume of the retrobulbar adipose tissue (Bahn and Heufelder, 1993; Bartalena et al., 2002; Feldon et al., 2005; Peros et al.,1995). Pathogenesis of the exophtalmus is determined by 3 consecutive processes: infiltration by immunocompetent cells, oedema of the retrobulbar tissue and fibrosis (Bartalena et al., 2000; 2002; 2004). Results of the studies on retrobulbar tissue morphology in patients with an active phase of TAO revealed presence of excessive amount of hydrophilic glycosaminoglycans (mainly hialuronic acid and chondroitin sulphur), increased volume of adipose tissue and massive infiltration with immune system cells (macrophages, lymphocytes and, to lesser extent, B lymphocytes), accompanied by numerous soluble inflammatory cytokines and tissue growth factors (Bahn and Heufelder, 1993; De Bellis et al., 1998; Heufelder, 1995; Komorowski, 2001; Komorowski et al., 1998, Vayasevi et al., 2001).

II. Immunopathogenesis of Graves' Orbitopathy

In the early phase of inflammation, external eye muscles extend, as a result of infiltration with hydrophilic glycosaminoglycans (GAG), which leads to their disfunction (Heufelder, 1995). Separate muscle fibres are isolated by rapidly growing volume of extracellular matrix containing GAG and water in the proliferating perymisium (Bahn and Heufelder, 1993; Kahaly et al., 1998; Wiersinga and Prummel, 2001).

There are also dysfunctions of contractility of the external eye muscles, which manifest in vision disorders (diplopia) in patients with TAO. In the later stages of the disease, fibrosis and permanent lesion of myocytes may occur (Heufelder, 1995). Many investigators suggest that orbital fibroblasts play a key role in the pathogenesis of TAO (Bartalena et al., 2004; Heufelder et al., 1992; Smith, 2002; Smith T et al., 2002; Smith R et al., 1997). Proliferation of the fibroblasts and increased release of GAG to the extracellular matrix leads to the growth of the orbital volume and consequently, exopthalmus. Unlike fibroblasts localized in different sites, orbital fibroblasts have specific metabolic phenotype (Pappa et al., 2000; Smith T et al., 2003; Smith T, 2002) and show higher expression of H and PGE2 prostaglandins synthase in the presence of locally secreted proinflammatory cytokines (Chen et al., 2004; Feldon et al., 2005). Extracellular matrix (ECM) containing collagen compounds, glicoproteins, glycosaminoglycans and proteoglycans forms a natural barrier and support structure for all tissues and organs also in the retrobulbar space. Intensive degradation and restructurization of ECM under the influence of tissue enzymes, called metaloproteinases - MMPs and their endogenous inhibitors (TIMPs) are the basic changes observed in all autoimmune diseases (Graves' disease) and neoplasms (Komorowski et al., 2002, 2003). Increased activity of MMP leads to ECM degradation, while prevalence of TIMP activity to fibrosis. Tissue expression of genes which regulate activity of these enzymes is directly controlled by a number of cytokines, hormones and tissue growth factors (Komorowski et al., 2002, 2003, Stępień et al., 2002).

Fibroblasts localized in the orbits of patients with an active phase of TAO show "inflammatory phenotype" (Chen et al., 2005). Activated orbital fibroblasts produce numerous cytokines appearing in the inflammation site: IL-1, Il-1, IL-8, IL-16, and RANTES (Cao et al., 1998; Sempowski et al., 1998; Wang et al., 1996). It was also reveled that in the presence of IL-1β fibroblasts release big amounts of proinflammatory IL-6 (and Il-6R) (Chen et al., 2005), which induces transformation of B lymphocytes into antibody-producing plasmocytes and fibroblasts into adipocytes.

Results of the recent studies suggest that dysfunction of Th1/Th2 system, pro- and anti-inflammatory cytokines and adhesion molecules which control vascular endothelium function play a key role in the pathogenesis of TAO (Chen et al., 2005; Eckstein et al., 2004; Feldon et al., 2005; Komorowski, 2001; Komorowski et al., 1998; Myśliwiec et al., 2001; Myśliwiec et al, 2001). Adhesion molecules (L-selectins, ICAM-1, VCAM-1, N-CAM) and vascular net controlling growth factors (VEGF and bFGF) together with endothelial cells determine immunocytes transport to the inflammation sites and activate fibroblasts functions in the orbits of patients with TAO (Asahara et al., 1995; De Bellis et al., 1995; Iitaka et al., 1998, Imhof and Dunon, 1995; Komorowski et al., 2003; Myśliwiec et al., 2001; Patey et al., 1996; Springer, 1990; Wenisch et al., 1995). Among mononuclear cells infiltrating retrobulbar space in patients with TOA high number of IL-1 and TNFα - producing macrophages and lymphocytes with the prevalence of T lymphocytes (CD4+, CD8+ and "memory cells" CD45RO+ with cytotoxic activity and increased release of Th1 profile cytokines) over B lymphocytes (CD20+) was found. (Aniszewski et al., 2004; DeCarli et al., 1993; Eckstein et al., 2004; Grubeck-Loebenstein et al., 1994; Heufelder and Bahn, 1994; Pappa et al., 2000; Yang et al., 2000). In the orbital space of patients with the active phase of TAO presence of TNFα, INFγ and IL-1, TGFβ, PDGF stimulating GAG production from orbital fibroblasts were observed (Bahn and Heufelder, 1992; 1993; Cawood et al., 2006). Furthermore, it was shown that IL-1 receptor antagonist (IL-1Ra) is an effective inhibitor of IL-1 and GAG synthesis by fibroblasts. The aforementioned authors of clinical and experimental researches believe that Th1 profile cytokines which control cell-type reactions are one of the essential factors in the early phase of TAO. In the chronic phase, however, mechanisms of humoral response controlled by Th2 lymphocytes are involved. Recently, a new subpopulation of IL-17-producing cytokine, called a Th-17 line differing functionally from classical Th1 and Th2 lines was distinguished (Mangan et al., 2006). Increased activity of Th17 subpopulation seems to be responsible for development of autoimmune diseases.

It was revealed that TGFβ (a cytokine previously known for its immunosuppressive action) together with IL-23 or IL-6 (Bettelli et al., 2006) influenced "naive lymphocytes" (Th0) and induce their differentiation towards Th16 subpopulation (production of Th-17 subpopulation is antagonized by INFγ and IL-4). Action of INFγ and IL-12 on T0 cells induces production of Th1 subpopulation.

In 2005 Eckstein et al. proved that in the orbital tissue of patients with the active phase of TAO there were no dendritic cells. Moreover, increased number of macrophages ($CD14^+$ and RFD7+), expression of γ δ TCR receptors (TCR-γ δ $^+/CD4^+$) in almost 27%of local lymphocytes $CD45^+$ and low number of α β TCR cells (TCR-α β $^+/CD4^+$) were observed. It is supposed that lymphocytes with TCR γ δ $^+/CD4^+$ phenotype may play role in the pathogenesis of Graves' disease and TAO (Eckstein et al., 2005; Krętowski et al., 2000). Large population of TCR- γ δ +/CD4+ lymphocytes secreting Th1 profile cytokines is observed in tissues with inflammatory changes in the course of other autoimmune diseases (Eckstein et al., 2005). In the retrobulbar space in patients with Graves' disease and without thyroid orbitopathy, lymphocytes with TCR-γ δ $^+/CD4^+$ phenotype are practically not observed (Eckstein et al., 2005).

Investigations of bioptates from the retrobulbr space in patients with an active phase of TAO revealed higher proportion of mononuclear cells containing molecules of major histocompatibility complex class II (HLA DR^+), which are expressed on the antigen-presenting cells (lymphoctes, dendritic cells, Langerhans cells and other cells) under the influence of INFγ , released by T lymphocytes (Pappa et al., 2000). When induced by other cytokines (eg. IFNγ), HLA DR class II molecules may be present on the activated T lymphocytes, fibroblasts, thyroid epithelium and other cells. In the orbital fibroblasts, expression of CD40 molecule, enabling direct signal receiving from T lymphocytes and secretion of IL-6 together with IL-8 from fibroblasts, was discovered (Jakóbisiak, 1995; Pappa et al., 2000). Expression of this molecule also depends on IFNγ effects (Pappa et al., 2000). CD40 molecule present on the B lymphocytes belongs to the gp39 glicoprotein (L-Cd40), similar to TNF and found on the activated T lymphocytes. Through CD40 B lymphocyte receives signal enabling class shift of the produced antibodies including antibodies against TSH receptor, from IgM to IgG, IgA or IgM (Jakóbisiak, 1995). Not only is TSH receptor protein (TSH-R) present on the thyroid epithelium and lymphocytes, which leads to the excessive secretion of proinflammatory cytokines (Komorowski, 1992; Komorowski et al., 1993a; 1993b; 1994; Pawlikowski et al., 1994), but it also can be found on the fibroblasts and adipocytes in the orbits. Significant increase in TSH-R expression in the course of fibroblasts differentiation into adipocytes was also observed (Myśliwiec et al., 2002, Khoo et al., 1999; Noh et al., 2000). Induction of cytokine secretion by activated T lymphocytes intensifies proliferative activity of the fibroblasts (Barnard et al., 2002) and GAG production (Pappa et al., 2000). Mature autoreactive B lymphocytes, showing expression of BAFF-R receptors (B-cell maturation antigen receptor) and APRIL (proliferation-inducing ligand) which binds receptors for TNF, are also believed to play role in the pathogenesis of Graves' disease (Wang and Baker, 2006). Overexpression of BAFF-R receptor is connected with an "autoimmune phenotype" of B lymphocytes in different autoimmune disease. In the Graves' disease such a phenotype of B cells is connected with overproduction of antibodies against TSH receptor (TRAb) (Wang and Baker, 2006; Gilbert et al., 2006). The role of PPARγ in the pathogenesis of TAO has been recently considered. It was revealed that medications acting as agonists for these receptors intensify mechanisms of adipogenesis in the patients with TAO (Starkey et al., 2003). Thus, it is believed, that drugs which are antagonists of PPARγ receptors could be used in the therapy of thyroid orbitopathy in the future (Cawood et al., 2004).

Summarizing data from the literature, it should be emphasized that results of the studies performed in the recent 10 years suggest predominant role of the proinflammatory cytokines (secreted by macrophges, Th1/Th2 lymphocytes and TCR-$\gamma\delta^{+}$/$CD4^{+}$) and excessive number of stimulating TRAb - type antibodies, released by B lymphocytes and circulating in the bloodstream in the pathogenesis of TAO. Therefore, attempts of selective immunomodulation have been lately taken in patients in the active infiltratve-oedematous phase of TAO. Experimental therapy was based on the application of monoclonal antibodies against cytokines and lymphocytes. According to the current standards of immunomodulatory treatment of patients with the active phase of infiltrative-oedematous exophtalmus, massive doses of gluocorticosteroids are used. Gluocorticosteroids, due to their anti-inflammatory and immunomodulatory properties, were introduced to the TAO treatment in the early 50's (through suppressed expression of genes for TNFα and other Th1-profile cytokines and intensified transcription mechanisms for genes, coding for IL-1Ra and IL-10) [Barnes, 1998; Guy et al., 1989; Kazim et al., 199; Myśliwiec et al., 2001; Nagayama et al., 1987; Prummel and Wiersinga, 1998; Wiersinga and Prummel, 2001]. It was also shown that glucocorticosteoid therapy leads to the inhibited GAG synthesis and secretion from fibroblasts, suppressed expression of HLA-DR molecules, caused by the effects of INFγ (Heufelder1995; 1997; Heufelder, Bahn and Smith, 1992; Smith et al., 1989).

Although majority of leading endocrinological centres advise to use methylprednisolon pulses at large doses in patients with TAO (Krassas and Heufelder, 2001), this method does not always restore proper vision and may cause harmful side effects. Results of in vitro studies on tissues collected from orbital space from patients with TAO suggest that anticytokine therapy (anti-TNFα and anti-IL-1) could be a treatment of choice in some patients with thyroid orbithopathy (Avanduk et al., 2005; Cawood et al., 2006).

III. New Immunomodulators in the Treatment of Graves' Ophthalmopathy

In 2005, a team of investigators from the University in Birmingham first published data on the use of monoclonal antibodies against TNFα (infliximab) in the experimental treatment of 46-year female with an active phase of TAO and the symptoms of optic nerve compression. (Durrani et al., 2005). One-off intravenous infusion with infliximab at a dose of 5mg/kg body weight (lasting for an hour) significantly improved function of the sight organ, which was reflected by the reduction in CAS scale from 10/10 to 3/10 and regression of the optic nerve compression within 72 hours after the therapy implementation. Infliximab-chimeric monoclonal human/mice IgG-class antibody is directed towards TNF (Rutgeerts et al., 2004). So far, in Europe infliximab (Remicade, Schering-Plough) has been registered for treatment of serious active form of Crohn's disease in patients who had not responded to the corticosteroid and immunosuppressive therapy (Rutgeetrs et al., 2004). Infliximab was also effective in the treatment of acute choroidoretinitis (El-Shabrawi and Hermann, 2002). Its mechanism of action has not been explained yet. Similarly to other antibodies against TNF, including humanized IgG4 CDp571 antibody and etanercept - a chimeric fusion protein, neutralizing TNFα, which consists of extracellular part of the p75 receptor for TNF, bound with fragments of a receptor participating in the phagocytosis (Fc) of the human type 1 antibody (IgG1). Infliximab influences neutralization of the soluble fraction of TNF. It was also proved that infliximab, dose-dependingly, in therapeutic concentration, induced apoptosis of the lymphocytes in peripheral blood in healthy volunteers and subjects with Crohn's disease (Lugering et al., 2001; Rutgeerts et al., 2004).

In 2006 in the Department of Endocrinology of the Medical University in Łódź, antibodies against TNFα (intravenous infusion of infliximab at a dose of 3,7 mg/kg body weight for 2 hours) were used in the treatment of thyroid ophtalmopathy in 58-year old female patient with Graves' disease (Komorowski et al., 2007). Basing on the results of ophtalmological (CAS and NO SPECS scales) and radiological examinations (MRI), efficacy of infliximab was confirmed in the reduction of exophtalmus by 2 mm within 5 weeks after therapy implementation, in limitation of the inflammatory process (reduction by 3 points in CAS scale), reduction of the external eye muscles volume and restriction of the inflammation in MRI (T2 time) within 10 weeks after commencement of the treatment (Laitt et al., 1994; Hosten et al., 2001; Prummel et al., 2001, Utech et al., 1995, Yokohama et al., 2002). Cytokine treatment implemented by us did not cause any undesirable side effects.

In 2005 results of the study on the efficacy of treatment of TAO with another anti-TNFα drug – etanercept were published (Paridaenes et al., 2005). The drug was given to 10 patients with an active phase of TAO subcutaneously at a dose of 25 mg twice a week for 12 weeks. Clinical effects were visible within 6 weeks after therapy implementation. No side effects were recorded. Etanercept (Enbrel, Wyeth) is also efficient in the treatment of rheumatoid arthritis (Moreland et al., 1997; Weinblatt et al., 1999).

Two years ago, a group of Italian investigators presented an interesting case study of a 45-year old female patient with an active phase of TAO, treated with rituximab (RTX, MabThera, Roche) (Salvi et al., 2006). Rutiximb is a humanized chimeric antibody against CD20 (El Fassi et al., 2006). Binding of the RTX to the CD20 antigen on B lymphocytes blocks their activation and differentiation, saving stem cells, pro-B lymphocytes and plasmocytes at the same time (Tsokos, 2004). The mechanisms of action of RTX is depletion of CD20+ cells by antibody- and complement-dependent cytotoxicity as well as by induction of apoptosis (El Fassi et al., 2006). It was also shown that antibodies against TSH (TRAb) are produced by mature B lymphocytes and higher TRAb concentration in blood of patients with an active phase of TAO is correlated with clinical symptoms of thyroid orbitopathy (Gerding et al., 2000). In the aforementioned case there was long–lasting (12 months) distinct improvement of infiltrative-oedematous lesions in the orbits (CAS) after double use of RTX at a dose of 1000 mg (iv). Salvi et al. (2006) had a unique opportunity to investigate lymphocyte subpopulation in blood, thyroid tissue and orbits with a flow cytometry method and assess their morphology based on histological and immunohistochemical techniques. Obtained results were compared to the TRAb concentrations in blood and clinical course of the disease in the patient with TAO. After second administration of RTX only transitory 50%-reduction of plasma TRAb concentration, not correlated with long-lasting very low levels of B lymphocytes in blood, was observed. No B and T lymphocytes were found in the retrobulbar tissue. Despite considerable deficiency in B lymphocytes in the bloodstream, within 2 months after intravenous infusion of RTX TRAb concentration increased (the patient was subjected to the subtotal strumectomy to decrease the number of antigens against TSH receptors). In spite of the increase in the TRAb concentration in blood, no recurrence of oedematous-infiltrative lesions was recorded. The authors of the study explained the improvement of the optic lesions with the suppression of an autoimmune process resultant from hindrance of antigen presentation to B lymphocytes (Salvi et al., 2006). Last year, Salvi et al. (2007) documented that RTX administration positively affected the clinical course of TAO in nine patients with active Graves' ophthalmopathy, independently of either thyroid function or circulating antithyroid antibodies, including TRAb. In another case of patient with GD and TAO treated by RTX infusion (in CAS scale improvement) leading to peripheral blood B-cell depletion without decrease of TRAb levels as well as underwent total thyroidectomy and orbital decompression Bonara et al. (2008) found the existence of B-cells in the thyroid tissue specimens only. At that times they did not find lymphocytes in any of the orbital tissue specimens. Authors concluded that RTX therapy in GD may cause amelioration of ophthalmopathy by depleting total lymphocyte population in the orbit, but not lymphocyte depletion in thyroid tissue with consequent unchanged serum TRAb levels.

IV. Conclusions

Summarizing the review of literature on the experimental immunomodulatory treatment of patients with an active phase of TAO, it should be clearly emphasized that further randomized prospective studies are necessary to assess safety, and efficacy of anticytokine (infliximab, etanercept) and antilymphocyte (rutiximab; RTX) drugs in the more distant future.

References

[1] Cawood T, Moriarty P, O/Shea D. Recent development in thyroid eye disease. *Br. Med. J.* 2004: 329: 385-390.

[2] Heufelder AE, Weetman AP, Ludget M, Bahn RS. Pathogenesis of Graves' ophthalmopathy. Prummel MF ed. Recent Developments in Gaves' Ophthalmopathy. 2000; 15-37. Kluwer Academic Publishers, Boston, USA.

[3] Bahn RS, Heufelder A E: Pathogenesis of Graves' ophthalmopathy. *New Engl. J. Med.* 329: 1468-1475, 1993.

[4] Feldon EF, Park DJJ, O'Lughlin CW, Nguyen VT, Landskroner-Eiger S, Chang D, Thatcher TH, Phipps RP. Autologous T-lymphocytes stimulate proliferation of orbital fibroblasts derived from patients with Graves' ophthalmopathy. I*nvest.Ophtalmol. Vis. Sci.* 2005; 46: 3913-3921.

[5] Perros P, Crombie AL, Kendall-Taylor P. Natural history of thyroid associated ophthalmopathy. *Clin. Endocrinol.* 1995; 42: 45-50.

[6] Bartalena L, Pinchera A, Marcocci C. Management of Graves' ophthalmopathy: reality and perspectives. *Endocr .Rev.* 2000; 21: 168-199.

[7] Bartalena L, Marocci C, Pinchera A. Graves' ophthalmopathy: a preventable disease? *Eur. J. Endocrnol.* 2002; 146: 457-461.

[8] Bartalena L, Wiersinga WM, Pinchera A.Graves' ophthalmopathy: state of the art and perspectives. *J. Endocrinol. Invest.* 2004; 27: 295-301.

[9] De Bellis A, Di Martino S, Fiordelisi F, Muccitelli V, Sinisi A, Abbate GF, Gargano D, Bellastella A, Bizarro A. Soluble intracellular adhesion molecule-1 (sICAM-1) concentrations in Graves' disease patients followed up for development of ophthalmopathy. *J. Clin. Endocrinol. Metab.*1998; 83: 1222-12126.

[10] Heufelder AE. Pathogenesis of Graves' ophthalmopathy: recent controversies and progress. *Eur. J. Endocrinol.* 1995; 132: 532-541.

[11] Kahaly G, Forster G, Hansen C. Glycosaminoglycans in thyroid eye disease. *Thyroid* 1998; 8: 429-432.

[12] Heufelder AE, Smith TJ, Gorman CA, Bahn RS. Increased induction of HLA-DR by interferon gamma in cultured fibroblasts derived from patients with Graves' ophthalmopathy and pretibial dermopathy. J Clin Endocrinol Metab 1991; 73: 307-313.

[13] Wiersinga MW, Prummel MF. Editorial: Pathogenesis of Graves' ophthalmopathy – current understanding. *J. Clin. Endocrinol. Metabol.* 2001; 86: 501-503.

[14] Smith RS, Smith TJ, Blieden TM, Phipps RP. Fibroblasts as sentinel cells: synthesis of chemokines and regulation of inflammation. *Am. J. Pathol.* 1997; 151: 317-322.

[15] Smith TJ, Koumas L, Gagnon A, Bell A, Sempowski GD, Phipps RP, Sirosky A.Orbital fibroblast heterogenity may determine the clinical presentation of thyroid-associated ophthalmopathy. *J. Clin. Endocrinol. Metab.* 2002; 87; 385-392.

[16] Smith TJ. Orbital fibroblasts exhibit a novel pattern of responses to proinflammatory cytokines: potential basis for the pathogenesis of thyroid-associated ophthalmopathy. *Thyroid* 2002; 12: 197-203.

[17] Vayasevi R W, Jyonouchi S C, Dutton C M, Munsakul N, Bahn R S. Effect of tumor necrosis factor-alpha, interferon-gamma, and transforming growth factor-ss on

adipogenesis and expression of thyrotropin receptor in human orbital preadipocyte fibroblasts. *J. Clin. Endocrinol. Metabol.* 2001; 86: 903-908.

[18] Heufelder A E, Bahn R S. Graves' immunoglobulins and cytokines stimulate the expression of intracellular adhesion molecule-1 (ICAM-1) in cultured Graves' orbital fibroblasts. *Eur. J. Clin. Invest* 1992; 22: 529-537.

[19] Pappa A, Lawson JMM, Calder V, Fells P, Lightman S. T cells and fibroblasts in affected extraocular muscles in early and late thyroid associated ophthalmopathy. *Br. J. Ophthalmol.* 2000; 84: 517-522.

[20] Komorowski J, Jankiewicz J, Robak T, Błasińska-Morawiec M, Stępień H. Cytokines serum levels as the markers of thyroid activation in Graves' disease. *Immunol. Lett.* 1998; 60: 143-148.

[21] Komorowski J., Jankiewicz-Wika J., Suprunowicz I., Góraj B., Ścibór J., Stępień H.: Effects of methylprednisolone treatment on peripheral blood levels of matrix metalloproteinases (MMP-1,-2,-3,-8,-9) tissue inhibitors of MMPs (TIMP-1, TIMP-2), angiogenic cytokines (VEGF, bFGF) and adhesion molecules (sICAM-1, sVCAM-1) in patients with thyroid-associated ophthalmopathy (TAO). *Endokr. Pol.* 2003; 54: 13-21.

[22] Komorowski J, Pasieka Z, Jankiewicz-Wika J, Stępień H. Matrix metalloproteinases (MMP 1, -2, -3, -8, -9), tissue inhibitors of MMPs (TIMP-1, -2) and angiogenic cytokines (VEGF, bFGF) in peripheral blood of thyroid cancer patients. *Thyroid* 2002; 12: 655-662.

[23] Komorowski J. Interleukins in Graves' disease. In: O'Neill L A J and Bowie A (eds.) Methods in molecular medicine. Interleukin protocols. Humana Press, Totova, New Jersey, 2001, vol. 60, pp. 251—261.

[24] Stępień H M, Kołomecki K, Pasieka Z, Komorowski J, Stępień T, Kuzdak K. Review: Angiogenesis of endocrine glands tumours – new molecular targets in diagnostics and therapy. *Eur. J. Endocrinol.* 2002; 146: 143-151.

[25] Chen B, Shanli T, Smith TJ. IL-1β induces IL-6 expression in human orbital fibroblasts: identification of an anatomic-site specific phenotypic attribute revelant to thyroid-associated ophthalmopathy. *J. Immunol.* 2005;175: 1310-1319.

[26] Cao HJ, Wang HS, Zhang Y, Lin H-Y, Phipps RP, Smith TJ. Activation of human orbital fibroblast through CD40 engagement results in a dramatic induction of hyaluronan synthesis and prostoglandin endoperoxide H synthase-2 expression: insights into potential pathogenic mechanisms of thyroid associated ophthalmopathy. *J. Biol. Chem.* 1998; 273: 29615-29625.

[27] Eckstein AK, Quadbeck B, Tews T, Mann K, Kruger C, Mohr CH, Steuhl K-P, Esser J, Gieseler. Thyroid associated ophthalmopathy: evidence for $CD4^{+}\gamma\delta$ T cells; de novo differentation of $RFD7^{+}$ macrophages, but not of $RFD1^{+}$ dendric cells; and loss of γδ and αβ T cell receptor expression. *Br. J. Ophthalmol.* 2004; 88: 803-808.

[28] Myśliwiec J, Krętowski A, Szelachowska M, Topolska J, Mikita A, Kinalska I. Serum L-selectin and ICAM-1 in patients with Graves' ophthalmopathy during treatment with corticosteroids. *Immunol. Lett.* 2001;123: 123-126.

[29] Myśliwiec J, Krętowski A, Topolska J, Siewko K, Jakubczyk D., Szelachowska M, Mikita A, Kinalska I. Serum Th1 and TH2 profile cytokine level changes in patients

with Graves' ophthalmopathy treated with corticosteroids. *Horm. Metab. Res.* 2001; 33: 739-743.

[30] Wang H-S, Cao HJ, Winn VD, Rezanka LJ, Frobert Y, Evans CH, Sciaky D, Young DA, Smith TJ. Leukoregulin induction of prostaglandin endoperoxide H synthase=2 in human orbital fibroblasts: an in vitro model for connective tissue inflamation, *J. Biol. Chem.*1996; 271: 22718-22728.

[31] Sempowski GD, Rozenblit J, Smith TJ, Phipps RP. Human orbital fibroblasts are activated through CD40 to induce pro-inflammatory cytokine production. *Am. J. Physiol.* 1998; 274; C707-C714.

[32] Iitaka M, Miura S, Yamanaka K, Kawasaki S, Kitahama S, Kawakami Y, Kakinuma S, Oosuga I, Wada S, Katayama S: Increased serum vascular endothelial growth factor levels and intrathyroidal vascular area in patients with Graves' disease and Hashimo's thyroiditis. *J. Endocrinol. Metabol.* 1998; 83: 3908-3912.

[33] Asahara T, Bauters C, Zheng L P, Takeshita S, Bunting S, Ferrara N, Symes J F, Isner J M: Synergistic effect of vascular endothelial growth factor and basic fibroblast growth factor on angiogenesis in vivo. *Circulation* 1995; 92: 365-371.

[34] Imhof B A, Dunon D. Leukocyte migration and adhesion. *Adv. Immunol.* 1995; 58: 345-416.

[35] Springer T A: Adhesion receptors of the immune system. Nature 1990; 346: 425-434.

[36] Patey N, Vaseux R, Canioni D, Potter T, Gallatin W M, Brousse N: Intracellular adhesion molecule-3 on endothelial cells. Expression in tumors but not in inflammatory responses. *Am. J. Pathol.* 1996; 148: 465-472.

[37] Wenisch C, Myskiw D, Gessl A, Graninger W: Circulating selectins, intracellular adhesion molecule-1, and vascular cell adhesion molecule-1. *J. Clin. Endocrinol. Metab.* 1995; 80:2122-2126.

[38] Aniszewski JP, Valyasevi RW, Bahn RS. Relationship between disease duration and predominant orbital T cell subset in Graves' ophthalmopathy. *J. Clin. Endocrinol. Metab.* 2000; 85: 776-780.

[39] De Carli, D'Elios M, Maritti S, Marocci C, Pinchera A, Ricci M. Cytolitic T cells with TH-1 like cytokine profile predominate in retroorbital lymphocytic infiltrates of Graves' ophthalmopathy. *J. Clin Endoccrinol. Metab.* 1993; 77: 1120-1124.

[40] Heufelder AE, Bahn RS. Modulation of Graves', orbital fibroblast proliferation by cytokines and corticosteroids receptor agonist. *Invest. Ophthalmol. Vis. Sci.* 1994; 35: 120-127.

[41] Grubeck-Loebenstein B, Trieb K, Sztankay A, Holter W, Andrl H, Wick G. Retrobulbar T cells from patients with Graves' ophthalmopathy are CD8+ and specifically recognize autologous fibroblasts. *J. Clin. Invest.* 1994; 3: 2738-2743.

[42] Bahn R, Heufelder AE. Role of connective tissue autoimmunity in Graves ophthalmopathy. *Autoimmunity* 1992; 13: 75-79.

[43] Bahn R, Heufelder AE. Mechanisms of disease: pathogenesis of Graves' ophthalmopathy. *N. Engl. J. Med.* 1993; 329:1468-1475.

[44] Cawood TJ, Moriarty P, O'Farrelly C, O'Shea D. The effects of tumour necrosis factor-alpha and interleukin 1 on an in vitro model of thyroid-associated ophthalmopathy; contrasting effects on adipogenesis. *Eur. J. Endocrinol.* 2006; 155: 395-403.

[45] Mangan PR, Harrington LE, O'Quinn DB, Helms WS, Bullard DC, Olson CO, Hatton RD, Wahl SM, Schoeb TR, Weaver CT. Transforming growth factor-β induces development of the TH17 lineage. *Nature* 2006; 441: 231-234.

[46] Bettelli E, Carrier Y, Gao W, Korn T, Strom TB, Oukka M, Weiner HL, Kuchroo VK. Reciprocal development pathways for the generation of pathogenic effector TH17 and regulatory T cells. *Nature* 2006; 441: 235-238.

[47] Kretowski A, Myśliwiec J, Kinalska I. Abnormal distribution of gammadelta T lymphocytes in Graves' disease and insulin-dependent diabetes type 1.*Arch. Immunol. Ther. Exp.* (Warsz). 2000;48(1):39-42.

[48] Jakóbisiak M. Immunologia. Wydawnictwo Naukowe PWN, Warszawa 1995.

[49] Komorowski J. Increased interleukin-2 level in patients with primary hypothyroidism. *Clin. Immunol. Immunopatol.* 1992; 63: 200-2002.

[50] Komorowski J, Stępień H, Pawlikowski M. The evidence of thyroliberin/triiodothyronin control of TSH secretory response from human peripheral blood monocytes cultured in vitro. *Neuropeptides* 1993; 25: 31-34.

[51] Komorowski J, Żylińska K, Pawlikowski M, Stępień H. Stimulatory effect of thyrotropin (TSH) on interleukin-2 (IL-2) release from human blood lymphocytes. A dose-response study in vitro. *Horm. Metab. Res .1*993; 25: 598-599.

[52] Komorowski J, Stępień H, Pawlikowski M. Increased interleukin-2 during standard TRH test in man. *Neuropeptides* 1994; 27: 151-156.

[53] Pawlikowski M, Stępień H, Komorowski J. Hypothalamic-pituitary-thyroid axis in the immune system. *Neuroimmunomodulation* 1994; 1: 149-152.

[54] Myśliwiec J, Krętowski A, Stępień A, Mirończuk K, Kinalska I. Thyrotropin receptor antibodies detected by the human recombinant TBII assay – a surrogate marker for autoimmune activity in Graves' ophthalmopathy? *Med. Sci. Monit.* 2002; 8: MT159-162.

[55] Khoo DHC, Ho SC, Seah LL, Fong KS, Tai ES, Chee SP, Eng PHK, Aw SE, Fok ACK. The combination of absent thyroid peroxidase antibodies and high thyroid-stimulating immunoglobulin levels in Graves' disease identifies a group at markedly increased risk of ophthalmopathy. *Thyroid* 1999; 9: 1175-1180.

[56] Noh JY, Hamada N, Inoue Y, Abe Y. Thyroid-stimulating antibody is related to Graves ophthalmopathy, but thyrotropin-binding inhibitor immunoglobulin is related to hyperthyroidism in patients with Graves' disease. *Thyroid* 2000; 10: 809-813.

[57] Bernard A, Lamy AL, Alberti I. The two-signal model of T-cell activation after 30 years. Transplantation 2002; 73: S31-S35.

[58] Wang SH, Baker JR. Targeting B cells in Graves' disease. *Endocrinology* 2006; 147: 4559-4560.

[59] Gilbert JA, Kalled SL, Moorhead J, Hess DM, Rennert P, Li Z, Khan MZ, Banga JP. Treatment of autoimmune hyperthyroidism in a murine model of Graves' disease with TNF-family ligand inhibitors suggest a key role for B cell activating factor in disease pathology. *Endocrinology* 2006; 147: 4561-4586.

[60] Starkey K, Heufelder A, Baker G, Joba W, Evans M, Davies S Ludgate M. Perixisome proliferator-activated receptor-gamma in thyroid eye disease: contraindication for thiazolidinedione use? *J. Clin. Endocrinol. Metab.* 2003; 88: 55-59.

[61] Barnes BJ. Antiinflammatory actions of corticosteroids: molecular mechanisms. *Clin. Sci.* 1998; 84: 557-572.

[62] Kazim M, Trokel S, Moore S. Treatment of acute Graves' ophthalmopathy. *Ophthalmology* 1991; 98: 1443-1448.

[63] Nagayama Y, Izumi M, Kiriyama T. Treatment of Graves' ophthalmopathy with high-dose intravenous methylprednisolone pulse therapy. *Acta Endocrinol.* 1987; 116: 513-518.

[64] Guy JR, Fagien B, Donovan J, Rubin ML. Methylprednisolone pulse therapy in severe thyroid optic neuropathy. *Ophthalmology* 1989; 96: 1048-1053.

[65] Heufelder A E: Retro-orbital autoimmunity. *Bailliers Clin. Endocrinol. Metab.* 1997; 11: 499-520.

[66] Smith TJ, Bahn RS, Gorman CA. Connective tissue, glycosaminoglycans, and diseases of the thyroid. *Endocr. Rev. 1*989; 10: 366-391.

[67] Krassas G, E, Heufelder A E: Immunosuppressive therapy in patients with thyroid eye disease: an overview of current concepts. *Eur. J. Endocrinol.* 2001; 144: 311-318.

[68] Heufelder AE, Bahn RS, Smith TJ. Regulation by corticosteroids of interferon gamma-induced HLA-DR antigen expression in cultured human orbital fibroblasts. Cli *Endocrinol.* 1992;37: 643-659.

[69] Avanduk AM, Avanduk MC, Pazarli H, Oguz V, Varnell ED, Kaufman HE, Aksoy F. Immunohisochemical analysis of orbital connective tissue specimens of patients with active Graves ophthalmopathy. *Curr. Eye Res.* 2005; 30: 631-638.

[70] Rutgeerts P, Sandborn WJ, Feagan BG Reinisch W, Olson A, Travers S, Rachmilewitz D, Hanauer SB, Lichtenstein GR, de Viliers WJ, Present D, Sands BE and Colombel JF. Infliximab for induction and maintenance therapy for ulcerative colitis. *N. Engl. J. Med.* 2005; 353: 2462-2476.

[71] Durrani OM., Reuser TQ and Murray PI.. Infliximab: a novel treatment for sight-threatening thyroid associated ophthalmopathy. *Orbit* 2005; 24: 117-119.

[72] El-Shabrawi Y, Hermann J. Anti-tumor necrosis factor-alpha therapy with infliximab as an alternative to corticosteroids in the treatmentof human leukocyte antigen B27 – associated acute anterior uveitis. *Ophthalmology* 2002; 109: 2342-2346.

[73] Lugering A, Schmidt M, Lugering N, Pauels HG, Domschke W, Kucharzik T. Infliximab induces apoptosis in monocytes from patients with chronic active Crohn's disease by using a caspasedependent pathway. *Gastroenterology* 2001; 121: 1145-1157.

[74] Komorowski J, Jankiewicz-Wika J, Siejka A, Ławnicka H, Kłysik A, Goś R, Majos A, Stefańczyk L, Stępień H. Monoclonal anti-TNFα antibody (infliximab) in the treatment of patient with thyroid associated ophthalmopathy. *Klinika Oczna* 2007, 109: 457-460.

[75] Laitt RD, Hoh B, Wakeley C, Kabala J Harrad R, Potts M and Goddard P. The value of the short tau inversion recovery sequence in magnetic resonance imaging of thyroid eye disease. *Brit. J. Radiol.* 1994; 67: 244-247.

[76] Yokohama N, Nagataki S, Ashizawa K and Eguch K. Role of magnetic resonance imaging in the assessment of disease activity in thyroid-associated ophtalmopathy. *Thyroid* 2002; 12: 223-227.

[77] Hosten N, Sander B, Cordes M, Schubert CJ, Schorner W and Felix R. Graves` ophtalmopathy. MR imaging of the orbits. *Radiology* 1989; 172: 759-762.

[78] Prummel M, Gerding MN, Zonneveld FW and Wiersinga WM. The usefulness of quantitative orbital magnetic resonance imaging in Graves` ophtalmopathy. *Clin. Endocrinol.* 2001; 54: 205-209.

[79] Utech CI, Khatibnia U, Winter PF and Wulle KG. MR T2 relaxation time for the assessment of retrobulbar inflammation in Graves` ophtalmopathy. *Thyroid* 1995; 5: 185-193.

[80] Paridaenes D, Van den Bosch WA, Van der Loos TL Krenning EP, Van Hagen PM. The effect of etanercept on Graves' ophthalmopathy: a pilot study. *Eye* 2005; 19: 1286-1289.

[81] Moreland LW, Baumgartner SW, Scgiff MH, Tindall EA, Fleischmann RW, Weaver AL, Ettlinger RE, Cohen S, Koopman WJ, Mohler K, Widmer MB, Blosch CM. Treatment of rheumatoid arthritis with a recombinant human necrosis factor receptor (p75)-Fc fusion protein. *N. Engl. J. Med.* 1997; 337: 141-147.

[82] Weinblatt ME, Kremer JM, Bankhurst AD, Bulpitt KJ, Fleishmann RM, Fox RI, Jackson CG, Lange M, Burge DJ. A trial of etanercept, a recombinant tumor necrosis factor receptor: Fc fusion protein, in patients with rheumatoid arthritis receiving methotrexate. *N. Engl. J. Med.* 1999; 340: 253-260.

[83] Salvi M, Vannucchi G, Campi I, Rossi S, Bonara P, Sbrozzi F, Guastella C, Avignone S, Pirola G, Ratiglia R and Beck-Peccoz P. Efficacy of rituximab treatment for thyroid-associated ophthalmopathy as a result of intraorbital B-cell depletion in one patient unresponsive to steroid immunosuppression. *Eur. J. Endocrinol.*, 2006; 154: 511-517.

[84] El Fassi D, Nielsen CH, Hasselbalch HC and HegedUs L. The rationale for B lymphocyte depletion in Graves' disease. Monoclonal anti-CD20 antibody as a novel treatment option. *Eur. J. Endocrinol.* 2006; 154: 623-632.

[85] Gerding MN, van der Meer JW, Broenink M, Bakker O, Wiersinga WM, Prummel ME. Associationof thyrotrophin receptor antibodies with the clinical features of Graves' ophthalmopathy. *Clin. Endocrinol.* 2000; 52: 267-271.

[86] Tsokos GC. B-cells, be gone-- B-cell depletion in the treatment of rheumatoid arthritis. New Engl J Med 2004; 350: 2546-2548.

[87] Salvi M, Vannucchi G, Campi I, Curro N, Dazzi D, Simonetta S, Bonara P, Rossi S, Sina C, Guastella S, Guastella C, Ratglia R, Beck-Peccoz P. Treatment of Graves' disease and associated ophthalmopathy with the anti-CD20 monoclonal antibody rituximab: an open study. *Eur. J. Endocrinol.* 2007; 156: 33-40.

[88] Bonara P, Vannucchi G, Campi I, Rossi S, Cantoni F, Frugoni C, Sbrozzi F, Guastella C, Avignone S, Beck-Peccoz P, Salvi M. Rituximab induces distinct intraorbital and intrathyroidal efects in one patient satisfactory treated for Graves' ophthalmopathy. *Clin. Rev. Allergy Immunol.* 2008; 34: 118-123.

In: Thyroid Hormones: Functions, Related Diseases and Uses ISBN: 978-1-60741-080-5
Editors: F. S. Kuehn, M. P. Lozada

Chapter VII

Managing Moderate to Severe Graves Ophthalmopathy: An Up-to-Date Review

Christopher I. Zoumalan[1,3], Kimberly P. Cockerham[2], and Michael Kazim[3]

[1] Division of Ophthalmic Plastic and Reconstructive Surgery, Department of Ophthalmology, New York University Langone School of Medicine, New York, New York, USA

[2] Department of Ophthalmology, Stanford University School of Medicine, Stanford, California, USA

[3] Departments of Ophthalmology and Surgery, Columbia University, New York, New York, USA

Abstract

Graves ophthalmopathy (GO) is the most common cause of orbital inflammation and proptosis in adults. There is however, no agreement on its management. Corticosteroids and external beam orbital radiation (XRT) have been used to treat active inflammation. Other immunomodulatory agents, including azathioprine, cyclosporine, intravenous immunoglobulin (IVIG), and plasmapheresis have not proved to be effective. Newer agents including anti-CD20 monoclonal antibodies (rituximab) and TNF blockers hold potential therapeutic value but have not been formally investigated. Moreover, the lack of standard study design, treatment protocols, and outcome measures limits comparison of studies. Despite these limitations, there is evidence that the combination of corticosteroids and orbital radiation therapy is more effective than corticosteroids alone in the treatment of moderate to severe GO. In order to evaluate the management of GO, the design and funding of a multi-center trial is required.

Graves ophthalmopathy (GO, thyroid eye disease, thyroid orbitopathy) is an autoimmune disorder characterized by inflammation and expansion of the orbital fat and extraocular muscles. It is associated with Graves disease (GD) in over 80% of cases and [1-3]. Although it is seen in all age groups, it most commonly affects adults in the fourth and fifth decades. The pathophysiology of GO is not completely understood, but there is evidence for both humoral and cell-mediated immune processes [4-7]. It is known that both Th1 and Th2 cytokine pathways are involved, resulting in the release of numerous cytokines which stimulate cell proliferation, hydrophilic glycosaminoglycans synthesis, and adipogenesis [8-10]. When significant enough, these cytokine-mediated processes can result in a clinically apparent active phase. The active phase generally persists for six months to one year in non-smokers may last two to three years in smokers. However, the duration and severity of disease is unpredictable. After the active, inflammatory process ends, fibrosis and the associated disabling symptoms persist in the chronic, inactive phase [8,11,12].

The current lack of a universally accepted classification system for GO places limitations on the current review. The NOSPECS classification identifies and categorizes the signs and symptoms of GO, but only some criteria characterize active disease (Table 1). The clinical activity score (CAS) measures ten clinical signs and symptoms including retrobulbar pain, pain on eye movements, eyelid erythema, conjunctival injection, chemosis, swelling of the caruncle, eyelid edema or fullness as measures of active disease (Table 2). Mild GO is defined by ocular symptoms with little to no signs of ocular involvement (NOSPECS categories 0 or 1 and/or CAS less than 3). Moderate to severe GO include one or more of the following: soft-tissue signs (i.e. lid swelling, chemosis), proptosis, motility restriction, and vision changes due to corneal exposure or optic nerve compression (one or more of NOSPECS categories 2,3,4, and 6 and/or CAS of 3 or more).

Most patients experience mild disease and require supportive measures, such as frequent use of artificial tears, limiting salt intake, abstaining from smoking tobacco and sleeping with their head elevated. Medical treatment employed in cases of moderate to severe GO most commonly includes corticosteroids with or without external beam orbital radiation (XRT). However, disease management varies widely [13]. The goals of medical therapy are to shorten the duration and minimize the severity of the active phase, thereby reducing the chronic phase disfigurement and disability produced by irreversible fibrosis.

Table 1. NOSPECS classification of Graves ophthalmopathy

Class 0: No signs or symptoms
Class 1: Only signs (limited to upper lid retraction, with or without lid lag)
Class 2: Soft tissue involvement (chemosis and lid edema, conjunctival injection)
Class 3: Proptosis
Class 4: Extraocular muscle involvement
Class 5: Corneal involvement (primarily due to lagophthalmos)
Class 6: Sight loss (due to optic nerve involvement)

Table 2. Clinical activity score*

Pain
1 Painful, pressure-like feeling on or behind the globe during the last 4 weeks
2 Pain on attempted up, side or down gaze during the past 4 weeks
Redness
3 Redness of the eyelid(s)
4 Diffuse redness of the conjunctiva, covering at least one quadrant
Swelling
5 Swelling of the eyelid(s)
6 Chemosis
7 Swollen caruncle
8 Increase by 2 mm or more in proptosis during a period of one to three months
Impaired function
9 Decrease in eye movements in any direction of 5 degrees or more during a period of one to three months
10 Decrease in visual acuity (1 or more lines on Snellen chart, using a pinhole) during a period of one to three months

* A score of 1 is given for each feature present (3 or above indicates mild to moderate Graves ophthalmopathy).

Corticosteroids

Corticosteroids inhibit cyclooxygenase and phospholipase A2 in the arachidonic acid pathway, decreasing production of inflammatory mediators including leukotrienes, prostaglandins, and thromboxane. Corticosteroids also decrease antigen presentation to T cells and increase the breakdown of circulating antibodies. [4,11,14]

Corticosteroids are most commonly administered orally or intravenously (IV) to treat moderate to severe GO. Local injections of corticosteroids into the orbit have produced inconsistent results with some investigators reporting improvement in motility and reduction in extraocular muscle (EOM) size [15], while others have found no improvement in the orbitopathy [16,17]. In patients with contraindications to systemic corticosteroids, local injections may provide a therapeutic option [15,18].

Despite the efficacy of corticosteroids in managing moderate to severe GO, their chronic administration is associated with Cushingoid facies, weight gain, osteoporosis, gastric irritation, labile hypertension, elevated intraocular pressure, hyperglycemia, and mood alteration. Intravenous corticosteroid treatment is associated with a lower rate of adverse side effects [19], however single case reports have reported fatal cardiac events and hepatic necrosis associated with the use of IV corticosteroids to treat GO [20,21].

External Beam Therapy

XRT has been used to treat GO for over 90 years, but the current XRT protocol was reported in 1973 [22]. Though the mechanism of action is not fully understood, XRT (total dose = 20Gy) is biologically active against infiltrating lymphocytes, tissue-bound monocytes, and fibroblasts altering the local cellular matrix and interrupting the inflammatory process in a more permanent fashion than can be achieved with corticosteroids [14,16]. XRT is used to treat moderate to severe GO, however, its efficacy has not been established by a prospective randomized trial. One prospective, randomized trial found no value in treating mild to moderate GO with XRT [23,24].

Our review of literature found that XRT was well tolerated and produced few short-term or long-term side effects [19]. One particular study found that 15 (54%) of 28 patients surveyed had side effects, usually minor, including transient hair loss at temples, tiredness, myalgias, headaches, insomnia, and nausea [12].

Alternative Immunomodulatory Therapy

As an alternative to corticosteroids and XRT, azathioprine, cyclosporine, intravenous immunoglobulin (IVIG), and plasmapheresis have been proven of little therapeutic value [25-30]. The goal of steroid-sparing immunomodulatory therapy is to control disease while minimizing adverse effects. Their pharmacologic mechanisms of action are more specific than corticosteroids. While overall systemic side effects are lower, there are reports of multiple organ system complications (i.e. renal and liver toxicity, bone marrow suppression, and leukopenia). Although there are numerous clinical trials that support the use of immunomodulatory therapy in other autoimmune diseases such as rheumatoid arthritis and systemic lupus erythematosus (SLE), there is no prospective, randomized study of these agents used to treat GO. Efficacy studies that exist have not been well modeled, and are mainly small, retrospective, or uncontrolled [14,31-35].

Recent Advances in B-Cell Depletion and GO

Advances in the understanding of the pathogenesis of GO has led to the experimental use of therapeutic B-cell depletion in moderate to severe GO. B-cells play a role in the pathologic modulation of T-cells and orbital fibroblasts in patients with GO. Additionally, B-cells produce antibodies which may facilitate GO [36-38].

During the past ten years, therapeutic B-cell depletion using rituximab (RTX) has emerged as an effective treatment for non-Hodgkins lymphoma [36,37]. RTX is a monoclonal antibody that binds to CD-20, a surface protein expressed by both immature and mature B-cells but not by plasma cells, and results in transient B-cell depletion lasting approximately 4-6 months. RTX has been used to treat autoimmune diseases such as rheumatoid arthritis, SLE, giant cell arteritis, and dermatomyositis [37,38].

RTX's efficacy in other autoimmune disorders has prompted some investigators to treat patients with moderate to severe GO with RTX [39,40]. Though the studies are small, uncontrolled, and not randomized, the patients treated with RTX showed clinical improvement in GO shortly after RTX infusion. GO remained quiescent up to a year of follow up. However, the treatment is associated with risks consequent to six months of B-cell depletion. A well-designed, randomized study will be required to effectively evaluate RTX's role in managing moderate to severe GO.

Current Interpretation of Data

The first-line treatment for moderate to severe GO remains corticosteroids and/or XRT. [14,31,32]. The interpretation of the data from existing studies is limited by the lack of good natural history data and the highly variable nature of the disease. Furthermore, there is no uniformly accepted activity or severity index.

We have published a review article comparing the outcomes of GO patients treated with corticosteroids and/or XRT [19]. Subsequently, we have updated our review of publications in the English language to compare the outcomes of treatment using corticosteroids with or without XRT. We performed a review of published studies identified in a PubMed on-line review from January 1966 to June 2008 using the following key words: Graves ophthalmopathy, thyroid eye disease, Graves disease, and thyroid orbitopathy. Our inclusion criteria required at least eight enrolled subjects within a retrospective or prospective study published in the English language. Furthermore, we included only those studies that compared the outcomes through definable measures, orbital imaging studies (CT or MRI), self assessment surveys, or clinical examinations.

Results

Study Profiles

We identified twenty studies for review. Eight enrolled patients in randomized prospective studies [12,16,30,34,41-44], and the remainder were either prospective or retrospective case series.

General Patient Treatment Profile

We reviewed a total of 886 patients from twenty studies. The patient demographics, study inclusion and exclusion criteria varied. Some studies excluded patients who had had prior treatment for GO [12,16,41-45], while others included patients that had already been treated with XRT, immunomodulatory agents, or decompressive surgery [31,46-51]. Others failed to detail prior treatment [52-55].

Table 3. Studies Evaluating Corticosteroids in Managing GO

Publication	Pts.	Treatment/Study Type	Adjunctive treatment	Outcome Measures	Duration of follow up (wks)	Comment /conclusions
Aktaran et al (2007)[41]	52 (25 received IV steroids, 27 received PO steroids)	Prospective, randomized, single blind, 26 received IV steroids (500 mg/week for total 6 wks), 26 received PO (75mg/daily) steroids taper over 10 weeks	None	CAS	12	18/25 (72%) and 13/27 (49%) had an overall favorable response with IV and PO steroids, respectively.
Bartalena et al, (1983) [21]	48(36 PO steroids and XRT, 12 only PO steroids)	Prospective case series in 36 pts that received combined PO steroids (70-80mg tapered over 6 months) and XRT. 12 pts that received only PO steroids were part of a prospective randomized study.	36 received combined PO steroids and XRT (20Gy x 2wks)	Clinical activity index, clinical assessment	12	26/36 (72%) excellent or good response in combined group, 12/12 that received only PO steroids had regression or improvement in soft tissue changes, but only 33% had overall good results (no excellent results reported).
Bartalena et al, (1998)[31]	75	Prospective, randomized study. PO steroids (0.5 mg/kg/day prednisone x 1 month then with 8wk PO taper		CAS and patient's impression	52	50/75 (67%) improved/regressed by CAS.
Baschieri et al[34]	55 (30 received PO steroids, 25 received IVIG)	Prospective, randomized, blinded study. 80mg/day PO steroids x 2 wks then tapered over 5 months		Soft tissue changes, CT, proptosis, NOSPECS	24	76% favorable response to NOSPECS with IVIG, 66% response with PO steroids
Chang et al[42]	22	Prospective case series. IV steroids 0.5g/day x 3 then 5 month PO steroid taper (starting at 40mg PO/day then tapered)		NOSPECS, CAS, CT	17	12/22 (55%) good response esp lacrimation, soreness, soft tissue swelling, proptosis
Dandona et al[41]	37	Case series, (IV steroids 1gm or 0.5gm/day x3 with three week PO oral taper		Self assessment, eye exam, muscle size on CT	Not clearly stated	32/37 (86.5%) improved with reduction in proptosis.

Publication	Pts.	Treatment/Study Type	Adjunctive treatment	Outcome Measures	Duration of follow up (wks)	Comment /conclusions
Hiromatsu et al[44]	23	Prospective case series. 1 gm/day IV steroids x3, repeat 3-5 times over 5 weeks (total 9-12gm) followed by 30 mg/day PO steroids x 1 month, then taper		NOSPECS class, MRI muscle size	24	12/23 (52.2%) improved diplopia and soft tissue swelling, decrease in mean proptosis values, 13/23 (56.5%) decrease muscle size on MRI.
Kahaly et al[33]	70 (35 IV steroids and 35 PO steroids)	Randomized, single blind study. 35 received IV steroids 0.5gm/day x 6wks (once weekly), then down to 0.25gm/pulse IV steroids x6wks (once weekly); 35 received PO steroids 0.1gm/day then taper for 12 wks by 0.01g/wk (cumulative dose of 4.5gm and 4.0gm, respectively)		Proptosis and lid width, visual acuity, IOP in upgaze, diplopia, B-U/S, CAS, self assessment survey	12	Favorable response in 27/35 (77%) of patients receiving IV steroids vs 18/35 (51%) with PO steroids on CAS; rapid improvement seen in IV group,
Kazim et al[43]	30	Retrospective case series. 80-120 mg/day PO steroids tapered "over many months"		Subjective improvement, improved fusion, proptosis, clinical exam	24	10/30 (33%) improved in some way.
Kendall-Taylor et al[38]	11	Prospective case series. IV steroid (500mg /day x 2) then with 40mg PO steroid taper x4wks		Eye exam with IOP, CT EOM size, photos,	24	6/7 (85.7%) with optic neuropathy improved, 9/11 (81.8%) improved soft tissue swelling, proptosis persisted in all patients, 8/9 (88.9%) improved EOM size on CT
Koshiyama et al[36]	8	Prospective case series. IV steroids 1gm/day x 3 then tapered to 30-40mg/day PO steroids with variable tapered length (6-14wks)	XRT (20Gy x 2wks) given after completion of pulse IV steroids	Diplopia, muscle size on MRI, NOSPECS class	3 yr (156wks)	7/8 (88%) excellent result

Table 3. Continued

Publication	Pts.	Treatment/Study Type	Adjunctive treatment	Outcome Measures	Duration of follow up (wks)	Comment /conclusions
Macchia et al[32]	51 (26 received PO steroids and 25 received IV steroids)	Randomized, prospective study 60-80mg PO steroids with 4-6 month taper. IV group received 1000mg/day for two consecutive days each week for total of 6 weeks.	None	NOSPECS, self assessment survey, proptosis	2yrs	21/25 (84%) had improvement with IV steroids, and 15/26 (57%) had improvement with PO steroids.
Marcocci et al, (1987)[14]	60 (30 were treated with XRT and PO steroids, 30 were treated with combined XRT and retrobulbar steroids	Prospective, randomized, controlled study. PO steroids group: 70-80 mg/day PO steroids x 3wks then tapered over 5-6 months, Retrobulbar steroids group: 14 injections (methylprednisolone, 40mg/1.5ml) q20-30days x9months	XRT (20Gy x2wks), started at same time as steroids	Clinical exam, NOSPECS	78	Overall excellent response in 18/30 (60%). Retrobulbar steroid and XRT group had overall improvement in 80%
Marcocci et al, (2001)[30]	82 (41 received PO steroids, 41 received IV steroids)	Prospective, single blind, randomized study. 100 mg/day PO steroid with taper over 22 wks, (total dose 6g) vs IV steroids 15mg/kg/day x 2 days every 2 weeks for 4 cycles, repeat with 7.5mg/kg IV steroids x 2 every 2 wks for 4 cycles (total dose 9-12gm)	XRT (20Gy x 2wks) started one week after onset of steroids	Proptosis, lid fissure width, diplopia, CAS	52	Overall improvement of 36/41 (88%) with IV steroids, (26/41) 63% with PO steroids; less side effects with IV (23/41 vs 35/41 in PO, optic neuropathy better result with IV (11/14 vs 3/9)

Publication	Pts.	Treatment/Study Type	Adjunctive treatment	Outcome Measures	Duration of follow up (wks)	Comment /conclusions
Matejka et al[37]	8	Prospective case series. IV 12.5mg/kg q 1 mo), then repeated 3-6 times monthly, given PO steroids interpulse (0.5mg/kg/day) then 4 wk PO steroid taper after last pulse IV dose.		Self assessment, NOSPECS, EOM and proptosis on CT	24	7/8 (87.5%) had improvement in all parameters
Noth et al[35]	19	Prospective case series. 20-60mg/day PO steroids x 3months	+/- XRT (20Gy x2wks)	Clinical exam, NOS PECS	~3yrs (156wks)	5/11 (45.5%) had good result with PO steroids only, 6 went on to have XRT and 1 went on to have XRT and decompressive surgery.
Prummel et al, (1989)[28]	18	Prospective, single blind, randomized study. 60 mg PO steroids/day vs cyclosporine x12wks	Vs Cyclosporine	NOSPECS, proptosis, EOM size on CT	52	11/18 (61.1%) responded by EOM size on CT, clinical scores and proptosis at 12 wks
Prummel et al, (1993)[12]	56 (28 received PO steroids, 28 received XRT)	Prospective, double blind randomized trial. 60mg PO steroids/day for 4wks then taper down over 20wks	Vs XRT (20Gy x2wks)	Highest NOSPECS class, CT	24	14/28 (50%) responded to steroids, 13/28 (46%) responded to XRT
Staar et al[39]	225	Partly retrospective and prospective case series. 60 mg PO steroids simultaneously started with onset of XRT, PO steroids tapered over 6wks	With XRT (16-19Gy over 6wks)	Subjective impression, NOSPECS	52	Overall, 153/225 (68%) improved.

Table 3. Continued

Publication	Pts.	Treatment/Study Type	Adjunctive treatment	Outcome Measures	Duration of follow up (wks)	Comment /conclusions
Tagami et al[40]	27 (11 received XRT and IV steroids, 16 received only IV steroids)	Prospective case series. 1 gm/pulse IV steroids x 3, repeat q1 week x 4 (if clinically indicated), then followed by 40-50mg/day PO steroids, tapered over next 3-12 months	12 pts received XRT (followed 2wks after pulse IV steroids were completed)	Clinical score, CT or MRI of EOM, NOSPECS	2yrs (104wks)	overall 9/11 (81.8%) improved in XRT and IV steroids group, and 12/16 (75%) improved in IV steroids group, NOSPECS improved as average across the group;

CAS= clinical activity score, RAI=radioactive iodine treatment, XRT= external beam orbital radiation, GO= Graves ophthalmopathy, PO=oral, IV=intravenous, IVIG=intravenous immunoglobin therapy, EOM=extraocular muscles.

Of the 886 patients, 624 (70.4%) from 14 studies were treated with oral corticosteroids with or without XRT. Of the 624 patients, 292 had received only oral prednisone (average of 76 +/- 26 mg/day). The length of oral corticosteroid treatment (including taper) averaged 17.5 +/-5.4 weeks. In 11 studies, 262 patients (29.6%) were treated predominantly with IV corticosteroids (methylprednisolone) with or without XRT. The average number of pulses received was 5.8 +/-3.8 over an average length of 13 +/-1.5 weeks of treatment. Most of the patients receiving IV corticosteroids (n=202) without XRT also received oral corticosteroids between pulses of IV corticosteroids and were given a tapered course of oral corticosteroids that averaged 37.9 +/- 4.9 mg/day over 14 +/-17 weeks. (Table 3)

Clinical Measurement of Disease Severity and Treatment Response

The studies we reviewed measured severity and activity using different scoring systems including NOSPECS classification system, clinical activity score (CAS), American Thyroid Association classification, Stanford Score, International Index, and self-assessment surveys. Additional data was acquired from the clinical examination findings including proptosis, gaze-evoked changes in intraocular pressure (IOP), and neuroimaging abnormalities (Table 3).

The NOSPECS classification system was most commonly used (12 of 20 studies). The CAS was used in 7 of 20 studies. Many studies included self-assessment patient surveys to further evaluate treatment response. (Table 3).

Intravenous vs. Oral Corticosteroids

Because of dissimilar assessment measures between the studies, we judged the results as favorable if the author reported the results as either good or excellent.

Corticosteroids were the primary medical therapy used to treat active GO. Overall 66.6% of the 886 patients responded favorably to corticosteroid treatment, which included those also treated with XRT. A total of 494 patients were treated with oral or predominantly IV corticosteroids alone. A total of 164 (56.0%) of 292 patients treated with oral corticosteroids alone had a favorable response, and 150 (74.3%) of 202 patients treated with IV corticosteroids alone had a favorable response (Table 4).

Only four of the studies compared IV to oral corticosteroid treatment in a prospective and randomized method [34, 41-43]. None of the studies used a tapering regimen of oral corticosteroids following a regimen of IV corticosteroids. All four showed patients treated with IV corticosteroids faired better than those treated with oral corticosteroids. Kahaly et al [42] showed an improvement in the CAS by at least three points in 27 (77%) of 35 patients treated with IV corticosteroids as compared to 18 (51%) of 35 patients treated with oral corticosteroids. Macchia et al [43] reported similar results using NOSPECS; 21 (84%) of 25 patients treated with IV corticosteroids had a favorable response as compared to 15 (57%) of 26 treated with oral corticosteroids.

Table 4. Outcomes Following Treatment of Patients with Active Thyroid Eye Disease

	Cort PO only	Cort IV only	Cort PO and XRT	Cort IV and XRT	Cort PO (+/- XRT)	Cort IV (+/- XRT)
Total patients	292	202	332	60	624	262
Overall favorable response	162/292 (56.0%)	150/202 (74.3%)	223/332 (67.2%)	52/60 (86.7%)	388/624 (62.2%)	202/262 (77.1%)
Improvement in diplopia	50/135 (37.0%)	61/122 (50.0%)	133/169 (78.7%)	14/19 (73.7%)	40/105 (38.1%)	75/141 (53.2%)
Improvement in motility	20/53 (37.7%)	32/54 (59.3%)			20/53 (37.7%)	32/64 (50.0%)
Improvement in proptosis	40/94 (42.6%)	100/163 (61.3%)	170/273 (62.3%)		31/48 (64.6%)	79/117 (67.5%)
Improvement in extraocular muscle thickness	35/42 (83.3%)	27/38 (71.1%)	20/30 (66.6%)	6/8 (75%)	50/60 (83.3%)	33/46 (71.2%)

Cort = corticosteroid; XRT = external beam x-irradiation; IV = intravenous administration; PO = oral administration.

Combined Corticosteroid and XRT Treatment

The cumulative radiation dose and the radiation field were similar in nearly all studies (20Gy delivered to each orbit over a two-week period). There was an overall 70.2% favorable response in the 392 patients who underwent both XRT and IV or oral corticosteroid treatment. Patients that received IV corticosteroids with or without XRT responded more favorably (86.7% favorable response, n=60) than those receiving oral corticosteroids and XRT (67.2% favorable response, n=332).

Summary of Outcomes

Given the limitations of our study, the updated review of the published English literature suggests that corticosteroid-mediated treatment produces benefit in 66.6% in GO patients who have moderate to severe disease. IV corticosteroids used in repeated daily or weekly pulses (average of 5.8 pulses/treatment) may be more effective than daily oral corticosteroids. Furthermore, a combination of corticosteroids and XRT was more effective than corticosteroids alone. When combined with XRT, IV administration of corticosteroids was more effective than oral administration.

Among the four prospective randomized studies, IV corticosteroids had an advantage in treatment outcome over oral corticosteroids [34,41-43]. The treatment outcomes were more substantial in those treated with IV corticosteroids (over 77% favorable outcome) than with oral corticosteroids (up to 62% favorable outcome). Nevertheless, patients treated with IV or oral corticosteroids showed improvement in proptosis, diplopia, ocular motility, and in self assessment of benefit.

Limitations to our Review

The reviewed studies differed in design, treatment protocol, and outcome measures. As a result, the potential clinical impact of corticosteroids and XRT in the treatment of GO was difficult to reliably assess.

We found it particularly difficult to interpret the results of GO severity and activity among different scoring systems. Although NOSPECS was the most commonly used scoring system, it does not accurately evaluate disease activity of GO. Clinical worsening may not represent increased inflammatory activity but rather progressive fibrosis associated with resolving inflammation. CAS measures the activity of the disease but does not provide information regarding overall progression or severity of GO. Many studies used self-assessment surveys to document improvements in quality of life; however, these are non-standardized and difficult to interpret across studies.

Conclusion

Our review of the literature suggests that there is inadequate case-based evidence to reliably assess the efficacy of corticosteroids or XRT in shortening the active phase of GO or improving long-term disfigurement and disability in patients with moderate to severe GO. Ongoing research continues to inspire clinicians to embark on new immunomodulatory therapy for patients with refractory or difficult to manage cases of GO. In order to evaluate the management of GO, the design and funding of a multi- center trial are required.

References

[1] Dickinson AJ, Perros P. Controversies in the clinical evaluation of active thyroid-associated orbitopathy: use of a detailed protocol with comparative photographs for objective assessment. *Clin Endocrinol (Oxf).* Sep 2001;55(3):283-303.

[2] Mourits MP, Koornneef L, Wiersinga WM, Prummel MF, Berghout A, van der Gaag R. Clinical criteria for the assessment of disease activity in Graves' ophthalmopathy: a novel approach. *Br J Ophthalmol.* Aug 1989;73(8):639-644.

[3] Bartley GB, Fatourechi V, Kadrmas EF, et al. Clinical features of Graves' ophthalmopathy in an incidence cohort. *Am J Ophthalmol.* Mar 1996;121(3):284-290.

[4] Bahn RS, Heufelder AE. Pathogenesis of Graves' ophthalmopathy. *N Engl J Med.* Nov 11 1993;329(20):1468-1475.

[5] Jacobson DM. Dysthyroid orbitopathy. *Semin Neurol.* 2000;20(1):43-54.

[6] Kazim M, Goldberg RA, Smith TJ. Insights into the pathogenesis of thyroid-associated orbitopathy: evolving rationale for therapy. *Arch Ophthalmol.* Mar 2002;120(3):380-386.

[7] Werner SC. Classification of the eye changes of Graves' disease. *Am J Ophthalmol.* Oct 1969;68(4):646-648.

[8] Kennerdell C, Maroon et al. Dysthyroid Orbitopathy. *Practical Diagnosis and Management of Orbital Disease.* Boston: Butterworth/Heinemann Press; 2001:53-75.

[9] Clauser L, Galie M, Sarti E, Dallera V. Rationale of treatment in Graves ophthalmopathy. *Plast Reconstr Surg.* Dec 2001;108(7):1880-1894.

[10] Eckstein A, Quadbeck B, Mueller G, et al. Impact of smoking on the response to treatment of thyroid associated ophthalmopathy. *Br J Ophthalmol.* Jun 2003;87(6):773-776.

[11] Sergott RC, Glaser JS. Graves' ophthalmopathy. A clinical and immunologic review. *Surv Ophthalmol.* Jul-Aug 1981;26(1):1-21.

[12] Prummel MF, Mourits MP, Blank L, Berghout A, Koornneef L, Wiersinga WM. Randomized double-blind trial of prednisone versus radiotherapy in Graves' ophthalmopathy. *Lancet.* Oct 16 1993;342(8877):949-954.

[13] Weetman AP, Wiersinga WM. Current management of thyroid-associated ophthalmopathy in Europe. Results of an international survey. *Clin Endocrinol (Oxf).* Jul 1998;49(1):21-28.

[14] Hatton MP, Rubin PA. The pathophysiology of thyroid-associated ophthalmopathy. *Ophthalmol Clin North Am.* Mar 2002;15(1):113-119.

[15] Ebner R, Devoto MH, Weil D, et al. Treatment of thyroid associated ophthalmopathy with periocular injections of triamcinolone. *Br J Ophthalmol.* Nov 2004;88(11):1380-1386.

[16] Marcocci C, Bartalena L, Panicucci M, et al. Orbital cobalt irradiation combined with retrobulbar or systemic corticosteroids for Graves' ophthalmopathy: a comparative study. *Clin Endocrinol (Oxf).* Jul 1987;27(1):33-42.

[17] Trobe JD, Glaser JS, Laflamme P. Dysthyroid optic neuropathy. Clinical profile and rationale for management. *Arch Ophthalmol.* Jul 1978;96(7):1199-1209.

[18] Garber MI. Methylprednisolone in the treatment of exophthalmos. *Lancet.* Apr 30 1966;1(7444):958-960.

[19] Zoumalan CI, Cockerham KP, Turbin RE, et al. Efficacy of corticosteroids and external beam radiation in the management of moderate to severe thyroid eye disease. *J Neuroophthalmol.* Sep 2007;27(3):205-214.

[20] Gursoy A, Cesur M, Erdogan MF, Corapcioglu D, Kamel N. New-onset acute heart failure after intravenous glucocorticoid pulse therapy in a patient with Graves' ophthalmopathy. *Endocrine.* Jun 2006;29(3):513-516.

[21] Weissel M, Hauff W. Fatal liver failure after high-dose glucocorticoid pulse therapy in a patient with severe thyroid eye disease. *Thyroid.* Jun 2000;10(6):521.

[22] Donaldson SS, Bagshaw MA, Kriss JP. Supervoltage orbital radiotherapy for Graves' ophthalmopathy. *J Clin Endocrinol Metab.* Aug 1973;37(2):276-285.

[23] Gorman CA, Garrity JA, Fatourechi V, et al. A prospective, randomized, double-blind, placebo-controlled study of orbital radiotherapy for Graves' ophthalmopathy. *Ophthalmology.* Sep 2001;108(9):1523-1534.

[24] Gorman CA, Garrity JA, Fatourechi V, et al. The aftermath of orbital radiotherapy for graves' ophthalmopathy. *Ophthalmology.* Nov 2002;109(11):2100-2107.

[25] Atabay C, Schrooyen M, Zhang ZG, Salvi M, Glinoer D, Wall JR. Use of eye muscle antibody measurements to monitor response to plasmapheresis in patients with thyroid-associated ophthalmopathy. *J Endocrinol Invest.* Oct 1993;16(9):669-674.

[26] Burrow GN, Mitchell MS, Howard RO, Morrow LB. Immunosuppressive therapy for the eye changes of Graves' disease. *J Clin Endocrinol Metab.* Sep 1970;31(3):307-311.

[27] Claridge KG, Ghabrial R, Davis G, et al. Combined radiotherapy and medical immunosuppression in the management of thyroid eye disease. *Eye.* 1997;11 (Pt 5):717-722.

[28] Yamamoto K, Saito K, Takai T, Yoshida S. Treatment of Graves' ophthalmopathy by steroid therapy, orbital radiation therapy, plasmapheresis and thyroxine replacement. *Endocrinol Jpn.* Aug 1982;29(4):495-501.

[29] Antonelli A, Saracino A, Alberti B, et al. High-dose intravenous immunoglobulin treatment in Graves' ophthalmopathy. *Acta Endocrinol (Copenh).* Jan 1992;126(1):13-23.

[30] Prummel MF, Mourits MP, Berghout A, et al. Prednisone and cyclosporine in the treatment of severe Graves' ophthalmopathy. *N Engl J Med.* Nov 16 1989;321(20):1353-1359.

[31] Bartalena L, Marcocci C, Chiovato L, et al. Orbital cobalt irradiation combined with systemic corticosteroids for Graves' ophthalmopathy: comparison with systemic corticosteroids alone. *J Clin Endocrinol Metab.* Jun 1983;56(6):1139-1144.

[32] Prummel MF, Bakker A, Wiersinga WM, et al. Multi-center study on the characteristics and treatment strategies of patients with Graves' orbitopathy: the first European Group on Graves' Orbitopathy experience. *Eur J Endocrinol.* May 2003;148(5):491-495.

[33] Bartalena L, Marocci C, Bogazzi F, Bruno-Bossio G, Pinchera A. Glucocorticoid therapy of Graves' ophthalmopathy. *Exp Clin Endocrinol.* May 1991;97(2-3):320-327.

[34] Marcocci C, Bartalena L, Tanda ML, et al. Comparison of the effectiveness and tolerability of intravenous or oral glucocorticoids associated with orbital radiotherapy in the management of severe Graves' ophthalmopathy: results of a prospective, single-blind, randomized study. *J Clin Endocrinol Metab.* Aug 2001;86(8):3562-3567.

[35] Kapadia MK, Rubin PA. The emerging use of TNF-alpha inhibitors in orbital inflammatory disease. *Int Ophthalmol Clin.* Spring 2006;46(2):165-181.

[36] Boye J, Elter T, Engert A. An overview of the current clinical use of the anti-CD20 monoclonal antibody rituximab. *Ann Oncol.* Apr 2003;14(4):520-535.

[37] Kimby E. Tolerability and safety of rituximab (MabThera). *Cancer Treat Rev.* Oct 2005;31(6):456-473.

[38] Leandro MJ, Cambridge G, Ehrenstein MR, Edwards JC. Reconstitution of peripheral blood B cells after depletion with rituximab in patients with rheumatoid arthritis. *Arthritis Rheum.* Feb 2006;54(2):613-620.

[39] El Fassi D, Nielsen CH, Hasselbalch HC, Hegedus L. Treatment-resistant severe, active Graves' ophthalmopathy successfully treated with B lymphocyte depletion. *Thyroid.* Jul 2006;16(7):709-710.

[40] Salvi M, Vannucchi G, Campi I, et al. Treatment of Graves' disease and associated ophthalmopathy with the anti-CD20 monoclonal antibody rituximab: an open study. *Eur J Endocrinol.* Jan 2007;156(1):33-40.

[41] Aktaran S, Akarsu E, Erbagci I, Araz M, Okumus S, Kartal M. Comparison of intravenous methylprednisolone therapy vs. oral methylprednisolone therapy in patients with Graves' ophthalmopathy. *Int J Clin Pract.* Jan 2007;61(1):45-51.

[42] Kahaly GJ, Pitz S, Hommel G, Dittmar M. Randomized, single blind trial of intravenous versus oral steroid monotherapy in Graves' orbitopathy. *J Clin Endocrinol Metab.* Sep 2005;90(9):5234-5240.

[43] Macchia PE, Bagattini M, Lupoli G, Vitale M, Vitale G, Fenzi G. High-dose intravenous corticosteroid therapy for Graves' ophthalmopathy. *J Endocrinol Invest.* Mar 2001;24(3):152-158.

[44] Bartalena L, Marcocci C, Bogazzi F, et al. Relation between therapy for hyperthyroidism and the course of Graves' ophthalmopathy. *N Engl J Med.* Jan 8 1998;338(2):73-78.

[45] Baschieri L, Antonelli A, Nardi S, et al. Intravenous immunoglobulin versus corticosteroid in treatment of Graves' ophthalmopathy. *Thyroid.* Aug 1997;7(4):579-585.

[46] Noth D, Gebauer M, Muller B, Burgi U, Diem P. Graves' ophthalmopathy: natural history and treatment outcomes. *Swiss Med Wkly.* Oct 20 2001;131(41-42):603-609.

[47] Matejka G, Verges B, Vaillant G, et al. Intravenous methylprednisolone pulse therapy in the treatment of Graves' ophthalmopathy. *Horm Metab Res.* Feb 1998;30(2):93-98.

[48] Kendall-Taylor P, Crombie AL, Stephenson AM, Hardwick M, Hall K. Intravenous methylprednisolone in the treatment of Graves' ophthalmopathy. *Bmj.* Dec 17 1988;297(6663):1574-1578.

[49] Staar S, Muller RP, Hammer M, Nolte M. Results and prognostic factors in retrobulbar radiotherapy combined with systemic corticosteroids for endocrine orbitopathy (Graves' disease). *Front Radiat Ther Oncol.* 1997;30:206-217.

[50] Tagami T, Tanaka K, Sugawa H, et al. High-dose intravenous steroid pulse therapy in thyroid-associated ophthalmopathy. *Endocr J.* Dec 1996;43(6):689-699.

[51] Koshiyama H, Koh T, Fujiwara K, Hayakawa K, Shimbo S, Misaki T. Therapy of Graves' ophthalmopathy with intravenous high-dose steroid followed by orbital irradiation. *Thyroid.* Winter 1994;4(4):409-413.

[52] Dandona P, Havard CW, Mier A. Methylprednisolone and Graves' ophthalmopathy. *Bmj.* Mar 25 1989;298(6676):830.

[53] Chang TC, Huang KM, Hsiao YL, Tzeng SS, Kao SC. Relationships of orbital computed tomographic findings and activity scores to the prognosis of corticosteroid therapy in patients with Graves' ophthalmopathy. *Acta Ophthalmol Scand.* Jun 1997;75(3):301-304.

[54] Hiromatsu Y, Kojima K, Ishisaka N, et al. Role of magnetic resonance imaging in thyroid-associated ophthalmopathy: its predictive value for therapeutic outcome of immunosuppressive therapy. *Thyroid.* Winter 1992;2(4):299-305.

[55] Kazim M, Trokel S, Moore S. Treatment of acute Graves orbitopathy. *Ophthalmology.* Sep 1991;98(9):1443-1448.

In: Thyroid Hormones: Functions, Related Diseases and Uses ISBN: 978-1-60741-080-5
Editors: F. S. Kuehn, M. P. Lozada

Chapter VIII

Thyroid Function in Infants of Mothers with Graves' Disease and Hyperthyroidism During Pregnancy

***Ryuzo Higuchi*[*,1] and *Sawako Minami*[2]**
[1]Department of Perinatal Medicine, Divisions of NICU and [2]Obstetrics, Wakayama Medical University, 811-1 Kimiidera, Wakayama, 641-0012 Japan

Abstract

We report a retrospective study of thyroid function in seven infants whose mothers had Graves' disease and hyperthyroidism during the gestational period due to onset, relapse, instability, or poor compliance. Three infants showed transient central hypothyroidism, one of whom had short-term neonatal thyrotoxicosis before central hypothyroidism. These infants had TRAb < 50% and TSAb < 400% at birth, and maternal hyperthyroidism appeared before 32 weeks gestation. Three other infants had neonatal Graves' disease until 1, 2 and 3 months of age, respectively, with TRAb > 70% and TSAb > 700% at birth, and maternal hyperthyroidism appeared after 28 weeks gestation. One infant whose mother had hyperthyroidism until 10 weeks gestation was euthyroid after birth. These cases suggest that passage of thyroid hormones from mother to fetus occurs when the maternal level of thyroid hormones is high. Maternal hyperthyroidism before 32 weeks gestation and relatively high autoantibodies in the neonate are related to development of central hypothyroidism. In addition, maternal hyperthyroidism after 28 weeks gestation may not be related to development of central hypothyroidism.

Keywords: Central hypothyroidism, Graves' disease, pregnancy, TSH receptor antibodies, thyroid- stimulating antibodies

* E-mail: rhiguchi@wakayama-med.ac.jp

Introduction

Transient central hypothyroidism is a rare condition seen in infants born to mothers with hyperthyroidism in the gestational period. However, it is unknown how maternal hyperthyroidism leads to development of central hypothyroidism in offspring. Therefore, we performed a retrospective study of thyroid function in infants whose mothers had Graves' disease and hyperthyroidism during the gestational period due to onset, relapse, instability, or poor compliance.

Patients and Methods

We have previously reported transient central hypothyroidism in three infants whose mothers had Graves' disease and hyperthyroidism in the gestational period [1]. The maximum levels of maternal free T4 (FT4) during pregnancy were 8.4, 7.65 and 3.92 ng/dL, respectively, which led us to hypothesize that hyperthyroidism with FT4 > 3.0 ng/dL could affect fetuses and lead to development of central hypothyroidism. Data for thyroid function tests were collected for infants whose mothers with Graves' disease had hyperthyroidism with FT4 > 3.0 ng/dL during pregnancy. Three of the infants showed central hypothyroidism, one of whom had prior short-term neonatal thyrotoxicosis [2], and three had neonatal Graves' disease, one of whom had congenital Graves' disease. The seventh infant was euthyroid. Follow-up study confirmed that these tests were within the reference range without use of medication by two-year old. Maternal and neonatal FT4 was sampled within3 days before delivery and within 24 hours after birth, respectively. Neonatal TSH receptor antibodies (TRAb) and thyroid stimulating antibodies (TSAb) were sampled from cord blood or within 3 days after birth. The reference ranges for TRAb and TSAb are < 15% and < 180%, respectively.

Results

Case 1: Transient central hypothyroidism after short-term thyrotoxicosis in an infant whose mother was non-compliant with medication [2]. A male infant was born at 27 weeks gestation with a birth weight of 1152 g. His 27-year-old G2P0 mother had been diagnosed with Graves' disease at age 13 years old. However, she had been non-compliant with medication and was transferred to our hospital because of threatened preterm labor and suspected abruptio placentae. Her thyroid function data were free T3 (FT3) 21.1 pg/mL, FT4 8.1 ng/dL, TSH < 0.03 μIU/mL, TRAb 52%, and TSAb 294%. The infant was born via caesarean section on the day the mother was transferred to our hospital. TRAb in the cord blood was 16% and the infant showed tachycardia of approximately 200/min after birth, with the following hyperthyroid function 1 h after birth: FT_3 7.0 pg/mL, FT_4 4.7 ng/dL, and TSH 0.12 μIU/mL. We administered propylthiouracil (PTU) orally at a dose of 10 mg/kg/day, but the thyroid function data returned to the euthyroid state within five days, faster than PTU usually displays effect (Figure 1). We stopped PTU at 5 days of age. Subsequently, a hypothyroid state was observed at 12 days of age: FT3 2.1 pg/ml, FT4 0.4 ng/dl, and TSH 0.03 μIU/ml. The reference ranges for serum FT4 and TSH during the first week of life after 25-27 weeks' gestation are 0.6-2.2 ng/dL and 0.2-30.3 mU/L, respectively [3]. The TSH response to TSH-releasing hormone (TRH) (10 μg/kg) was almost nothing (0.04 μIU/ml after 30 min) and administration of oral l-thyroxine (5 μg/kg/day) was started at two weeks of age (Table 1). The TRH test normalized at 6 months of age and thyroxine supplementation was stopped (Table 2).

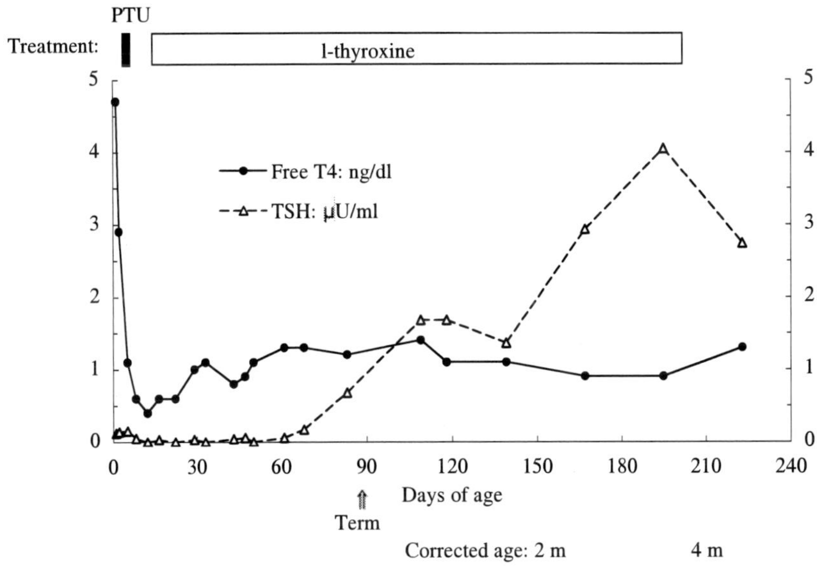

Figure 1. Clinical course of Case 1.

Case 2: Failure of screening for congenital hypothyroidism in an infant with transient central hypothyroidism whose mother was non-compliant with medication. A male infant was born at 34 weeks gestation with a birth weight of 2445 g. His 23-year-old G1P1 mother had been diagnosed with Graves' disease at age 21 years old. However, she had been non-compliant with medication and was transferred to a local hospital because of the possibility of preterm labor complicated with thyrotoxicosis in week 31 of gestation. Her thyroid function data were FT_3 21.1 pg/mL, FT_4 7.65 ng/dL, TSH < 0.05 μIU/mL, and TRAb 41.9%. PTU was administered orally at a dose of 300 mg/day, and her serum FT_4 had decreased to 3.23 ng/dL at 34 weeks gestation, when the infant was spontaneously delivered vaginally after premature rupture of the membranes (PROM). TRAb in the cord blood was 42.7%. Radiography demonstrated formation of distal femoral epiphyses. The infant showed poor sucking and hyperbilirubinemia from 2 days after birth and was treated with phototherapy. Thyroid function data at 4 days of age were FT_3 1.05 pg/mL, FT_4 0.65 ng/dL and TSH 0.25 μIU/mL, and a neonatal screening test performed at 8 days of age was passed. The reference ranges for serum FT4 and TSH during the first week of life after 34-36 weeks gestation are 1.2-4.4 ng/dL and 1.2-21.6 mU/L, respectively [3]. Subsequently, constipation appeared. Hypothyroid function was still observed at four weeks of age (FT_3 3.16 pg/mL, FT_4 0.75 ng/dL and TSH 1.33 μIU/mL) with the maximal TSH response in the TRH test ranging from 1.79 to 5.55 μIU/mL after 30 min (Tables 1 and 2). Hence, oral l-thyroxine (10 μg/kg) supplementation was started. The TRH test normalized at 13 months of age and thyroxin supplementation was stopped.

Case 3: An infant with transient central hypothyroidism whose mother developed Graves' disease during pregnancy and became euthyroid at delivery. A male infant was born at 37 weeks gestation with a birth weight of 3244 g. His 26-year-old G0P0 mother had been diagnosed with thyrotoxicosis attributable to Graves' disease at 31 weeks of gestation. Her thyroid function data were FT_3 16.04 pg/mL, FT_4 3.92 ng/dL, TSH 0.01 μIU/mL, and TRAb 62.3%. PTU was administered orally at a dose of 300 mg/day and she became euthyroid (FT_4 1.74 ng/dL, TSH 0.03 μIU/mL, and TRAb 50%) two days before an elective caesarean section. Thyroid function data in the cord blood were FT_4 1.00 ng/dl, TSH 0.84 μIU/ml, and TRAb 20.3%. Radiography demonstrated formation of distal femoral epiphyses. Two days after birth, the infant's thyroid function decreased (FT_3 0.98 pg/mL, FT_4 0.66 ng/dL, TSH 0.4 μIU/mL) and oral l-thyroxine (5 μg/kg) supplementation was started. The reference ranges for serum FT4 and TSH during the first week of life after 37-42 weeks of gestation are 2.0-5.3 ng/dL and 1.0-39 mU/L, respectively [3]. The maximal TSH response in the TRH test ranged from 0.18 to 1.58 μIU/mL after 30 min at 3 months of age (Tables 1 and 2). The TRH test normalized at 20 months of age and thyroxine supplementation was stopped.

Table 1. Thyroid function tests and TRAb and TSAb levels in mothers with hyperthyroidism during pregnancy and in offspring with central hypothyroidism

Maternal thyroid function and autoantibodies during gestation

Case	*Gestation (weeks)*	*free T3 (pg/mL)*	*free T4 (ng/dL)*	*TSH (μIU/mL)*	*TRAb[a] (%)*	*TSAb[b] (%)*
1	27	21.1	8.1	<0.03	52	294
2	31	21.1	7.65	<0.005	41.9	504
3	31	16.04	3.92	0.01	62.3	

Neonatal thyroid function data and levels of TRAb and TSAb at birth

Case	*Gestation (weeks)*	*free T3 (pg/mL)*	*free T4 (ng/dL)*	*TSH (μIU/mL)*	*TRAb[a] (%)*	*TSAb[b] (%)*
1	27	7	4.7	0.12	16	370
2	34			<0.005	42.7	
3	37	0.82	1	0.84	20.3	384

Neonatal thyroid function data before l-thyroxin supplementation

Case	*Age (days)*	*free T3 (pg/mL)*	*free T4 (ng/dL)*	*TSH (μIU/mL)*

Maternal thyroid function and autoantibodies during gestation

Case	*Gestation (weeks)*	*free T3 (pg/mL)*	*free T4 (ng/dL)*	*TSH (μIU/mL)*	*TRAb*[a] *(%)*	*TSAb*[b] *(%)*
1	12	2.1	0.4	0.03		
2	4	1.05	0.65	0.025		
3	2	0.98	0.66	0.4		

[a] TRAb: TSH receptor antibodies (normal range < 15 %)

[b] TSAb: thyroid-stimulating antibodies (normal range < 180 %)

Table 2. Serial TRH tests (10 μg/kg, i.v.) in infants with transient central hypothyroidism

Case	*Age*	*TSH levels (μIU/mL)*				
		0 min.	*30 min.*	*60 min.*	*90 min.*	*120 min.*
1	12 days	0.03	0.04			
	4 months	1.68	6.02			
	6 months	4.05	18.05			
2	4 weeks	1.79	5.55	4.15	3.41	2.92
	4 months	0.277	1.63	0.873	0.553	0.390
	13 months	0.664	13.17			
3	3 months	0.18	1.58	0.98	0.64	0.43
	20 months	5.93	30.03	18.86	12.70	7.81

Case 4: An infant with congenital and neonatal Graves' disease whose mother had onset of Graves' disease during pregnancy. The 25-year-old G1P0 mother showed struma from 8 weeks gestation, and leg edema, weight gain (6.9 kg in 2 weeks), dyspnea, and cough from 28 weeks gestation. Her thyroid function data were FT_4 3.7 ng/dL, TSH <0.1 μIU/mL and TRAb 70.0%, and fetal heart rate monitoring showed fetal tachycardia of 180/min at 29 weeks gestation. She was diagnosed with thyrotoxic cardiac failure due to Graves' disease and administered digoxin and furosemide. A female neonate was born vaginally at 30 weeks gestation with a birth weight of 1740 g, and showed jittery movement, struma, exophthalmus, cardiomegaly (CTR: 75%) (Figure 1), tachycardia (199/min) and cleft palate. The thyroid function data in cord blood were FT_4 5.7 ng/dL, TSH <0.1 μIU/mL, and TRAb 72.0%. The neonate was administered three intravenous shots of propranolol, inorganic iodide for 14 days, digoxin for 30 days, and PTU for 62 days. Thereafter, the infant remained euthyroid.

Case 5: An infant with neonatal Graves' disease whose mother had relapsing Graves' disease during pregnancy. A male infant was born at 36 weeks gestation with a birth weight of 2729 g. His 26-year-old G0P0 mother had been diagnosed with hyperthyroidism due to Graves' disease at 22 years old. Her thyroid function became euthyroid after administration of methimazole (MMI), and MMI was discontinued before pregnancy. Early in the gestation she was euthyroid: FT_4 1.21 ng/dL and TRAb 0%. She became hyperthyroid at 19 weeks gestation, when propylthiouracil (PTU) was started, but her FT_4 increased to 3.82 ng/dL and the fetal heart rate increased to 170-180/min at 28 weeks gestation. Oral inorganic iodine and prednisolone were added, but thyroid function tests worsened at 30 weeks gestation, as follows: FT_3 9.21 pg/mL, FT_4 4.39 ng/dL, TSH 0.01 μIU/mL, and TRAb 80.0%. Subsequently, she became almost euthyroid (FT_4 1.94 ng/dL and TRAb 85%) at 36 weeks gestation and a baby boy was born vaginally. Thyroid function data in cord blood were FT_3 2.02 pg/mL, FT_4 0.9 ng/dL, TSH 12.9 μIU/mL, and TRAb 81.0%. The infant became irritable and his heart rate during quiet sleep increased from 120/min to 170/min. PTU was started 7 days after birth and inorganic iodine and propranolol were added 11 days after birth because thyroid function tests indicated FT_3 15.10 pg/mL, FT_4 6.35 ng/dL, and TSH 0.88 μIU/mL. Antithyroid treatment was stopped on day 128.

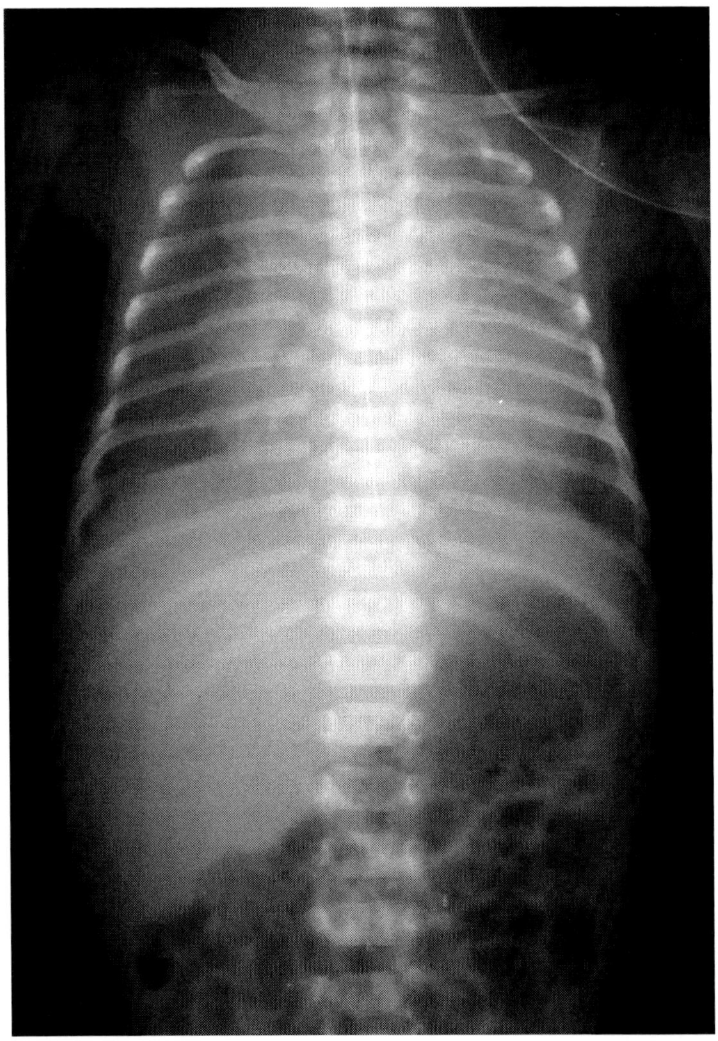

Figure 2. Chest x-ray on admission of Case 4 shows cardiomegaly and hepatomegaly.

Case 6: An infant with neonatal Graves' disease whose mother had uncontrolled Graves' disease during pregnancy. A female infant was born at 36 weeks gestation with a birth weight of 2729 g. Her 24-year-old G0P0 mother had been diagnosed with hyperthyroidism due to Graves' disease at 15 years old. Maternal thyroid function became euthyroid after administration of methimazole (MMI). PTU was introduced at 4 weeks gestation to replace MMI. At 6 weeks gestation, she was euthyroid (FT_4 0.9 ng/dL and TSH 0.08 μIU/mL), but became hyperthyroid at 20 weeks gestation (FT_4 2.84 ng/dL and TSH 0.02 μIU/mL). Despite an increase in the dose of PTU (600 mg/day), maternal FT_4 rose to 3.14 ng/dL at 27 weeks gestation, and MMI was restarted at 29 weeks gestation because FT_4 increased to 3.38 ng/dL. Thyroid function tests in cord blood showed FT_3 1.53 pg/mL, FT_4 0.86 ng/dL, TSH 22.11 μIU/mL, and TRAb 85.1%. The newborn infant had jittery movement, tachycardia (170/min) from day 14, and elevated FT_4 to 4.51 ng/dL. PTU was administered for 20 days.

Case 7: A euthyroid neonate whose mother had relapse of Graves' disease in the first trimester. A male infant was born at 41 weeks gestation with a birth weight of 3045 g. His 24-year-old G0P0 mother had been diagnosed with Graves' disease at 18 years old. Her thyroid function became euthyroid after administration of MMI, which was stopped at 21 years old. Graves' disease relapsed with TRAb of 57% at 10 weeks gestation at age 23 years old and MMI was restarted. Thyroid function tests normalized in 12 days and those in cord blood showed FT_3 1.38 pg/mL, FT_4 0.80 ng/dL, TSH 2.849 μIU/mL, and TRAb 36.0%. The infant remained euthyroid.

Summary of the Seven Cases

Neonatal transient central hypothyroidism was observed in Cases 1 (combined with short-term neonatal thyrotoxicosis), 2 and 3. The gestation periods for these three infants were 27, 31 and 31 weeks, respectively. One of the mothers was diagnosed with hyperthyroidism at 27 weeks gestation and gave birth without treatment to an infant with thyrotoxicosis, which alternated with hypothyroidism for 5 days in the neonate. In the other two mothers, hyperthyroidism was diagnosed at 31 weeks gestation and controlled thereafter either partially or completely prior to birth of infants without thyrotoxicosis but with central hypothyroidism. The maximum TRAb and TSAb levels in the infants with central hypothyroidism were 42.7% and 384%, respectively.

Neonatal Graves' disease and hyperthyroidism were observed in Cases 4 (congenital Graves' disease), 5 and 6. The gestation periods of these three infants were 27, 29 and 29 weeks, respectively, and the TRAb and TSAb levels in the infants were at least 72% and 734%, respectively. One mother who had onset of Graves' disease during pregnancy gave birth at 30 weeks gestation without treatment for hyperthyroidism to a neonate who had congenital and neonatal Graves' disease. The level of FT4 was higher in the cord blood (5.7 ng/dL) than in the mother close to the time of delivery (3.7 ng/dL), and the TSAb level in cord blood was the highest among the three infants with neonatal Graves' disease. The other two mothers had hyperthyroidism at 27 and 29 weeks gestation, respectively, that was subsequently controlled prior to birth of infants with neither thyrotoxicosis nor hypothyroidism. In these two neonates, neonatal Graves' disease appeared at 1 or 2 weeks after birth. After stopping the antithyroid medication in the three cases at 63, 128 and 39 days after birth, respectively, the infants showed neither hypothyroidism nor hyperthyroidism. The required duration of antithyroid medication was not necessarily correlated with the level of neonatal TRAb or TSAb.

Case 7 was a euthyroid infant. Maternal hyperthyroidism observed up to 10 weeks gestation and neonatal TRAb of 36% did not affect the thyroid state in the neonate.

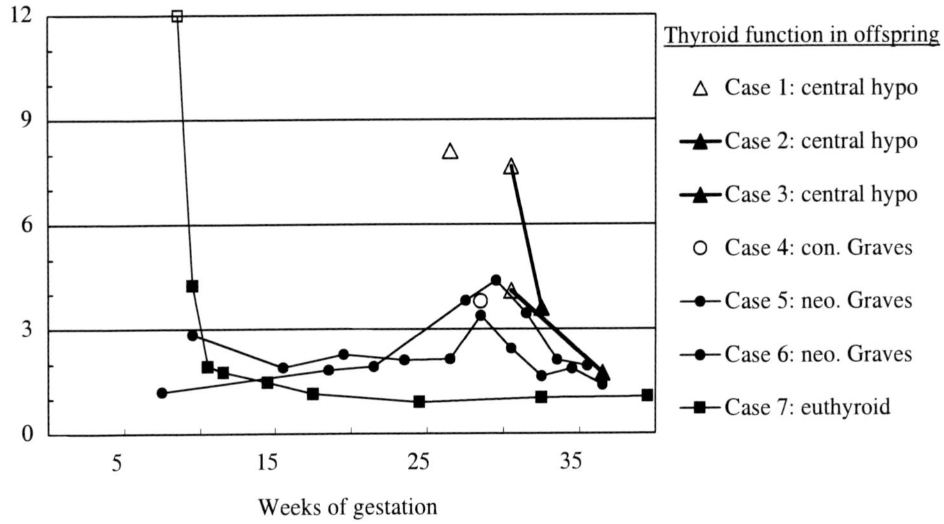

Figure 2. Free T4 level during pregnancy in mothers whose offspring showed transient central hypothyroidism (▲), congenital or neonatal Graves' disease (●), or a euthyroid state (■). Open marks and dotted lines indicate the periods without medication for hyperthyroidism, and closed marks and solid lines indicate those under medication for hyperthyroidism. Reference range for free T4: 0.95-1.74 ng/dL. Hypo: hypothyroidism, con: congenital, neo: neonatal, Graves: Graves' disease.

Table 3. Summary of seven infants whose mothers showed hyperthyroidism during pregnancy. Cases 1, 2, 3: transient central hypothyroidism; Cases 4, 5, 6: neonatal Graves' disease; Case 7: euthyroid

Case	Maternal Graves' disease			Neonate		
	Onset age	hyperthyroidism in pregnancy age/cause/duration	FT4 *	FT4 *	Gestation/BW	TRAb/TSAb
1	13y	27y/low compliance/…27w	8.10	4.70	27w/1152 g	16.0%/370%
2	21y	23y/low compliance/31-34w	3.23	ND	34w/2445 g	42.7%/ND
3	26y	26y/onset/31-35w	1.74	1.00	37w/3244 g	20.3%/384%

	Maternal Graves' disease			Neonate		
		hyperthyroidism in pregnancy				
4	25y	25y/onset/29-30w	3.70	5.70	30w/1740 g	72%/2233%
5	22y	26y/relapse/29-32w	1.94	0.90	36w/2729 g	81%/1386%
6	15y	24y/uncontrolled/27-29w	1.56	0.86	36w/2092 g	85.0%/734%
7	18y	24y/relapse/…10w	1.07	0.80	41w/3045 g	36%/ND

ND: not determined, *: ng/dL, BW: birth weight.

Discussion

Transient hypothyroxinemia in infants born to mothers with poorly controlled Graves' disease was first reported in 1988 [4]. The FT4 levels at birth in such infants are higher than at 5 days of age, suggesting that the FT4 level before birth was higher than in the period immediately after birth, probably due to passive transfer during the last trimester [5]. Low FT4 concentrations in combination with suppressed TSH levels and a blunted TSH response following TRH administration confirmed that the thyroid regulatory system was impaired in three of the cases described in this report. We hypothesized that maternal hyperthyroidism during pregnancy leads to thyrotoxicosis in a fetal environment, as seen in Case 1 [2]. Another report has described an infant in whom central hypothyroidism developed after neonatal thyrotoxicosis persisted for only a few days after birth [6]. The condition is thought to be due to passive transfer of maternal thyroxine from a mother with hyperthyroidism. The fetal thyroid responds to TSH or TRAb from 20 weeks gestation, and undetectable TSH in the fetal cord serum in the presence of markedly elevated FT4 suggests pituitary negative feedback at as early as 20 weeks gestation [7]. The major negative feedback effect of thyroid hormone on TSH secretion is mediated by serum FT4 that is monodeiodinated to T3 by type II deiodinase in the hypothalamus and pituitary thyrotroph cells [8]. There is a continuous significant decrease in the TSH/FT4 ratio from the midgestation fetus to young adults [9], and passively transferred FT4 is thought to affect secretion of TSH to the largest extent in the midgestation fetus. However, the time in pregnancy when maternal thyrotoxicosis might lead to development of central hypothyroidism in offspring is unknown. In Case 3, a full-term normal birth weight infant was born to a mother who had euthyroid function at the time of delivery, and in Case 2 maternal thyroid function was improving at the time of delivery after antithyroid drug therapy had been introduced in week 31 of gestation. Hence, the most unusual maternal thyroid hormone concentration in each of the three cases was concluded to be before 32 weeks of gestation, at the time when passage of thyroid hormones from a mother with hyperthyroidism to the fetus is likely to occur. Three other cases of central hypothyroidism have been reported in term or near-term infants born to mothers who were non-compliant with medication or in whom Graves' disease was undiagnosed during pregnancy [10]

Immunoglobulins move transplacentally, mainly during the late-gestational period. TRAb and TSAb were both positive but were not high enough to provoke neonatal hyperthyroidism in the cord blood in Cases 1-3 (Table 1). Therefore, it is likely that thyroxine, and not autoantibodies transferred from the mother, affected the maturation of the fetal hypothalamic-pituitary-thyroid system. One case has been reported of a premature infant showing central hypothyroidism after 3 months of neonatal Graves' disease due to TRAb transferred from a mother with Graves' disease [11], and a second report described seven premature infants with congenital thyrotoxicosis who developed hypothyroidism and required T4 treatment from day 64 [12]. A review of the available case reports (Table 4) indicates that central hypothyroidism may develop in three different ways: by way of short-term (a few days) thyrotoxicosis due to passively transferred thyroxine; by way of long-term (more than 1 month) hyperthyroidism due to passively transferred TRAb; and directly after birth. High levels of thyroid hormones produced by fetal thyroids due to maternal TRAb transfer may also impair the fetal hypothalamic-pituitary-thyroid system.

The gestation periods of the 3 infants with neonatal Graves' disease whose mothers had hyperthyroidism were 27, 29 and 29 weeks, respectively, and the TRAb and TSAb levels in these infants were high. After stopping antithyroid medication at 63, 128 and 39 days after birth, respectively, the infants showed neither hypothyroidism nor hyperthyroidism. Therefore, if hypothesis that hyperthyroidism with FT4 more than 3 ng/dl is related to development of central hypothyroidism would be true and if the duration of hyperthyroidism would not be taken into account maternal hyperthyroidism after 28 weeks gestation might not be related to development of central hypothyroidism in offspring.

In Graves' disease after 20 weeks gestation, the objective is disease control in the mother and the fetus. Prevention of congenital Graves' disease, such as that in Case 4, requires protection of the fetal thyroid from stimulation by maternal TRAb transfer, and antithyroid drugs should be adjusted based not only on maternal thyroid function but also on the fetal thyroid function. Here is a need to evaluate the fetal thyroid function, for example, by echo monitoring of the thyroid gland [13]. We once experienced a case of congenital Graves' disease in an infant born to a euthyroid mother who had been treated with subtotal thyroidectomy and had highly stimulative receptor antibodies (TRAb=69%, TSAb=3,263%) [14], and it is now apparent that we should have treated the mother with both antithyroid drugs and l-thyroxine. Both mothers of two infants with congenital Graves' disease who we have experienced so far had highly stimulative receptor antibodies.

The cases shown in Table 3 suggest that maternal thyrotoxicosis before 32 weeks gestation may be critical for development of central hypothyroidism in offspring, except for the last case [10] in Table 4 in which diagnosis was not confirmed in a TRH test. Furthermore, Case 3 indicates that the possibility of central hypothyroidism cannot be excluded in cases where term infants born to euthyroid mothers with Graves' disease are exposed to maternal thyrotoxicosis before 32 weeks gestation. We also note one report of a very low birth weight infant who started l-thyroxine treatment at 1 year of age and showed developmental delay, suggesting that both fetal exposure to high thyroxine levels and infantile hypothyroidism may be causes of developmental delay [15]. Therefore, thyroxine supplementation during a period of central hypothyroidism is of importance. However, TSH-based neonatal screening cannot detect congenital central hypothyroidism, as shown in Case 2. T4-based screening may be useful for detecting central hypothyroidism, but the preferential strategy to prevent maternal Graves' disease-associated hypothyroidism is control of thyroid function throughout pregnancy [16].

Conclusion

Maternal hyperthyroidism before 32 weeks gestation may be related to development of transient central hypothyroidism in offspring.

Table 4. Summary of case reports of central hypothyroidism related to maternal thyrotoxicosis

Ga *Wks*	Bw *G*	Maternal Graves' Disease *Onset, Control At Delivery*	Thyrotoxicosis *Duration*	Trab (Tsab)	Hypothyroidism *Onset, Recovery*	Ref.
27	1152	Pre-Gestation, Poor	2 Days	16%	12 Days, 6 M	Case 1
30	1620	Pre-Gestation, Poor	2 Days	88.7%	16 Days, 15 M	6
31	1474	Pre-Gestation, Poor	3 M	(2438%)	7 M, >18 M	11
33	2016	23 Wks Gestation, Partial	-	45.2%	0 Day, 24 M	15
34	2455	Pre-Gestation, Partial	-	42.7%	4 Days, 13 M	Case 2
36	3250	Pre-Gestation, Partial	-	ND	4 Days, >4 M	10
37	3244	31 Wks Gestation, Good	-	20.3%	2 Days, 20 M	Case 3
38	2735	Pre-Gestation, Poor	-	Negative	4 Days, >3 M	10
38	3490	Around Delivery, Poor	-	Negative	7 Days,	10

GA, gestational age; BW, birth weight; ND, not determined.

References

[1] Higuchi R, Miyawaki M, Kumagai T, Okutani T, Shima Y, Yoshiyama M, Ban H, and Yoshikawa N. Central hypothyroidism in infants who were born to mothers with thyrotoxicosis before 32 weeks' gestation. *Pediatrics* 2005;115:e623-e625.

[2] Higuchi R, Kumagai T, Kobayashi M, Minami T, Koyama H, and Ishii Y. Short-term hyperthyroidism followed by transient pituitary hypothyroidism in a very low birth weight infant born to a mother with uncontrolled Graves' disease. *Pediatrics* 2001;107:e57.

[3] Adams LM, Emery JR, Clark SJ, Carlton EI, and Nelson JC. Reference ranges for newer thyroid function Tests in premature infants. *J. Pediatr.* 1995; 126:122-127.

[4] Matsuura N, Konishi J, Fujieda K, Kasagi K, Iida Y, Hagisawa M, Fujimoto S, Fukushi M, and Takasugi N. TSH receptor antibodies in mothers with Graves' disease and outcome in their offspring. *Lancet* 1988;1:14-17.

[5] Matsuura N, Harada S, Ohyama Y, Shibayama K, Fukushi M, Ishikawa N, Yuri K, Nakanishi M, Yokota Y, Kazahara K, and Oguchi H. The mechanism of transient hypothyroidism in infants born to mothers with Graves' disease. *Pediatric Res.* 1997;42:214-218.

[6] Hashimoto H, Maruyama M, Koshida R, Okuda N, and Sato T. Central hypothyroidism resulting from pituitary suppression and peripheral thyrotoxicosis in a premature infant born to a mother with Graves' disease. *J. Pediatr.* 1995;127:809-811.

[7] Rakover Y, Weiner E, Mosh N, Shalev E. Fetal pituitary negative feedback at early gestational age. *Clin. Endocrinol.* 1999;50:809-814.

[8] Larsen PR, Dick ET, Markovitz BP, Kaplan MM, and Gard TG. Inhibition of intrapituitary thyroxine to 3,5,3' triiodethyronine conversion prevents acute suppression of thyrotropin release by thyroxine in hypothyroid rats. *J. Clin. Invest.* 1979;64:117-128.

[9] Fisher DA, Nelson JC, Carlton EI, Wilcox RB. Maturation of human hypothalamic-pituitary-thyroid function and control. *Thyroid* 2000;10:229-234

[10] Lee YS, Loke KY, Ng SCY, Joseph R. HJ. Maternal thyrotoxicosis causing central hypothyroidism in infants. *Paediatr. Child Health* 2002;38:206-208.

[11] Aida T, Egashira M, Itou M, et al. A case of central hypothyroidism following transient neonatal hyperthyroidism. *Jap. J. Pediatr.* 2002;106:1020-1024.

[12] Smith C, Thomsett M, Choong C, et al. Congenital thyrotoxicosis in premature infants. *Clin. Endocrinol.* 2001;54:371-376.

[13] Luton D, Le Gac I, Vuillard E, Castanet M, Guibourdenche J, Noel M, Toubert ME, Leger J, Boissinot C, Schlageter MH, Garel C, Tebeka B, Oury JF, Czernichow P. and Polak M. Management of Graves' disease during pregnancy: The key role of fetal thyroid gland monitoring. *J. Clin. Endcrinol. Metab.* 2005;90:6093-6098.

[14] Ohmori H, Higuchi R, Hiraishi E, Hiraishi S, Kobayashi S, and Kashii K. A case of neonatal hyperthyroidism with fetal cardiac failure. *J. Jpn. Society Neo.* 1988; 23(1): 298-293.

[15] Nishizawa K, Hosaka A, and Yamashiro Y. A case of transient pituitary hypothyroidism secondary to poorly controlled maternal Graves' disease. *Jpn. J. Pre neo. Med.* 2004;16:23-28

[16] Kempers MJ, van Tijin DA, van Trotsenburg AS, de Vijlder JJ, Wiedijk BM, Vulsma T. Central congenital hypothyroidism due to gestational hyperthyroidism: detection where prevention failed. *J. Clin. Endocrinol. Metab.* 2003;88:5851-5857.

In: Thyroid Hormones: Functions, Related Diseases and Uses ISBN: 978-1-60741-080-5
Editors: F. S. Kuehn, M. P. Lozada

Chapter IX

Thyroid Hormone and Neuro-Astrocyte Interactions

Andréa Gonçalves Trentin*
Dept. Biologia Celular, Embriologia e Genética,
Centro de Ciências Biológicas, Universidade Federal de Santa Catarina,
Campus Universitário, 88040-900, Trindade, Florianópolis, S.C., Brazil

Abstract

The role of thyroid hormone (T3) in astrocyte morphogenesis is clearly demonstrated. T3 regulates several aspects of astrocyte differentiation and maturation, including the production of cytoskeleton, extracellular matrix (ECM) molecules and growth factors. T3 induces astrocytes to secrete a combination of growth factors including fibroblast growth factor-2 (FGF2) and epidermal growth factor (EGF) that act autocrinally influencing different aspects of astrocyte and neuronal differentiation and function. In addition, T3 alters the expression and organization of the glial fibrillary acidic protein (GFAP) and the ECM proteins laminin and fibronectin, and regulates the expression of the proteoglycans syndecans, thus producing a high-quality substrate for neuronal differentiation. In fact, T3-treated astrocytes promote neural growth and neuritogenesis. Indeed, and indirect mechanism of thyroid hormone on neuronal development mediated by astrocytes has been proposed. Moreover, an important and additional role of T3 in regulating glutamate uptake by cerebellar astrocytes was recently demonstrated. This effect is promoted by the up regulation of astrocytic glutamate transporters GLAST and GLT-1 that result in glial and neuronal protection against glutamate toxicity. Therefore, T3 is involved in the control of most facets of functional neural networks, a large amount of them mediated by the improvement of astrocytic microenvironment.

Keywords: glial cell, T3, neuronal development, neuronal differentiation

* Phone: 55 48 3721 6905 ; Fax: 55 48 3721 5148 ; e-mail: atrentin@ccb.ufsc.br.

Introduction

Astrocytes correspond to a heterogeneous class of cells that have many different roles and make up 20 to 50% of the volume of most brain areas. Differentiated astrocytes are classically recognized by the expression of the glial fibrillary acidic protein (GFAP) Astrocyte functions include the regulation of neuronal metabolism and activity, glucose supply, extracellular ion concentrations, cerebral blood flow, and neurotransmitter levels, in addition to the secretion of neuroactive substances and the production of most of the extracellular matrix components in the central nervous system (CNS). Astrocytes express voltage-gated ion channels and neurotransmitter receptors that are co-activated at synapses and then participate in removing potentially toxic excitatory amino acids from synapses by high-affinity transporters thus participating in the regulation of synapse formation and synaptic transmission. During development, astrocytes are responsible for modulating neuronal differentiation and guiding neuronal migration and axon growth. In addition, it has been proposed that astrocytes retain stem cell characteristics (for review see Fields and Stevens-Graham, 2002; Trentin, 2006).

Thyroid Hormone and Astrocyte Morphogenesis

Thyroid hormone is essential for normal brain development (Santisteban and Bernal, 2005; Bernal, 2005a). The absence of thyroid hormone during the critical period of neurogenesis leads to multiple irreversible morphological abnormalities due mainly to defects in neuronal migration and nerve process outgrowth. Clinical observations describe the cerebral consequences of congenital hypothyroidism: cretinism. Neurological cretinism in its fully developed form is characterized by profound mental retardation, deaf-mutism, and spastic diplegia (Konig and Moura Neto, 2002; Trentin, 2006).

Despite the well known direct influence of thyroid hormone on neurons, a number of studies have demonstrated that thyroid hormone promotes astrocyte differentiation and maturation. Astrocytes express thyroid hormone receptors α and β subtypes suggesting that astrocytes are direct target cells of thyroid hormones. *In-vivo*, neonatal hypothyroidism results in an increased number of astrocytes and Bergmann glia in the rat cerebellum and *in-vitro*, thyroid hormone affects astrocyte morphology, GFAP organization, glutamine synthetase activity and expression and regulates the protein phosphorylation and glucose transport. In astrocytes, thyroid hormone is also involved in the regulation of extracellular matrix organization, growth factor secretion, and cell proliferation. Thyroid hormone regulates K+ buffering of the developing brain by regulating astrocyte NaKATPase expression (for review see Trentin, 2006). Thyroid hormone also controls the transition from radial glia to mature astrocytes, and from vimentin-positive to GFAP-positive cells in the basal forebrain and hippocampus (Gould *et al.,* 1990; Martinez-Galan *et al.,* 1997) and in cerebellar astrocytes (Manzano *et al.*, 2007), demonstrating the influence of thyroid hormone in astrocyte maturation.

Thyroid Hormone Influences the Astrocytic Production of Growth Factors and Extracellular Matrix (ECM) Components

We have previously demonstrated that thyroid hormone induces morphological alterations in astrocytes from cerebral hemispheres and mesencephalon of newborn rats. These cells underwent progressive transformation from flat polygonal cell to a process-bearing form, accompanied by re-organization of GFAP filaments and protein synthesis (Trentin et al.. 1995; Trentin and Moura Neto, 1995; Lima et al., 1997) and mediated by the synthesis and secretion of growth factors (Trentin et al., 2001). A similar effect of thyroid hormone on astrocyte morphology was reported by others (Gavaret et al., 1991; Paul et al., 1996; Aizenman and de Vellis, 1987) and suggested involving the activation of protein kinase A and ERK signaling pathway (Ghosh et al., 2005) in addition to the β-adrenergic receptor system (Ghosh and Das, 2007).

On the other hand, cerebellar astrocytes from newborn animals do not undergo morphological differentiation in response to T3 treatment, but proliferate instead (Trentin et al., 1995). This effect is also mediated by the autocrine secretion of a combination of growth factors, among which are fibroblast growth factor types 1 and 2 (FGF1 and FGF1, respectively), tumor necrosis factor-β (TNFβ) and interleukin-3 (IL-3), that autocrinally promote cell proliferation. FGF2 seems to be the principal one (Trentin et al., 2001). Moreover, epidermal growth factor (EGF) is also secreted by cerebellar astrocytes after T3 stimulation (Gomes et al., 1999; Martinez and Gomes, 2002).

The FGF2 secreted by cerebellar astrocytes after thyroid hormone stimulation, in addition to the proliferative effect, affects the extracellular matrix composition. T3 treatment stimulates the production of both laminin and fibronectin by astrocytes and promotes alterations in their organization from a puntate to a fibrillar pattern (Trentin et al., 2003). Furthermore, the EGF secreted by cerebellar astrocytes after T3 stimulation, autocrinally regulates the extracellular matrix production in these cells through MAPK/phosphatidylinositol 3-kinase pathways (Martinez and Gomes, 2002; Martinez and Gomes, 2005; Trentin, 2006).

Recently, we have investigated the expression of the proteglycans syndecans in cultures of T3-treated cerebellar astrocytes from newborn rats. Our results demonstrated reduced expression of syndecans 2 and 3 in T3-treated cerebellar astrocytes, when compared to control cultures (Mendes de Aguiar et al., 2008a). This balance of proteoglycans may be involved in T3 action mediated by FGF2 signaling, possibly affecting the formation of the trimeric signaling receptor complex composed by syndecan/FGF/FGF-receptor (FGFR), which is essential for FGFR dimerization, activation, and subsequent cell signaling (Ornitz, 2000; Turnbull et al., 2001).

Neuro-Astrocytes Interaction and Thyroid Hormone Metabolism in the Brain

Astrocytes exert a central role in the transport of thyroid hormone in brain and its conversion to the biological active form. In the brain, more than 80% of 3,5,3'-

triiodothyronine (T3) is produced by local conversion of thyroxine (T4) (Courtin *et al.,* 1986; Crantz *et al.,* 1982) in a reaction catalized by the selenoprotein type II iodothyronine 5'-deiodinase (D2) (Courtin *et al.,* 1988; Leonard, 1988; Pallud *et al.,* 1997) expressed in astrocytes through the brain and in tanycytes in the mediobasal hypothalamus (Guadano-Ferraz *et al.,* 1997; Bernal, 1999; Guadano-Ferraz *et al.,* 1999; Bernal, 2005b). In addition, the transport of T4 from the blood to the CNS has recently been suggested to be performed by the organic anion-transport polypeptide Oatp14 that is predominantly expressed in the brain, especially in the brain capillaries and choroid plexus (Sugiyama *et al.,* 2003). Furthermore, the monocarboxylate anion transporter (MCT8) was functionally characterized as a very active and specific thyroid hormone transporter (Friesema *et al.,* 2003). MCT8 was observed to be highly expressed in choroid plexus and olfactory bulb, cerebral cortex, hippocampus and amygdala. Since, MCT8 was found to be predominant in neurons, it was suggested that it plays a decisive role in the transport of T3 into them (Heuer *et al.,* 2005). Therefore, a general mechanism concerning thyroid hormone transport and distribution in the brain has been proposed in which T4 is captured by astrocytes and tanycyte from the blood-brain or blood-cerebrospinal fluid (CSF) barriers by the Oatp transporter. In these cells, T4 is converted into T3 that enters into neurons through MCT8. Neurons express type III deiodinase (D3) that degrades T3 to its inactive metabolite diiodothyronine (T2). This model suggests that neuro-astrocyte interaction exerts a central role in T3 homeostasis (Bernal, 2005; Santisteban and Bernal, 2005; Heuer *et al.*, 2005).

Non-genomic actions of thyroid hormone have been implicated in the regulation of thyroid hormone metabolism in the brain. These actions result in "acute" or "rapid onset" effects when compared to genomic mechanisms that require gene transcription and consequently translation of mRNA (for reviews see Davis *et al.*, 2008 and Leonard, 2008). Recently, a cell surface receptor for thyroid hormone has been described on the plasma membrane of virtually all cells and characterized as the integrin □V□3 (Berg *et al.*, 2005; Davis *et al.*, 2005). The thyroid hormone domain is at or near the Arg-Gly-Asp (RGD) binding site of the integrin. T4, and in a less stent T3, acting via this integrin receptor can activate the mitogen-activated protein kinase (MAPK, ERK1/2) signal transduction cascade (Berg *et al.*, 2005; Cody *et al.*, 2007). Thyroid hormone through the non-genomic mechanisms, have been implicated in the dynamic regulation of the number and quantity of actin fibers in astrocytes. T4 and its transcriptionally inactive metabolite 3',5',3 triiodothyronine (reverse T3) are responsible for modulating microfilament organization while T3 is inert (Leonard, 2008). In astrocytes the actin cytoskeleton is involved in laminin deposition and organization and consequently in astrocyte adhesion (Farwell *et al.*, 1999; Farwell *et al.*, 1995). Similar mechanisms are involved in the organization of actin cytoskeleton in granule neurons thus modulating granule cells migration on laminin substrate and neurite outgrowth (Farwell *et al.*, 2005). The biological consequence of the loss of the actin filaments is the inability of the cell to anchor laminin to its cell surface, and the loss of this key guidance molecule can interrupts neurite pathfinding and neuronal migration.

Thyroid Hormone Promotes Neuronal Development Mediated By Astrocytes

During brain development, thyroid hormone exerts significant influence on neuronal development. It has been implicated in the survival, proliferation, migration, and also arborization and expression of specific phenotypic markers of neurons (Heisenberg *et al.*, 1992; Muller *et al.*, 1995; Gomes *et al.*, 2001; Konig and Moura Neto, 2002). Thyroid hormone is directly involved in the development of granule neurons by affecting the survival and differentiation of these cells (Heisenberg *et al.*, 1992) in addition to preventing their apoptosis (Muller *et al.*, 1995). A recent study demonstrated that an acute administration of T_3 (at concentrations of 10, 50 or 100 μM) protects hippocampal neurons from glutamate toxicity through a rapid nongenomic regulation (Losi *et al.*, 2008). Besides this direct effect of thyroid hormone on granular neuron development, an indirect mechanism mediated by astrocytes has been proposed (Gomes *et al.*, 1999; Martinez and Gomes, 2002; Trentin *et al.*, 2003).

Consistent with this model, we verified that cerebellar neurons co-cultured on T3-treated astrocytes are more numerous and display longer neurites than those cultivated on control cells. This effect is related to the altered expression of extracellular matrix proteins induced by thyroid hormone and mediated by FGF2 that stimulates, in astrocytes, the production and re-organization of laminin and fibronectin from a punctuate to a fibrillar pattern (Trentin *et al.*, 2003). In fact, laminin and fibronectin organized in a fibrillar pattern have been demonstrated to promote neurite outgrowth (Garcia-Abreu *et al.*, 1995). Moreover, the EGF secreted after T3 stimulation has also been demonstrated to indirectly promote neurite outgrowth by the regulation of astrocyte extracellular matrix production involving MAPK/phosphatidylinositol 3-kinase pathways (Martinez and Gomes, 2002). In addition, thyroid hormone is involved in the astrocytic-production of syndecans that could also be implicated in neuronal migration, differentiation and maturation (Mendes de Aguiar *et al.*, 2008a).

Therefore, an indirect effect of the thyroid hormone on granular neuronal development mediated by astrocytes was proposed in which T3 induces the astrocyte secretion of growth factors, such as FGF2 and EGF, that autocrinally affects several astrocytic characteristics such as morphology, proliferation, adhesion and extracellular matrix production and organization, and thus influences neuronal development (Figure 1). These growth factors may directly influence neuronal growth and neuritogenesis by themselves (Trentin, 2006).

Thyroid Hormone Promotes Neuroprotection Mediated by Astrocytic-Glutamate Uptake

Glutamate is the main excitatory neurotransmitter in the mammalian CNS, but excessive activation of glutamate receptors can cause excitotoxicity (Meldrum, 2000; Danbolt, 2001). The removal of L-glutamate from the extracellular compartment occurs mainly through the activity of two high-affinity, sodium dependent astroglial glutamate transporters GLT-1 and GLAST (Rothstein *et al.*, 1996) that maintain low extracellular concentrations of glutamate, thereby protecting neurons against excitotoxicity *in-vivo* and modulating glutamate transmission (Rothstein *et al.*, 1996; Tanaka *et al.*, 1997; Watase *et al.*, 1998).

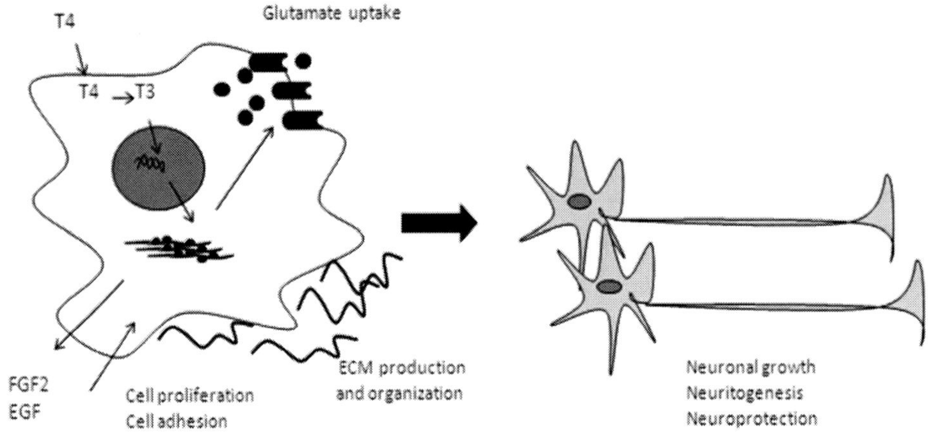

Figure 1. Model for thyroid hormone effect on neuronal development mediated by astrocytes. Thyroid hormone induces cerebellar astrocyte secretion of growth factors, such as FGF2 and EGF, that autocrinally promote astrocyte proliferation, adhesion, and extracellular matrix (ECM) production and organization. The T3 action on astrocyte metabolism indirectly influences neuronal growth and development (Trentin *et al.*, 2003; Martinez and Gomes, 2002; Trentin, 2006; Mendes de Aguiar *et al.*, 2008a). The growth factors secreted by astrocyte may also induce neuronal growth via the paracrine pathway. In addition, thyroid hormone increases the synthesis of the glutamate transporters GLAST and GLT-1 in cerebellar astrocytes, resulting in enhanced glutamate uptake by these cells and consequently promoting neuroprotection (Mendes de Aguiar *et al.*, 2008b).

This transport is also necessary for providing intracellular glutamate which supports essential metabolic pathways such as energy production and synthesis of glutathione, a tripeptide with crucial antioxidant functions in CNS (Danbolt, 2001; Re *et al.*, 2003). There are increasing evidences that the perturbation of glutamatergic transmission by a decrease/loss of glutamate transporters activity/expression can be regarded as a major cause for a number of neurological disorders being crucial for distinct neurodegenerative diseases (Danbolt, 2001). Although neuron degeneration and death are the ultimate consequences of the pathological process, it is now widely accepted that alterations in the function of surrounding glial cells are key features in the progression of these disorders. Recently, we demonstrated an additional role of thyroid hormone regulating glutamate uptake by cerebellar astrocytes. We showed that this effect is mediated through up-regulation of the astrocytic glutamate transporters GLAST and GLT-1 at both mRNA and protein levels. T3 treatment prevents the gliotoxic effect of glutamate in cultured astrocytes. In addition, increased neuronal viability against glutamate toxicity was observed when neurons were co-cultured on T3-treated astrocytes showing a protective effect (Mendes de Aguiar *et al.*, 2008b).

Stimulation of astrocytes with L-glutamate results in cell swelling triggered by oxidative stress which causes cellular damage to astrocytes (Chen *et al.*, 2000). Astrocyte death may also occur via an oxidative toxicity linked to depletion of a compartmentalized intracellular pool of glutamate specifically fed by glutamate uptake, essential for maintaining astrocytic glutathione levels and modulation of glutamate transporters activity is a key factor to astrocytic as well as neuronal survival (Re *et al.,* 2006). In addition, hypothyroidism was found to be associated with a marked oxidative stress related with an aberrant accumulation of neurofilament in hypothyroid neurons and to a decline in the activity of glutamate cysteine ligase, the rate limiting enzyme for the biosynthesis of glutathione (Rahaman *et al.*, 2001). Dasgupta and co-workers (2007) have demonstrated that the treatment of astrocytes with thyroid hormones increases the biosynthesis of glutathione by up-regulating glutamate cysteine ligase. In a recent paper, Lamirand and co-workers (2008) showed that the oxidative stress elicited by addition of H2O2 up regulates D3 and inhibits D2 by transcriptional mechanisms in cultured astrocytes. The oxidative stress might increases thyroid hormone degradation and inhibits the stimulated activation of T4 into T3 in astrocytes. This possibly results in decreased levels of T3 to surrounding neurons contributing to cellular injury of oxidative stress in brain. Therefore, the astrocytic protection against glutamate challenge induced by T_3 observed in our results (Mendes de Aguiar *et al.*, 2008b) could be related to an improved glutamate and cysteine uptake, or up regulation of glutathione synthesis, or both, thus increasing the antioxidant defenses in astrocytes.

Growth factors are involved in the regulation of the expression of glutamate transporters in astrocytes. EGF has been shown to induce GLT-1 expression in immature astrocytes through phosphatidylinositol 3-kinase and transcription factor NF-□B pathways (Zelenaia *et al.*, 2000). EGF, FGF and IGF enhance glutamate transport activity and the expression of GLAST mRNA and protein in neonatal rat astrocytes in culture (Suzuki *et al.,* 2001). Since, T_3 induces cerebellar astrocytes to secrete a combination of growth factors, including FGF_2 (Trentin *et al.,* 2001) and EGF (Gomes *et al.*, 1999) that act autocrinally, influencing different aspects of astrocyte and neuronal differentiation and function (Trentin, 2006), it is therefore possible that the T_3 effect in the regulation of GLAST and GLT-1 expression in cerebellar astrocytes could be an indirect effect of this hormone mediated by the secretion of these growth factors. Because the regulation of the extracellular glutamate levels represents an important mechanism in neuronal survival, we propose a new role for T_3 in neuroprotection mediated by astrocytes (Mendes de Aguiar *et al.*, 2008b).

Conclusion

Astrocytes can be considered as important mediators of the thyroid hormone actions in brain. Astrocytes regulate the transport of thyroid hormone from the blood to the CNS and its conversion into the active form and transport to neurons. Astrocyte differentiation and maturation are influenced by thyroid hormone in different aspects: morphological and biochemical alterations, proliferation, adhesion, extracellular matrix and cytoskeleton production and organization in addition to the upper regulation of astrocytic glutamate transporters. Most of these effects are mediated by autocrine secretion of growth factors such as FGF2 and EGF. However, non-genomic mechanisms of thyroid hormone are also involved. Therefore, thyroid hormone improves the astrocytic microenvironment in order to promote neuronal development and protection (Figure 1).

Acknowledgments

This work was supported by the, Coordenação de Aperfeiçoamento de Pessoal de Nivel Superior (CAPES/Brazil) Conselho Nacional de Desenvolvimento Científico e Tecnológico (CNPq/Brazil), Ministério da Ciência e Tecnologia (MCT/Brazil), PRONEX/CNPq and Fundação de Amparo à Pesquisa do Estado de Santa Catarina (FAPESC/Brazil). The author declares that there is no conflict of interest that would prejudice the impartiality of this scientific work.

References

Aizenman, Y. and de Vellis J. (1987). Synergistic Action of Thyroid-Hormone, Insulin and Hydrocortisone on Astrocyte Differentiation. *Brain Research, 414*, 301-308.

Bernal. J. (1999). Iodine and brain development. *Biofactors, 10*, 271-276.

Bernal, J. (2005a). Thyroid hormones and brain development. *Vitamins and Hormones, 71*, 95–122.

Bernal, J. (2005b). The significance of thyroid hormone transporters in the brain. *Endocrinology, 146*, 1698-1700.

Bergh, J. J., Lin, H. Y., Lansing, L., Mohamed, S. N., Davis, F. B., Mousa, S. and Davis, P. J. (2005). Integrin avb3 contains a cell surface receptor site for thyroid hormone that is linked to activation of mitogen-activated protein kinase and induction of angiogenesis. *Endocrinology, 146*, 2864–2871.

Chen, C. J., Liao, S.L., Kuo, J. S. (2000). Gliotoxic action of glutamate on cultured astrocytes. *Journal of Neurochemistry, 75*, 1557-1565.

Courtin F, Chantoux F and Francon J 1986 Thyroid-Hormone Metabolism by Glial-Cells in Primary Culture. *Molecular and Cellular Endocrinology* 48 167-178.

Courtin, F., Chantoux, F., Pierre, M. and Francon, J. (1988). Induction of Type-II 5'-Deiodinase Activity by Cyclic Adenosine 3', 5'-Monophosphate in Cultured Rat Astroglial Cells. *Endocrinology, 123*, 1577-1581.

Cody, V., Davis, P. J. and Davis, F. B. (2007). Molecular modeling of the thyroid hormone interactions with avb3 integrin. *Steroids, 72*, 165–170.

Crantz, F. R., Silva, J.E. and Larsen, P.R. (1982). An Analysis of the Sources and Quantity of 3,5,3'-Triiodothyronine Specifically Bound to Nuclear Receptors in Rat Cerebral-Cortex and Cerebellum. *Endocrinology, 110,* 367-375.

Danbolt, N.C. (2001). Glutamate uptake. *Progress in Neurobiology 65*, 1–105.

Dasgupta, A., Das, S. and Sarkar, P. K. (2007). Thyroid hormone promotes glutathione synthesis in astrocytes by up regulation of glutamate cystetine ligase through differential stimulation of its catalytic and modulator subunit mRNAs. *Free Radical Biology and Medicine, 42*, 617-626.

Davis, P.J., Leonard, J.L. and Davis, F.B. (2008). Mechanisms of nongenomic actions of thyroid hormone. *Frontiers in Neuroendocrinology, 29*, 211-218.

Davis, P. J., Davis, F. B. and Cody, V. (2005). Membrane receptors mediating thyroid hormone action. *Trends in Endocrinology and Metabolism, 16*, 429–435.

Farwell, A. P., Dubord-Tomasetti, S. A., Pietrzykowski, A.Z., Stachelek, S.J. and Leonard, J.L. (2005). Regulation of cerebellar neuronal migration and neurite outgrowth by thyroxine and 3,3_,5_-triiodothyronine. *Brain Research Devolmental Brain Research, 154*, 121–135.

Farwell, A.P., Tranter, M.P. and Leonard, J.L. (1995). Thyroxine-Dependent Regulation of Integrin-Laminin Interactions in Astrocytes. *Endocrinology, 136*, 3909-3915.

Fields, R.D. and Stevens-Graham, B. (2002). Neuroscience - New insights into neuron-glia communication. *Science, 298*, 556-562.

Friesema ECH, Ganguly S, Abdalla A, Fox JEM, Halestrap AP and Visser TJ 2003 Identification of monocarboxylate transporter 8 as a specific thyroid hormone transporter.

Garcia-Abreu, J., Cavalcante, L.A. and Moura Neto, V. (1995) Differential Patterns of Laminin Expression in Lateral and Medial Midbrain Glia. *Neuroreport, 6*, 761-764.

Gavaret, J.M., Toru-Delbauffe, D., Baghdassarian-Chalaye, D., Pomerance, M. and Pierre, M. (1991). Thyroid-Hormone Action - Induction of Morphological-Changes and Protein Secretion in Astroglial Cell-Cultures. *Developmental Brain Research, 58*, 43-49.

Ghosh, M. and Das, S. (2007). Increased beta(2)-adrenergic receptor activity by thyroid hormone possibly leads to differentiation and maturation of astrocytes in culture. *Cellular and Molecular Neurobiology. 27*, 1007-1021.

Ghosh, M., Gharami, K., Paul, S. and Das, S. (2005). Thyroid hormone-induced morphological differentiation and maturation of astrocytes involves activation of protein kinase A and ERK signalling pathway. *The European Journal of Neuroscience. 22*, 1609-1617.

Gomes, F.C., Lima, F.R., Trentin, A.G. and Moura Neto, V. (2001). Thyroid hormone role in nervous system morphogenesis. *Progress in Brain Research, 132*, 41-50.

Gomes, F.C.A., Maia, C.G., de Menezes, J.R.L. and Moura Neto, V. (1999). Cerebellar astrocytes treated by thyroid hormone modulate neuronal proliferation. *Glia, 25*, 247-255.

Gould , E., Frankfurt, M., Westlind-Danielsson, A. and McEwen, B. S. (1990). Developing Forebrain Astrocytes Are Sensitive to Thyroid-Hormone. *Glia, 3*, 283-292.

Guadano-Ferraz, A., Escamez, M. J., Rausell, E. and Bernal, J. (1999). Expression of type 2 iodothyronine deiodinase in hypothyroid rat brain indicates an important role of thyroid hormone in the development of specific primary sensory systems. *Journal of Neuroscience, 19*, 3430-3439.

Guadano-Ferraz, A., Obregon, M. J., St Germain, D. L. and Bernal, J. (1997). The type 2 iodothyronine deiodinase is expressed primarily in glial cells in the neonatal rat brain. *Proceedings of the National Academy of Sciences of the United States of America, 94*, 10391-10396.

Heisenberg, C. P., Thoenen, H. and Lindholm, D. (1992). Triiodothyronine Regulates Survival and Differentiation of Rat Cerebellar Granule Neurons. *Neuroreport, 3*, 685-688.

Heuer, H., Maier, M. K., Iden, S., Mittag, J., Friesema, E. C. H., Visser, T. J. and Bauer, K. (2005). The monocarboxylate transporter 8 linked to human psychomotor retardation is highly expressed in thyroid hormone-sensitive neuron populations. *Endocrinology, 146*, 1701-1706.

Konig, S. and Moura Neto, V. (2002). Thyroid hormone actions on neural cells. *Cellular and Molecular Neurobiology, 22*, 517-544.

Leonard, J.L. (1988). Dibutyryl Camp Induction of Type-II 5'-Deiodinase Activity in Rat-Brain Astrocytes in Culture. *Biochemical and Biophysical Research Communications, 151*, 1164-1172.

Leonard, J.L. (2008). Non-genomic actions of thyroid hormone in brain development. *Steroids, 73*,1008-1012.

Lima, F. R. S., Trentin, A. G., Rosenthal, D., Chagas, C. and Moura Neto, V. (1997). Thyroid hormone induces protein secretion and morphological changes in astroglial cells with an increase in expression of glial fibrillary acidic protein. *Journal of Endocrinology, 154*, 167-175.

Losi, G., Garzon, G. and Puia, G. (2008). Nongenomic regulation of glutamatergic neurotransmission in hippocampus by thyroid hormones. *Neuroscience, 2,***155-163**.

Manzano, J., Bernal, J. and Morte, B. (2007). Influence of thyroid hormones on maturation of rat cerebellar astrocytes. *International Journal of Developmental Neuroscience, 25,*171-179.

Martinez, R. and Gomes, F. C. A. (2002). Neuritogenesis induced by thyroid hormone-treated astrocytes is mediated by epidermal growth factor/mitogen-activated protein kinase-phosphatidylinositol 3-kinase pathways and involves modulation of extracellular matrix proteins. *Journal of Biological Chemistry, 277*, 49311-49318.

Martinez, R. and Gomes, F. C. A. (2005). Proliferation of cerebellar neurons induced by astrocytes treated with thyroid hormone is mediated by a cooperation between cell contact and soluble factors and involves the epidermal growth factor-protein kinase A pathway. *Journal of Neuroscience Research, 80*, 341-349.

Martinez-Galan, J. R., Pedraza, P., Santacana, M., Escobar del Rey, F., Morale de Escobar, G. and Ruiz-Marcos, A. (1997). Early effects of iodine deficiency on radial glial cells of the hippocampus of the rat fetus - A model of neurological cretinism. *Journal of Clinical Investigation, 99*, 2701-2709.

Meldrum, B. S. (2000). Glutamate as a neurotransmitter in the brain: review of physiology and pathology. *The Journal of Nutrition, 130*, 1007S-1015S.

Mendes-de-Aguiar, C. B., Costa-Silva, B., Alvarez-Silva, M., Tasca, C. I. and Trentin, A. G. (2008a). Thyroid Hormone Mediates Syndecan Expression in Rat Neonatal Cerebellum. *Cellular and Molecular Neurobiology, 28*, 795-801.

Mendes-de-Aguiar, C. B., Alchini, R., Decker, H., Alvarez-Silva, M., Tasca, C. I. and Trentin, A. G. (2008b). Thyroid hormone increases astrocytic glutamate uptake and protects astrocytes and neurons against glutamate toxicity. *Journal of Neuroscience Research*, DOI: 10.1002/jnr.21755.

Muller, Y., Rocchi, E., Lazaro, J. B. and Clos, J. (1995). Thyroid hormone promotes BCL-2 expression and prevents apoptosis of early differentiating cerebellar granule neurons. *International Journal of Developmental Neuroscience, 13*, 871-885.

Ornitz, D. M. (2000). FGFs, heparan sulfate and FGFRs: complex interactions essential for development. *Bioessays, 22*, 108–112.

Pallud, S., Lennon, A. M., Ramauge, M., Gavaret, J. M, Croteau, W., Pierre, M., Courtin, F, and St Germain, D. L. (1997). Expression of the type II iodothyronine deiodinase in cultured rat astrocytes is selenium-dependent. *Journal of Biological Chemistry, 272*, 18104-18110.

Paul. S., Das, S., Poddar, R. and Sarkar, P. K. (1996). Role of thyroid hormone in the morphological differentiation and maturation of astrocytes: temporal correlation with synthesis and organization of actin. *European Journal of Neuroscience 8*, 2361-2370.

Rahaman, S. O., Ghosh, S., Mohanakumar, K. P., Das, S. and Sarkar, P. K. (2001). Hypothyroidism in the developing rat brain is associated with marked oxidative stress and aberrant intraneuronal accumulation of neurofilaments. *Neuroscience Research, 40*, 273–279.

Re, D. B., Nafia, I., Melon, C., Shimamoto, K., Kerkerian-Le Goff, L. and Had-Aissouni, L. (2006). Glutamate leakage from a compartmentalized intracellular metabolic pool and activation of the lipoxygenase pathway mediate oxidative astrocyte death by reversed glutamate transport. *Glia, 54*, 47-57.

Re, D. B., Boucraut, J., Samuel, D., Birman, S., Kerkerian-Le Goff, L. and Had-Aissouni, L. (2003). Glutamate transport alteration triggers differentiation-state selective oxidative death of cultured astrocytes: a mechanism different from excitotoxicity depending on intracellular GSH contents. *Journal of Neurochemistry, 85*, 1159-1170.

Rothstein, J. D., Dykes-Hoberg, M., Pardo, C.A., Bristol, L.A., Jin, L., Kuncl, R. W., Kanai, Y., Hediger, M. A., Wang, Y., Schielke, J. P. and Welty, D.F. (1996). Knockout of glutamate transporters reveals a major role for astroglial transport in excitotoxicity and clearance of glutamate. Neuron 16(3):675-86.Santisteban P and Bernal J 2005 Thyroid development and effect on the nervous system. *Reviews in Endocrine and Metabolic Disorders, 6*, 217-228.

Sugiyama, D., Kusuhara, H., Taniguchi, H., Ishikawa, S., Nozaki, Y., Aburatani, H. and Sugiyama, Y. (2003). Functional characterization of rat brain-specific organic anion transporter (Oatp14) at the blood-brain barrier - High affinity transporter for thyroxine. *Journal of Biological Chemistry, 278*, 43489-43495.

Suzuki, K., Ikegaya, Y., Matsuura, S., Kanai, Y., Endou, H. and Matsuki, N. **(2001).** Transient upregulation of the glial glutamate transporter GLAST in response to fibroblast growth factor, insulin-like growth factor and epidermal growth factor in cultured astrocytes. *Journal of Cell Sci***ence, *114*, 3717-3725.**

Tanaka, K., Watase, K., Manabe, T., Yamada, K., Watanabe, M., Takahashi, K., Iwama, H., Nishikawa, T., Ichihara, N., Kikuchi. T., Okuyama, S., Kawashima, N., Hori, S., Takimoto, M. and Wada, K. **(1997).** Epilepsy and exacerbation of brain injury in mice lacking the glutamate transporter GLT-1. ***Science*, *276*,1699-1702.**

Trentin, A. G., Alvarez-Silva, M. and Moura Neto, V. (2001). Thyroid hormone induces cerebellar astrocytes and C6 glioma cells to secrete mitogenic growth factors. *American Journal of Physiology-Endocrinology and Metabolism, 281*, E1088-E1094.

Trentin, A. G., Mendes de Aguiar, C. B. N., Garcez, R. C. and Alvarez-Silva, M. (2003) Thyroid hormone modulates the extracellular matrix organization and expression in cerebellar astrocyte: Effects on astrocyte adhesion. *Glia,* 42, 359-369.

Trentin, A. G. and Moura Neto, V. (1995). T3 Affects Cerebellar Astrocyte Proliferation, GFAP and Fibronectin Organization. *Neuroreport, 6*, 293-296.

Trentin, A. G., Rosenthal, D. and Moura Neto, V. (1995). Thyroid-Hormone and Conditioned Medium Effects on Astroglial Cells from Hypothyroid and Normal Rat-Brain - Factor Secretion, Cell-Differentiation, and Proliferation. *Journal of Neuroscience Research, 41*, 409-417.

Trentin, A. G. (2006). Thyroid hormone and astrocyte morphogenesis. *Journal of Endocrinology, 189*,189-197.

Turnbull, J.,Powell, A. and Guimond, S. (2001). Heparan sulfate: decoding a dynamic multifunctional cell regulator. *Trends in Cell Biology, 11*,75–82.

Watase, K., Hashimoto, K., Kano, M., Yamada, K., Watanabe, M., Inoue, Y., Okuyama, S., Sakagawa, T., Ogawa, S., Kawashima, N., Hori, S., Takimoto, M., Wada, K. and Tanaka, K. (1998). Motor discoordination and increased susceptibility to cerebellar injury in GLAST mutant mice. *European Journal of Neuroscience, 10*, 976-988.

Zelenaia, O., Schlag, B. D., Gochenauer, G. E., Ganel, R., Song, W., Beesley, J. S., Grinspan, J. B., Rothstein, J. D. and Robinson, M. B. (2000). Epidermal growth factor receptor agonists increase expression of glutamate transporter GLT-1 in astrocytes through pathways dependent on phosphatidylinositol 3-kinase and transcription factor NF-kappaB. *Molecular Pharmacology, 57*, 667-678.

In: Thyroid Hormones: Functions, Related Diseases and Uses ISBN: 978-1-60741-080-5
Editors: F. S. Kuehn, M. P. Lozada

Chapter X

Amiodarone and Thyroid Dysfunction

***Sujoy Ghosh*[*,1] *and Andrew Collier*[2]**
[1]M.D., D.M. (Endocrinology), M.R.C.P. (U.K.), M.R.C.P.S (Glasgow)
Clinical Teaching and Clinical Research Fellow
The Ayr Hospital, Ayr KA6 6DX, Scotland, UK
[2]B.Sc (Hons), M.D, F.R.C.P (Edinburgh), F.R.C.P (Glasgow)
Honorary Senior Lecturer, Consultant Physician
The Ayr Hospital, Ayr KA6 6DX, Scotland, UK

Abstract

Amiodarone is a benzofuranic derivative, iodine-rich drug widely used for treatment of cardiac tachyarrhythmias. It often leads to transient changes in thyroid function tests, either due to the high iodine content of the drug or due to the direct toxic effect of the drug. The prevalence of amiodarone induced thyroid dysfunction depends on dietary iodine intake, age and sex of the patient and also presence of underlying thyroid disorder. Thyroid dysfunction occurs in about 15% of patients treated with amiodarone (Amiodarone induced hypothyroidism (AIH) or Amiodarone induced thyrotoxicosis (AIT)).

AIH is commoner in iodine sufficient areas and in patients with a background of Hashimoto's thyroiditis and is related to failure to escape from the acute Wolff Chaikoff effect. It may develop as early as 2 weeks or as late as 3 years following initiation of amiodarone therapy. Treatment of AIH consists of levothyroxine replacement, while continuing amiodarone therapy.

AIT is more complex and there are two varieties namely AIT type I and AIT type II. AIT type I is commoner in iodine deficient areas and typically occurs with underlying thyroid disease (due to Jod Basedow phenomenon). There is some benefit in stopping amiodarone in such a scenario and treating with thionamides with or without potassium perchlorate. AIT type II on the other hand is commoner in iodine sufficient areas and occurs due to the direct toxic effect of amiodarone on thyroid follicular cells. Withdrawal

* Corresponding Author: Address: Diabetes Day Centre, The Ayr Hospital, Dalmellington Road, Ayr, Post Code: KA6 6DX, Scotland, United Kingdom, Email: drsujoyghosh@rediffmail.com.

of amiodarone with or without glucorticoids is useful. Mixed forms are best treated with a combination of thionamides, potassium perchlorate and glucocorticoid. Thyroidectomy is contemplated in resistant cases. Radio-iodine is usually of little benefit due to low thyroidal radioiodine uptake.

Thyroid function tests should be performed at baseline prior to initiation of amiodarone therapy. Clinicians should also note presence of any goiter and document any history of autoimmune disorders. Thereafter thyroid function tests need to be repeated at 3-6 month interval initially and thereafter annually for at least a year following withdrawal of therapy. This is of utmost importance to detect amiodarone induced thyroid problems.

A significant proportion of patients on amiodarone are also on Warfarin and it is important to realize that amiodarone as well as thyroid dysfunction alters the pharmacokinetics of warfarin. Therefore adjustments of warfarin dosage have to be made accordingly.

A newer drug, namely dronedarone is currently under review. As dronedarone does not contain iodine it is hoped that it will have the same benefits but not the ill effects on thyroid function.

Keywords: Amiodarone, Thyroid function tests, Amiodarone induced hypothyroidism, Amiodarone induced thyrotoxicosis

Abbreviations

TFT: Thyroid Function Test
AIH: Amiodarone induced hypothyroidism
AIT: Amiodarone induced thyrotoxicosis

Quotation: "Our problems today have arisen with our solutions yesterday."

Introduction

Amiodarone is an anti-arrhythmic agent, used for various types of tachyarrhythmia's, both ventricular and supraventricular. It was initially developed in the early 1960's in Belgium and became popular in Europe as a treatment for angina pectoris. [1,2] It was later found to have anti-arrhythmic properties and belonged to a new class of anti-arrhythmic agents (Vaughan Williams Class III). Even today its mechanism of action is not clearly understood.[3]

During the 1970's and 1980's, amiodarone was increasingly used to treat patients with supraventricular and ventricular arrhythmias.[4] Despite being commonly prescribed throughout Europe amiodarone was not approved by the Food and Drug Administration (FDA) in the US until December 1985.[5] Amiodarone remains unusual for drugs approved by the FDA, as it was accepted without rigorous, randomised clinical trials.

Amiodarone has numerous reported side affects. Most individuals administered amiodarone on a long-term basis will experience at least one side effect. These side effects include lung, eye, gastrointestinal system and liver, skin and of course thyroid problems. The purpose of this chapter is to expand upon the different thyroid problems that can occur in people who take amiodarone long term.

Pharmacology of Amiodarone

Amiodarone is a class III anti-arrhythmic drug. In recent times it has been used extensively for the prophylaxis and the treatment of many cardiac rhythm disturbances, ranging from paroxysmal atrial fibrillation to life threatening ventricular tachyarrhythmias.[6] Probably because it seems to be safe in patients with significant left ventricular dysfunction and it has low pro-arrhythmic effects it is one of the most commonly used anti-arrhythmic drugs.[7,8]

Amiodarone is a benzofuranic derivative that bears a remarkable structural resemblance to thyroid hormones. [Figure 1] It also contains two iodine atoms and is almost 39% iodine by weight. When administered orally, the bioavailability of amiodarone is quite variable. Absorption ranges from 22 to 95%, with better absorption when it is given with food.[7] The average maintenance dose of amiodarone ranges from 200-600 mg and approximately 10% of the molecule is de-iodinated daily i.e. 3mg iodine released for every 100mg. This implies that approximately 7-21 mgs iodide is released daily. The normal and healthy daily intake of iodine is considered to be 150-200 mcg. [9,10] .Therefore patients on a maintenance dose of amiodarone have a marked increase in the daily iodine intake resulting in increased levels in plasma and urinary iodide levels, often as high as a 40 fold increase.[11]

Amiodarone is very lipophilic and is concentrated in the adipose tissue, liver, lung and to lesser extent the heart, kidney and brain.[12] Amiodarone is metabolized through different pathways, the most important of which is dealkylation, which leads to the formation of desethylamiodarone (DEA).[13] Amiodarone and its metabolites are primarily excreted through bile and feces. [14] The drug and its metabolites have a relatively long half life of approximately 100 days. [15] Therefore amiodarone toxicity can develop long after its withdrawal.

Amiodarone and Thyroid

Amiodarone affects normal thyroid hormone function and metabolism. The effects are traditionally divided into those that are due to intrinsic property of the drug and those effects that are due to raised iodine levels. [Table 1]

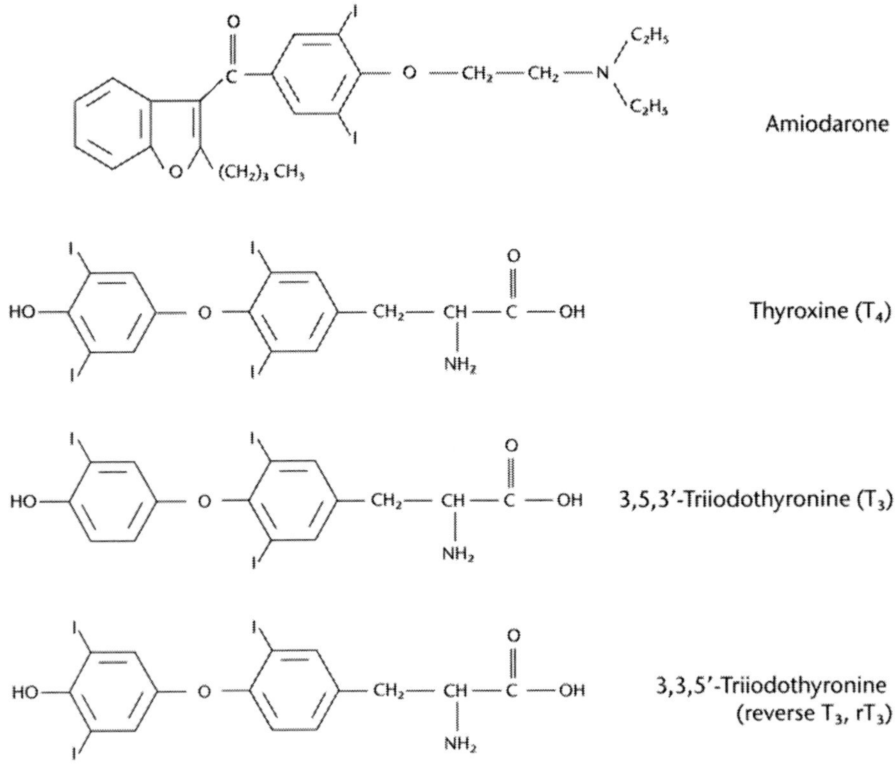

Figure 1. Structure of Amiodarone and Thyroid Hormones.

Table 1. Effects of Amiodarone on the Thyroid Gland

Intrinsic Drug Effect	Iodine-Induced Effects
Inhibition Of 5' De-Iodinase Enzyme	Potentiation Of Thyroid Autoimmunity
Decrease Binding Of T3 To Its Receptor	Failure To Escape From Wolff-Chaikoff Effect
Thyroid Cytotoxicity	Jod-Basedow Phenomenon

Effects Due to Inhibition of Enzymes Involved in Thyroid Hormone Metabolism

In peripheral tissues, particularly liver, amiodarone inhibits outer ring (type 1) 5'-deiodinase enzyme activity. This enzyme normally removes an atom from the outer ring of T4 to generate T3 and from the outer ring of rT3 to produce 3, 3'-diiodothyronine (T2). As a result of this, reduction in T3 production occurs with up to 30% lower levels of FT3 and rT3.[16] This inhibition may persist for months after withdrawal of the drug.[17,18,19] The reduced conversion of T4 to T3 may lead to a 20-40% rise in serum T4 concentrations. These changes are usually transient but may persist for months in some individuals, especially ones on higher doses of amiodarone. [20] [Table 2, 3]

Use of amiodarone is also associated with dose and time dependent changes in serum TSH concentrations. Often in the early period following initiation of amiodarone therapy, particularly with higher doses there is an increase in serum TSH levels. Generally these changes are transient [21, 22] and rarely reach levels greater than 20mU/l [23, 24].

In addition inhibition of type II 5'-deiodinase by amiodarone and desethylamiodarone results in decreased conversion of T4 to T3 in the pituitary. [25, 26] [Figure 2, 3]

Table 2. Effects of Amiodarone on Thyroid Function Tests in Euthyroid Patients

	First 3 Months (Acute Effects)	After 3 Months (Chronic Effects)
Total And Free T4	Modest Increase (↑ Upto 50%)	High Normal Or Raised (↑ Upto 20-40%)
Total And Free T3	Low Normal Or Decreased ↓ 15-20%	Low Normal Of Slightly Low ↓20%
TSH	Transient Increase (Upto 20mu/L)	Normal
rT3	Increased >200%	↑Increased >150%

Table 3. Reference ranges for serum thyroid hormones and TSH concentrations in euthyroid untreated subjects and in euthyroid patients receiving long-term amiodarone therapy

TEST	UNTREATED PATIENTS	ON AMIODARONE
Free T4 (pmol/l)	11-20	12-24.7
Free T3 (pmol/l)	3-5.6	2.5-5.1
TSH (mU/l)	0.35-4.3	0.35-4.3

Modified from: Newman CM, Price A, Davies DW, Gray TA, Weetman AP. Amiodarone and the thyroid: a practical guide to the management of thyroid dysfunction induced by amiodarone therapy. Heart 1998; 79: 121-127.

Effect of Amiodarone and its Metabolites on Thyroid Hormone Receptor Functioning:

Amiodarone and its metabolite DEA block T3 receptor binding to nuclear receptors. [27, 28] It has been shown that DEA behaves as a weak partial thyroid hormone receptor agonist and antagonizes effects of T3 when present in excess. [29] Higher tissue concentrations reached during chronic therapy may lead to antagonistic effects. [30]

At tissue level amiodarone may also induce a hypothyroid like picture by reducing the number and effectiveness of catecholamine receptors. [31, 32]

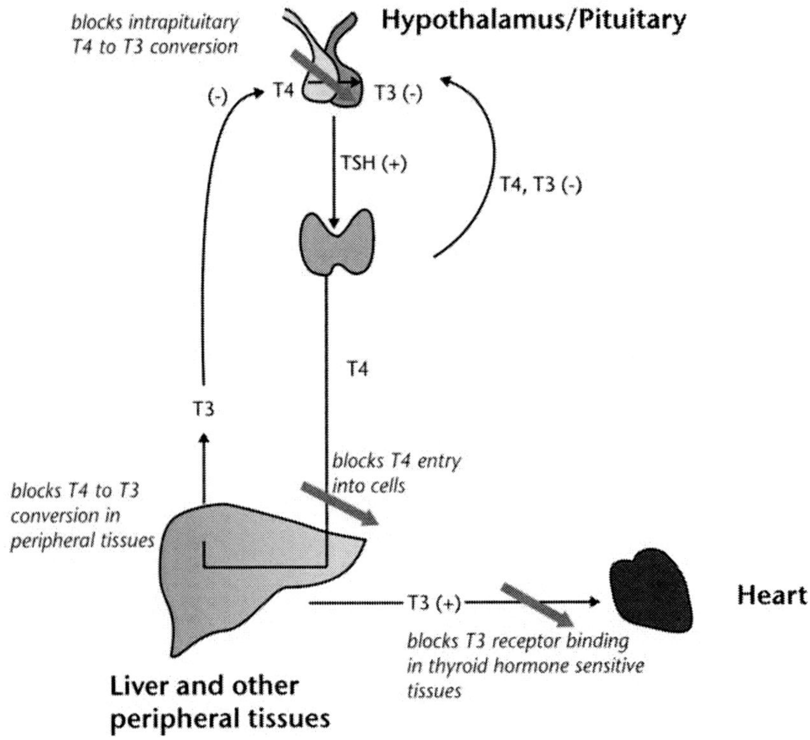

Figure 2. Effects of Amiodarone.

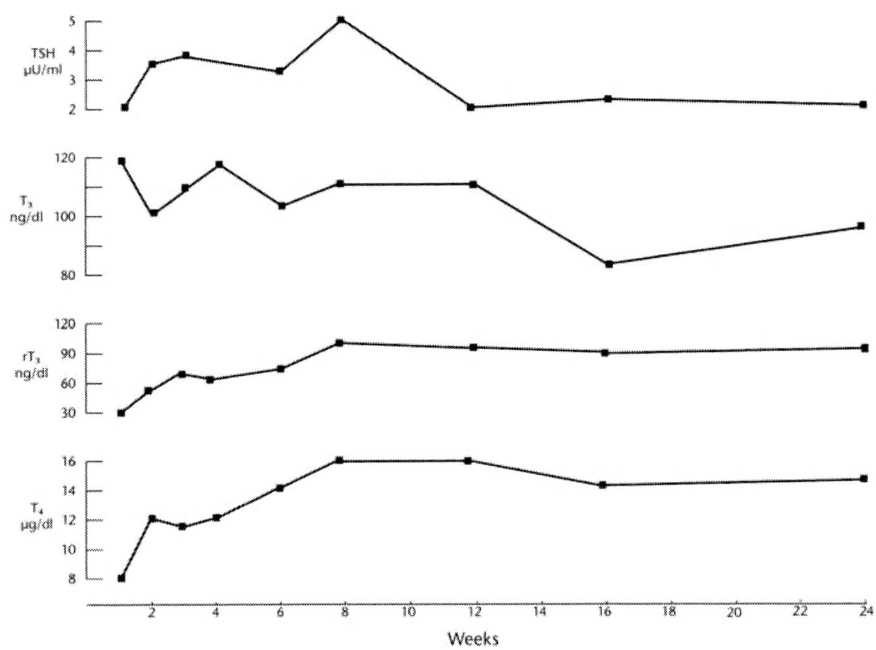

Figure 3. Effects of Amiodarone on TFTs [Adapted from Melmed S et al.Jcem1981; 53:997-1001.Thyroid Cytotoxicity:

Amiodarone and its metabolites also have direct cytotoxic effects on the thyroid. [33] Amiodarone-related thyroid cytotoxicity is mainly due to the direct effect of the drug in thyroid cells, though iodide excess may also contribute. DEA is thought to be more cytotoxic than amiodarone. [34] This cytotoxic damage tends to be associated with prolonged amiodarone treatment. [35]

Effect on Thyroid Autoimmunity:

The effect of amiodarone on thyroid autoimmunity remains contentious. Iodine is thought to induce thyroid autoimmunity in both humans and animals. [36, 37] In a small study treatment with amiodarone was shown to induce anti-thyroid auto antibodies. These auto antibodies seem to appear transiently during the early months following initiation of amiodarone treatment. Other studies have failed to confirm these findings. However amiodarone may be associated with an increase in certain sub-sets of lymphocytes which suggests that in susceptible individuals amiodarone may precipitate or exacerbate thyroid autoimmunity. [38] This may be of importance particularly in patients who develop amiodarone induced hypothyroidism.

Wolf-Chaikoff Effect:

Normally high doses of iodide blocks thyroid hormone synthesis through inhibition of the organification process. This phenomenon is called Wolff-Chaikoff effect.[39] This blockade is usually transient and is dependent on the intracellular iodide concentration.[40] The escape from the acute Wolff-Chaikoff effect involves a decrease in iodide transport into the thyrocytes leading to lower intracellular iodide concentrations, which are too low to maintain the inhibitory effects.[41] At the molecular level, an iodide induced down regulation of Sodium (Na)-iodide symporter (NIS) possibly by an increase in NIS protein turn-over and decrease in NIS activity is thought to be responsible for this complex auto-regulatory phenomenon induced by raised intracellular iodide concentrations.[42,43,44] [Figure 4]

Patients with a background of autoimmune thyroid disease are likely to “fail to escape” from the Wolff-Chaikoff effect. This may result in the development of hypothyroidism in patients with a background of Hashimoto’s disease. [45]

Jod-Basedow Phenomenon:

Patients with areas of autonomously functioning thyroid tissue do not autoregulate iodine. These patients particularly those living in iodine deficient areas may start producing excessive amounts of thyroid hormones as a result of the exposure to the large quantities of iodine available with the use of amiodarone.

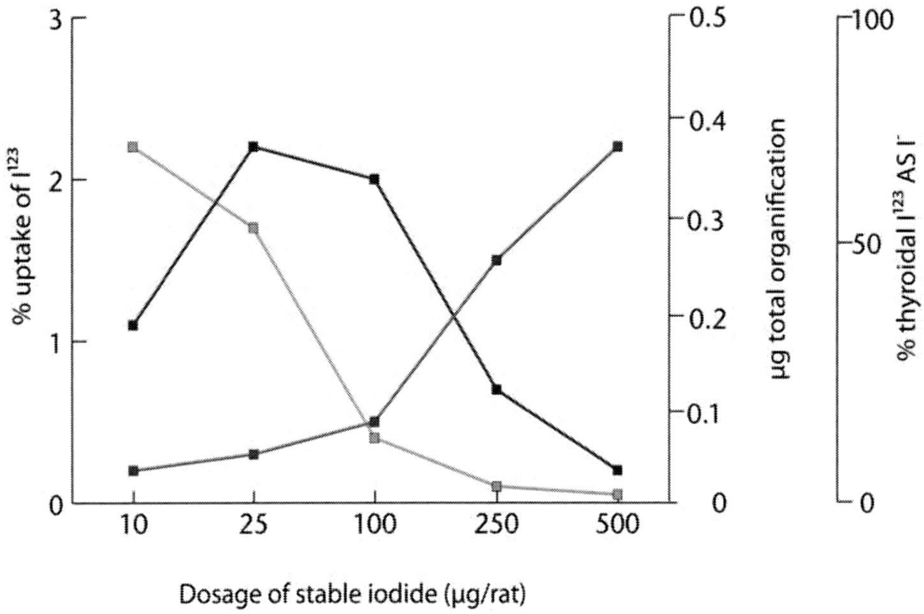

Demonstration of the Wolff-Chaikoff block induced by iodide in rat. With increasing doses of iodide intake there is at first an increase in total organification, but then, as the dose is increased further, a depression of organification of iodide and an increase in the free iodide present in the thyroid gland occurs.

Figure 4. WOLFF-CHAIKOFF EFFECT [Adapted from Wolff J, Chaikoff IL: Plasma inorganic iodide as a homeostatic regulator of thyroid function. J Biol Chem 174:555-564, 1948.]

This effect probably explains the occurrence of amiodarone induced hyperthyroidism that occurs in susceptible individuals living in iodine deficient areas.

Amiodarone Induced Hypothyroidism (AIH):

The incidence of amiodarone induced hypothyroidism varies widely ranging from as high as 13% in countries with high iodine intake such as UK and USA [46,47] to as low as 5% in countries with relatively low and intermediate iodine intake such as Italy and Spain [48,49] [Figure 5].

Failure to escape from the Wolff-Chaikoff effect and triggering of thyroid autoimmunity in susceptible individuals are thought to be the main mechanisms responsible for development of AIH. [50,51] As previously stated the risk of developing hypothyroidism is higher in individuals living in iodine sufficient areas It is also more likely in elderly and female patients and in patients with a positive family history of autoimmune thyroid diseases.[52,53,54]

As with other forms of hypothyroidism, clinical manifestations are often vague and varied. Patients may be entirely asymptomatic. Fatigue, lack of energy, intolerance to cold, mental and physical sluggishness along with dry skin is commonly reported.

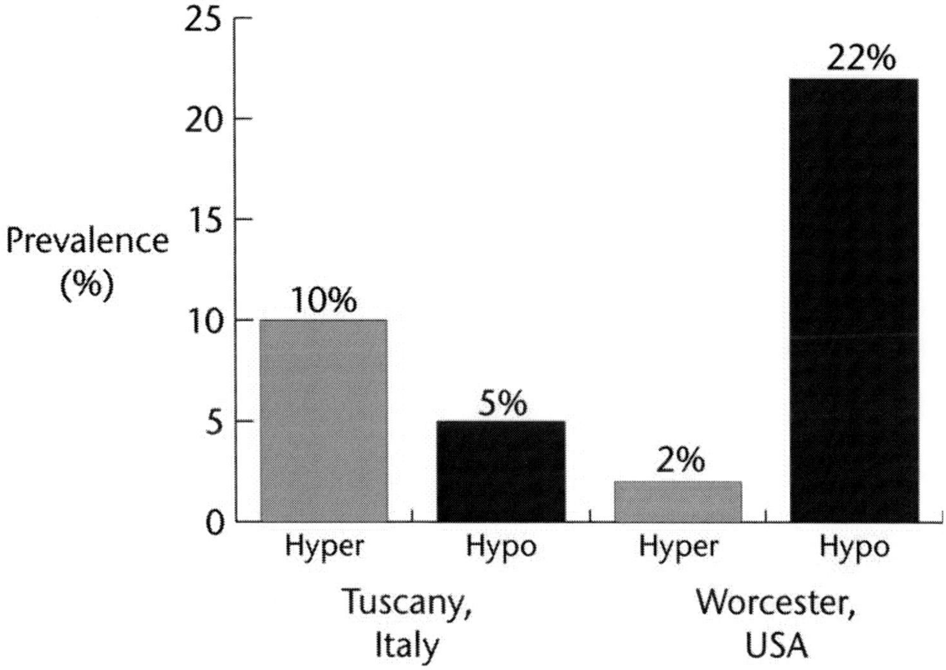

Figure 5. Prevalence of Amiodarone Induced Thyroid Dysfunction Depends of Iodine Intake [Adapted From E. Martino Et Al. Ann Intern Med (1984); 101: 28-34.

Goiter is uncommon. [55] Myxoedema coma has rarely been reported in patients taking amiodarone. [56] Hypothyroidism may develop as soon as two weeks or as late as 39 weeks after the initiation of amiodarone therapy. [57]

Biochemically the diagnosis is confirmed by the presence of a combination of low T4/Free T4, with raised TSH levels (preferably TSH>20 mU/l).[58] Low T3/ Free T3 concentrations are unreliable indicators of hypothyroidism as they may occur in euthyroid patients during amiodarone therapy. TSH values greater than normal but less than 20mU/L accompanied by near normal or slightly raised T4 values in individuals on amiodarone therapy are thought to represent sub-clinical hypothyroidism. Radio-iodine uptake is detectable in almost 80% of these patients although the exact mechanism is not well understood. [59] In addition perchlorate discharge test yields false positive results in most patients with amiodarone induced hypothyroidism. [60]

Treatment/Management: [Figure 6]

Purists may favour stopping amiodarone therapy or at least reducing the dose in patients with AIH.[61] In those in whom amiodarone therapy is stopped some become euthyroid within two to four months of stopping amiodarone therapy; however most, particularly the antibody positive patients remain hypothyroid and require levothyroxine replacement therapy.[62]

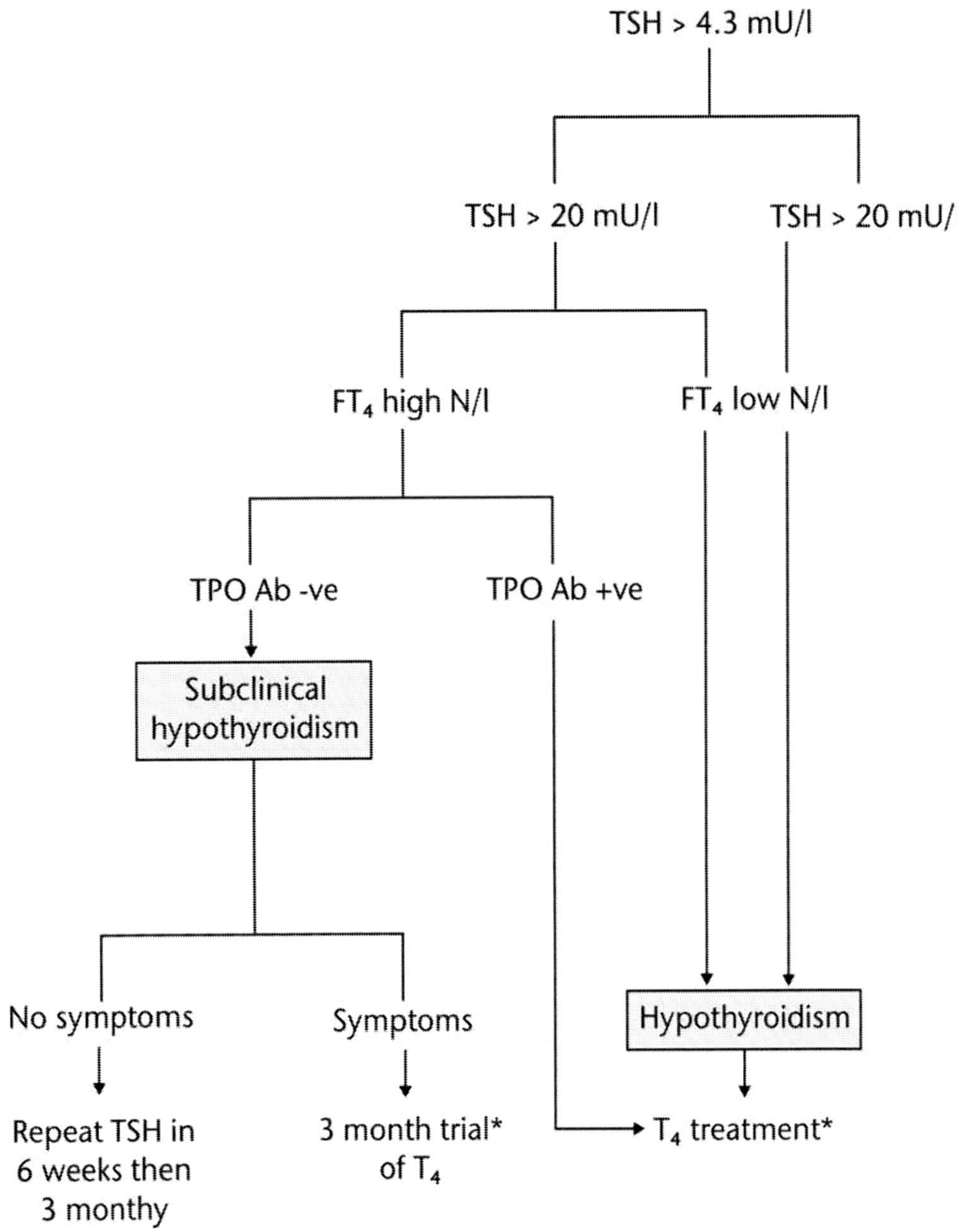

Figure 6. Management of AIH.

Restoration of euthyroidism following stoppage of amiodarone therapy can be accelerated in with the use of potassium perchlorate in single daily doses of 1 gm for up to 5 weeks. However within a few weeks, recurrence of hypothyroidism is common, possibly reflecting the long half-life of amiodarone. [63, 64]

In patients with AIH most physicians would continue amiodarone therapy. Indeed the safest, quickest and most reliable treatment of amiodarone-induced hypothyroidism is to continue amiodarone therapy and commence levothyroxine as replacement therapy. Levothyroxine is usually started at a low daily dose (25 to 50 mcg) and the dose is gradually increased (usually at 6 weekly interval) to achieve a high normal or slightly elevated TSH level. [65] Over-replacement should be avoided as it will undermine the anti-arrhythmic effects of amiodarone. It is also important to remember that TSH levels in euthyroid patients on amiodarone are often high normal or slightly elevated. [66]

Patients with sub-clinical hypothyroidism should be evaluated in a manner similar to subclinical hypothyroidism due to any other cause (including assessment of anti-TPO antibody status) and managed similarly. Most physicians would be inclined to treat those that either symptomatic or are positive for antibodies with levothyroxine replacement therapy. Whereas those who are negative should be followed up and thyroid function tests repeated at 3 monthly intervals. [67]

Amiodarone Induced Thyrotoxicosis: (AIT)

The incidence of AIT is less than that of amiodarone induced hypothyroidism, especially in iodine replete areas. In the UK and USA approximately 2% of patients receiving amiodarone develop AIT. [68, 69,] While in iodine deficient areas the incidence may be as high as 12%. [70]

The pathogenesis, clinical course and management of AIT is more complex than AIH.

AIT can occur any time during the course of use of amiodarone. The onset of thyrotoxicosis is often acute but may develop up to 2-3 years after the start of therapy. [71] Higher doses and larger cumulative doses of amiodarone are more likely to give rise to AIT and it can occur up to a year after stopping therapy.

AIT is usually suspected in patients with unexplained weight loss, muscle weakness, low grade fever, goiter and tremor. [72, 73]However the classical symptoms of thyrotoxicosis may be absent. Amiodarone is known to have antiadrenergic effects, beta-blocking activity and metabolites are known to block binding of T3 to its nuclear receptor. Thus amiodarone may mask some of the clinical features of thyrotoxicosis. [74] The presenting feature may be worsening of the underlying cardiac disorder or the appearance of new tachyarrhythmias. [75]

The biochemical diagnosis is made on the basis of presence of suppressed serum TSH levels accompanied by raised T3 or FT3 levels. In cases of subclinical thyrotoxicosis the TSH level will be suppressed with high normal or marginally raised T4 levels but with normal T3 or FT3 levels. [Figure: 7]

Traditionally AIT is subdivided into two types, Type I and Type II. The underlying pathogenesis and management differ for the two subtypes. [Table: 4]

Type I AIT

In type I AIT hyperthyroidism occurs due to an increased synthesis of T3 and T4 by the thyroid gland. These patients tend to have a pre-existing multi-nodular goiter or latent Graves' disease [76]. Type I AIT is more likely to occur in individuals living in iodine deficient areas. [77]

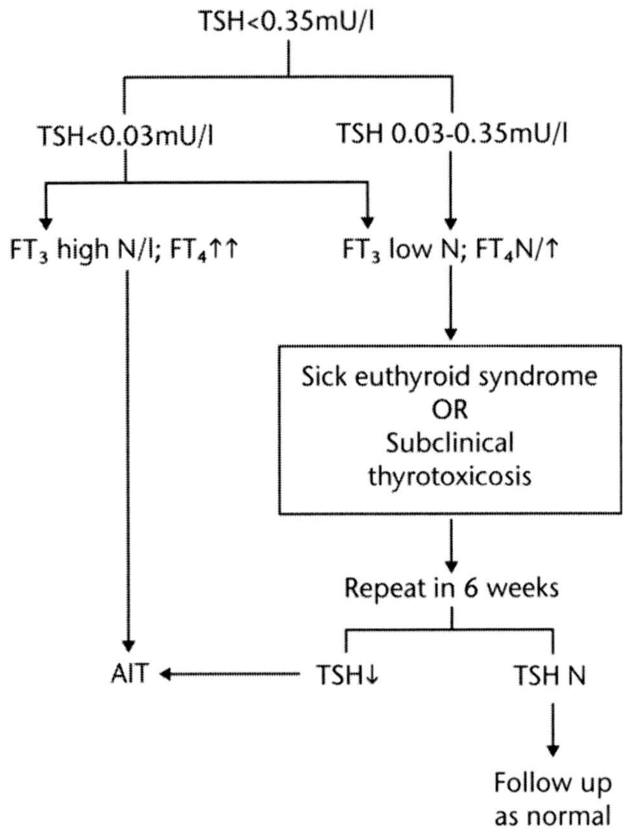

Figure 7. Management of AIT.

Table 4. Features differentiating type I from type II AIT

	TYPE I	TYPE II
Pre-existing thyroid abnormalities	Present	Absent
Goiter	Multinodular or diffuse goiter may be present	Absent or small tender goiter present
Thyrotoxic phase	Protracted	Transient
Thyroid antibodies	May be positive	Usually negative
Radioactive iodine uptake	Normal or raised	Low or absent
Serum IL-6 levels	Normal/slightly raised	Profoundly raised
Colour flow Doppler of thyroid parenchymal blood flow	High thyroidal blood flow	Low thyroidal blood flow
Response to thionamides	Yes	No
Response to glucocorticoids	No	Yes
Response to perchlorate	Yes	No
Subsequent hypothyroid phase	No	Possible

It is believed that there is alteration in the intrinsic auto-regulatory mechanism in the thyroid which normally prevents occurrence of hyperthyroidism in states of iodine excess. In these susceptible individuals iodine excess leads to production of excess thyroid hormones – the Jod-Basedow phenomenon. [78]

The clinical course of this form of thyrotoxicosis tends to be protracted as it results in triggering of autonomous over-activity in susceptible thyroid tissue. Presence of thyrotropin receptor antibody suggests that AIT type I has occurred in the presence of latent Graves' disease.

Unlike other causes of thyrotoxicosis the radioactive iodine uptake in these patients may not be raised. This is due to the high circulating levels of iodine caused by iodine released from amiodarone, coupled with the raised intrathyroidal iodine levels secondary to the effect of amiodarone on the NIS. Normal or high radioactive iodine uptake is more likely to occur in type I AIT.

Colour flow Doppler studies looking at blood flow in thyroid parenchyma has often been used to distinguish type I AIT from type II AIT. Being an overactive thyroid state colour flow Doppler in type I AIT is normal or increased. In type II AIT colour flow is usually absent due to the destruction of thyroid parenchyma.[79]

Amiodarone has a very long half life and therefore stopping amiodarone may have no immediate benefit. In fact amiodarone can ameliorate some of the features of thyrotoxicosis via mechanisms discussed earlier. Therefore stopping amiodarone in AIT type I may actually exacerbate the signs and symptoms of thyrotoxicosis.[80,81]

However for long term management of thyrotoxicosis one should consider stopping amiodarone particularly in the more severe cases of AIT type I. However one has to remember that withdrawal of amiodarone alone may not be of any benefit in the immediate management of the thyrotoxic state. The mainstay of management of patients with type I AIT is the use of thionamides such as carbimazole or methimazole.

Type II AIT

In type II AIT thyrotoxicosis occurs as a result of destructive thyroiditis. It is the commoner variety of AIT in iodine sufficient areas. It typically occurs in individuals without any underlying thyroid disease. It results from the direct toxic effects of amiodarone and its metabolite on thyroid follicular cells.[82,83] The destruction can occur anytime after start of therapy, even 2-3 years after starting amiodarone therapy.[84] The reasons for delayed toxicity in some cases are not clearly understood.

As a result of destructive thyroiditis there is release of pre-formed hormones into the circulation with resultant features of thyroid hormone excess. The thyrotoxic phase of type II AIT is understandably less protracted than AIT type I. The hyperthyroid phase may last from several weeks to several months and is often followed by a hypothyroid phase with spontaneous recovery in a significant proportion of patients.[85]

Apart from the general features of thyrotoxicosis patients with type II AIT may have a tender goiter similar to that of patients with sub-acute thyroiditis. The radioactive iodine uptake is low or absent as this is a state of destructive thyroiditis. Colour flow Doppler reveals little vascularity. Inflammatory markers such as IL-6 are elevated in patients with type II AIT. [86]

In vitro studies have shown that amiodarone is toxic to thyrocytes and this effect was inhibited by dexamethasone or perchlorate. [87] It has also been demonstrated that higher cumulative doses increases the risk of AIT type II. [88]

Discontinuation of amiodarone therapy (if possible) should be considered in cases of AIT type II. However the toxic effects of amiodarone persist for a long period even after stopping amiodarone due to its prolonged half life. However unlike type I AIT withdrawal of amiodarone therapy may suffice with the majority of patients becoming euthyroid within three to five months of amiodarone withdrawal. [89]

Glucocorticoid therapy accelerates recovery and should be considered in all patients with symptoms of thyrotoxicosis and/or worsening of their underlying arrhythmias. Prednisolone 40-60 mg daily is used in tapering doses over three months, depending on response. In most cases there is biochemical and clinical resolution of thyrotoxicosis within days of commencement of steroid therapy. [90] The steroid therapy may have to be maintained for up to 3 months as there can be clinical relapse following initial response in some patients.[91] Prolonged thyrotoxicosis was associated with higher serum free T4 levels and goiter.[92] Glucorticoids have been shown to be effective in patients in whom amiodarone therapy has been continued.[93,94]

Iopanoic acid has also been used to treat type II AIT. However glucocorticoids are more effective than iopanoic acid. [95]

Radioactive iodine therapy is ineffective in patients with type II AIT. The role of anti-thyroid thionamide drugs is also limited in these patients. [96] There may be a role for thionamide drugs in those patients with AIT type II in whom amiodarone therapy cannot be discontinued. [97]

Mixed AIT

Some patients with AIT may have a mixed form of thyrotoxicosis or the underlying subtype may not be easily identifiable even after detailed investigations. In such cases amiodarone therapy should be discontinued if possible. A combination of prednisolone and thionamide therapy should be started and the patient clinically and biochemically monitored. A rapid response suggests type II AIT and thionamide therapy should be stopped and if needed iopanoic acid added. On the other hand poor initial response suggests type I AIT, steroids are gradually reduced and depending on response perchlorate or lithium added. In resistant cases surgery may be necessary.

Patients on Warfarin

Patients on amiodarone are often on Warfarin as well. Amiodarone induced thyroid dysfunction may potentially interfere with the metabolism and action of amiodarone. The anticoagulant effects of warfarin is attenuated with hypothyroidism and exaggerated by thyrotoxic states. [98] In addition amiodarone may also interfere with the pharmacokinetics of warfarin directly (irrespective of its action via alteration of thyroid function). This effect may persist long after the withdrawal of amiodarone. It is thus essential that patients on amiodarone (especially those with amiodarone-induced thyroid dysfunction) should be monitored closely (with regular measurement of International Normalized Ratio) and dose adjustments are made accordingly.

Special Situations: Pregnancy

Amiodarone can be used in pregnant women if they have life threatening or refractory arrhythmias, that are resistant to other anti-arrhythmics. Infants of mothers taking amiodarone may develop hypothyroidism. This is usually transient and seldom requires thyroid hormone replacement therapy. [99]

Among a total of 64 pregnant women treated with amiodarone, abnormalities in thyroid function were found in 13 neonates. Two of whom had transient hyperthyroxinaemia and 11 had AIH (2 also had goiters).[100] In the follow-up of toddlers exposed transplacentally to amiodarone, all subjects had normal social competence and favorable global IQ scores, but showed some problems in reading, comprehension, written language and arithmetic, reminiscent of the Nonverbal Learning Disability syndrome [101].

Amiodarone is also secreted in breast milk. Although breast-feeding is not absolutely contraindicated it carries a risk because the baby is very sensitive to iodine induced hypothyroidism. Hence the thyroid function must be monitored in the neonate. [102]

Monitoring Thyroid Function Following Start of Amiodarone [Figure 8]

Prior to starting amiodarone therapy it is useful to document any previous history of thyroid dysfunction, presence of any autoimmune disorder and also to document any family history of thyroid dysfunction. Clinical examination to detect any goiter or clinical signs of an overactive or underactive thyroid should also be undertaken. Baseline investigations should include a thyroid function test and especially those with goiter or high normal TSH level should also have their antithyroid antibody status checked. The baseline results serve as a reference for comparison with future test results. They also serve to identify underlying thyroid dysfunction which may predispose the patient to abnormalities on thyroid function, once they are started on amiodarone.

The thyroid function test should be re-assessed 3 months after start of amiodarone therapy (earlier if clinically indicated). This should include an assessment of FrT3, FrT4 and TSH estimation. Thereafter thyroid function should be reassessed every 6 months (earlier if clinically indicated). Some authorities believe that TSH testing alone may suffice as the screening test in subsequent testing. Regular screening is undertaken to detect otherwise subtle/asymptomatic abnormalities of thyroid function induced by amiodarone therapy, especially AIH. The clinical onset of AIT type II is usually dramatic and difficult to predict, whereas AIT type I can occur months or years after stopping amiodarone therapy. Hence it is important to continue monitoring TFTs atleast for one year following withdrawal of amiodarone therapy.

However the cost-effectiveness of routine monitoring has never been fully evaluated

Future Hopes

A newer drug, namely dronedarone is currently under review. As dronedarone does not contain iodine it is hoped that it will have the same benefits but not the ill effects on thyroid function.

Conclusions

Amiodarone is a widely prescribed anti-arrhythmic, but its safe and effective use requires a firm understanding of its unusual pharmacokinetics as well as the potential for adverse events and drug interactions. It is outwith the remit of this chapter but clinicians should consider other antiarrhythmic drugs before choosing amiodarone recognising that the balance of risks and benefits depends on the clinical setting.

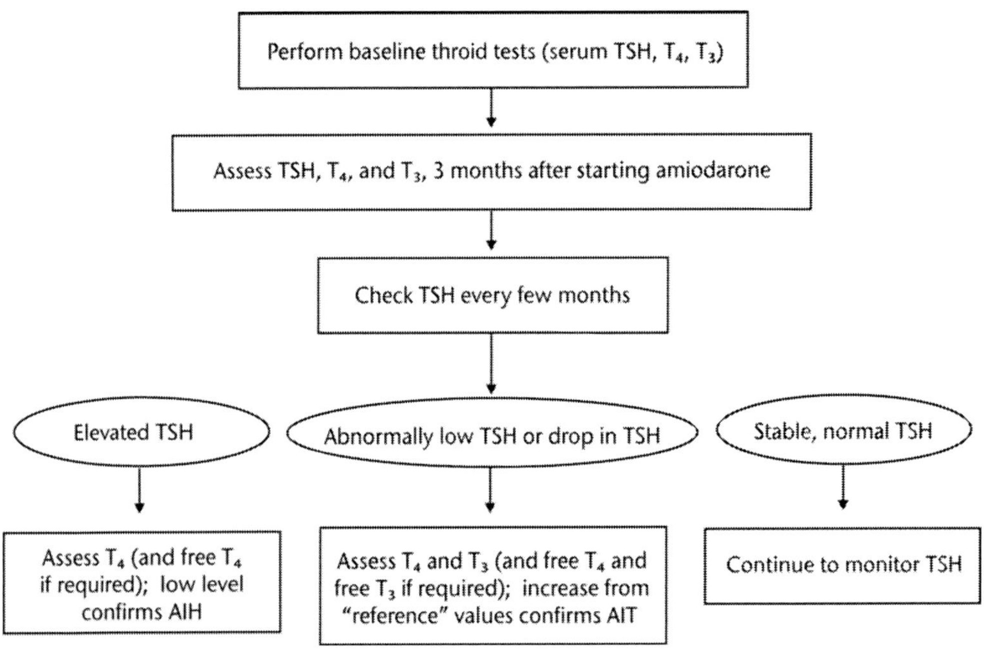

Figure 8. Monitoring Thyroid Function Following Start of Amiodarone.

Acknowledgments

We are indebted to Sarah Syme (Medical Photography) for her help.

References

[1] Deltour G, Binon F, Tondeur R, *et al* (1962). Studies in the benzofuran series. VI. Coronary-dilating activity of alkylated and aminoalkylated derivatives of 3-benzoylbenzofuran. (in French). *Archives internationales de pharmacodynamie et de thérapie* **139**: 247–54.

[2] Deltour G, Binon F, Tondeur R, *et al* (1962). Studies in the benzofuran series. VI. Coronary-dilating activity of alkylated and aminoalkylated derivatives of 3-benzoylbenzofuran. (in French). *Archives internationales de pharmacodynamie et de thérapie* **139**: 247–54.

[3] Charlier R, Deltour G, Tondeur R, Binon F (1962). Studies in the benzofuran series. VII. Preliminary pharmacological study of 2-butyl-3-(3,5-diiodo-4-beta-N-diethylaminoethoxybenzoyl)-benzofuran (in French). *Archives internationales de pharmacodynamie et de thérapie* **139**: 255–64.

[4] Singh BN, Vaughan Williams EM (1970). "The effect of amiodarone, a new anti-anginal drug, on cardiac muscle". *Br. J. Pharmacol.* **39** (4): 657–67.

[5] Rosenbaum MB, Chiale PA, Halpern MS, *et al* (1976). "Clinical efficacy of amiodarone as an antiarrhythmic agent". *Am. J. Cardiol.* **38** (7): 934–44

[6] Podrid PJ. Amiodarone—reevaluation of an old drug. *Ann Intern Med* 1995;122:689–700.

[7] Doval HC, Nul DR, Grancelli HO, *et al.* Randomized trial of low-dose amiodarone in severe congestive heart failure. *Lancet* 1994; 344:493–8.

[8] Julian DG, Camm AJ, Frangin G, *et al.* Randomised trial of effect of amiodarone on mortality in patients with left-ventricular dysfunction after recent myocardial infarction: EMIAT. *Lancet* 1997; 349:667–74.

[9] Delange FM, Ermans A-M 2000 Iodine deficiency. In: Braverman LE, Utiger RD (eds) Werner and Ingbar's The Thyroid—A Clinical and Fundamental Text, ed 8. Lippincott-Raven, Philadelphia, pp 295–315

[10] Delange FM, Ermans A-M 2000 Iodine deficiency. In: Braverman LE, Utiger RD (eds) Werner and Ingbar's The Thyroid—A Clinical and Fundamental Text, Ed 8. Lippincott-Raven, Philadelphia, pp 295–315

[11] Rao RH, McCready VR, Spathis GS. Iodine kinetic studies during amiodarone treatment. *J Clin Endocrinol Metab* 1986; 62:563–8.

[12] Holt DW, Tucker GT, Jackson PR, Storey GCA 1983 Amiodarone pharmacokinetics. Am Heart J 106:843–847

[13] Berger Y, Harris L 1986 Pharmacokinetics. In: Harris L, Roncucci R (eds) Amiodarone.Me`dicine et Sciences Internationales, Paris, pp 45–98

[14] Rao RH, McReady VR, Spathis GS 1986 Iodine kinetic studies during amiodarone treatment J Clin Endocrinol Metab 62: 563–567

[15] Plomp TA, van Rossum JM, Robles de Medina EO, van Lier T, Maes RAA 1984 Pharmacokinetics and body distribution of amiodarone in man. Arzneimittelforschung/Drug Res 34:513–520

[16] Rao, H. Iodine kinetic studies during amiodarone treatment. J Clin Endocrinol Metab 1986; 62:563. (Same as ref 9)

[17] Wiersinga WM 1997 Amiodarone and the thyroid. In: Weetman AP, GrossmanA(eds) Pharmacotherapeutics of the Thyroid Gland. Springer Verlag, Berlin, pp 225–287

[18] Lombardi A, Martino E, Braverman LE 1990 Amiodarone and the thyroid. Thyroid Today 13:1–7

[19] Harjai KJ, Licata AA 1997 Effects of amiodarone on thyroid function. Ann Intern Med 126:63–73

[20] Amico JA, Richardson V, Alpert B, Klein I 1984 Clinical and chemical assessment of thyroid function during therapy with amiodarone. Arch Intern Med 144:487–490

[21] Burger A, Dinichert D, Nicod P, Jenny M, Lemarchand-Beraud T, Vallotton MB 1976 Effect of amiodarone on serum triiodothyronine, reverse triiodothyronine, thyroxin, and thyrotropin. J Clin Invest 58:255–259

[22] Melmed S, Nademanee K, Reed AW, Hendrickson JA, Singh BN, Hershman JM 1981 Hyperthyroxinemia with bradycardia and normal thyrotropin secretion after chronic amiodarone administration. J Clin Endocrinol Metab 53:997–1001

[23] Nademanee K, Singh BN, Callahan B, *et al.* Amiodarone, thyroid hormone indexes, and altered thyroid function: long-term serial effects in patients with cardiac arrhythmias. *Am J Cardiol* 1986; 58: 981–6.

[24] Melmed S, Nademanee K, Reed AW, *et al.* Hyperthyroxinemia with bradycardia and normal thyrotropin secretion after chronic amiodarone administration. *J Clin Endocrinol Metab* 1981; 53: 997–1001.

[25] Franklyn JA, Davis JR, Gammage MD, Littler WA, Ramsden DB, Sheppard MC 1985 Amiodarone and thyroid hormone function. Clin Endocrinol (Oxf) 22:257–264

[26] Safran M, Fang S-L, Bambini G, Pinchera A, Martino E, Braverman LE 1986 Effects of amiodarone and desethylamiodarone on pituitary deiodinase activity and thyrotropin secretion in the rat. Am J Med Sci 29:136–141

[27] Gotzsche LB, Orskov H 1994 Cardiac triiodothyronine nuclear receptor binding capacities in amiodarone-treated, hypo- and hyperthyroid rats. Eur J Endocrinol 130:281–290

[28] Franklyn, JA. Amiodarone and thyroid hormone action. Clin Endocrinol 1985; 22:257.

[29] Bogazzi F, Bartalena L, Brogioni S, Burelli A, Cecconi E, Campomori A, Raggi F, Martino E 1998 Desethylamiodarone antagonizes the effect of T3 at the molecular level. J Endocrinol Invest 21 [Suppl]:93 (Abstract)

[30] Wiersinga WM 1997 Amiodarone and the thyroid. In: Weetman AP, Grossman (eds) Pharmacotherapeutics of the Thyroid Gland. Springer Verlag, Berlin, pp 225–287

[31] Rani CS 1990 Amiodarone effects on thyrotropin receptors and responses stimulated by thyrotropin and carbachol in cultured dog thyroid cells. Endocrinology 127:2930–2937

[32] Disatnik MH, Shainberg A 1991 Regulation of beta-adrenoceptors by thyroid hormone and amiodarone in rat myocardiac cells in culture. Biochem Pharmacol 41:1039–1044

[33] Chiovato L, Martino E, Tonacchera M, Santini F, Lapi P, Mammoli C, Braverman LE, PincheraA1994 Studies on the *in vitro* cytotoxic effect of amiodarone. Endocrinology 134:2277–2282

[34] Beddows SA, Page SR, Taylor AH, McNerney R, Whitley GSJ, Johnstone AP, Nussey SS 1989 Cytotoxic effects of amiodarone and desethylamiodarone on human thyrocytes. Biochem Pharmacol38:4397–4403

[35] Gross SA, Somani P. Amiodarone-induced ultrastructural changes in canine myocardial fibers. Am Heart J 112:771–779

[36] Bagchi N, Brown TR, Urdanivia E, Sundick RS 1985 Induction of autoimmune thyroiditis by dietary iodine. Science 230:325–328

[37] Allen EM, Appel MC, Braverman LE 1986 The effect of iodide ingestion on the development of spontaneous lymphocytic thyroiditis in the diabetes-prone BB/W rat. Endocrinology 118:1977–1981

[38] Rabinowe SL, Larsen PR, Antman EM, George KL, Friedman PL, Jackson RA, Eisenbarth GS 1986 Amiodarone therapy and autoimmune thyroid disease. Increase in a new monoclonal antibody defined T cell subset. Am J Med 81:53–57

[39] Wolff J, Chaikoff I. Plasma inorganic iodide as homeostatic regulator of thyroid function. J Biol Chem 1948; 174: 555.

[40] Wolff J, Chaikoff I, Goldberg R, et al. The temporary nature of the inhibitory action of excess iodide on organic iodide synthesis in the normal thyroid. Endocrinology 1949; 45: 504.

[41] Braverman LE, Ingbar SH. Changes in thyroidal function during adaptation to large doses of iodide. J Clin Invest 1963; 42:1216.

[42] Spitzweg C, Joba W, Morris JC et al. Regulation of sodium iodide symporter gene expression in FRTL-5 rat thyroid cells. Thyroid 1999; 9: 821.

[43] Eng PH, Cardona GR, Fang SL et al. Escape from the acute Wolff-Chaikoff effect is associated with a decrease in thyroid sodium/iodide symporter messenger ribonucleic acid and protein. Endocrinology 199; 140: 3404.

[44] Eng PH, Cardona GR, Previti MC, et al. Regulation of the sodium iodide symporter by iodide in FRTL-5 cells. Eur J Endocrinol 2001; 144: 139.

[45] Braverman, LE, Ingbar, SH, Vagenakis, AG, et al. Enhanced susceptibility to iodide myxedema in patients with Hashimoto's disease. J Clin Endocrinol Metab 1971; 32:515.

[46] Amico JA, Richardson V, Alpert B, *et al.* Clinical and chemical assessment of thyroid function during therapy with amiodarone. *Arch Intern Med* 1984;144:487–90.

[47] Shukla R, Jowett NI, Thompson DR, *et al.* Side effects with amiodarone therapy. *Postgrad Med J* 1994;70:492–8.

[48] Martino E, Safran M, Aghini-Lombardi F, *et al.* Environmental iodine intake and thyroid dysfunction during chronic amiodarone therapy. *Ann InternMed* 1984;101:28–34.

[49] Sanmarti A, Permanyer-Miralda G, Castellanos JM, *et al.* Chronic administration of amiodarone and thyroid function: a follow-up study. *Am Heart J* 1984;108:1262–8.

[50] Martino E, Aghini-Lombardi F, Mariotti S, Bartalena L, Lenziardi M, Ceccarelli C, et al. Amiodarone iodine-induced hypothyroidism: risk factors and follow-up in 28 cases. Clin Endocrinol (Oxf). 1987;26:227-37.

[51] Martino E, Aghini-Lombardi F, Bartalena L, Grasso L, Loviselli A, Velluzzi F, et al. Enhanced susceptibility to amiodarone-induced hypothyroidism in patients with thyroid autoimmune disease. Arch Intern Med. 1994;154:2722-6.

[52] WiersingaW. Amiodarone and the thyroid. In:Weetman AP, Grossman A, eds. *Handbook of experimental pharmacology, Vol 128: pharmacotherapeutics of the thyroid gland.* Heidelberg: Springer-Verlag, 1997:225–87.

[53] Franklyn JA, Davis JR, Gammage MD, *et al.* Amiodarone and thyroid hormone action. *Clin Endocrinol* 1985;22:257–64.

[54] Trip MD, Wiersinga WM, Plomp TA. Incidence, predictability, and pathogenesis of thyrotoxicosis and hypothyroidism. *Am J Med* 1991;91:

[55] Hawthorne GC, Campbell NP, Geddes JS, Ferguson WR, Postlethwaite W, Sheridan B, et al. Amiodarone-induced hypothyoidism. A commom complication of prolonged therapy: a report of eight cases. Arch Intern Med 1985;145:1016-9.

[56] Mazonson PD, Williams ML, Cantley LK, Daldorf LG, Utiger RD, Foster JR. Myxedema coma during long-term amiodarone therapy. Am J Med 1984; 77: 751-754.

[57] Nademanee, K. Amiodarone and thyroid function. Prog Cardiovasc Dis 1989; 31:427.

[58] Wiersinga WM, Trip MD. Amiodarone and thyroid hormone metabolism. *Postgrad Med J* 1986; 62:909–14.

[59] Martino E, Aghini-Lombardi F, Mariotti S, Bartalena L, Lenziardi M, Ceccarelli C, et al. Amiodarone iodine-induced hypothyroidism: risk factors and follow-up in 28 cases. Clin Endocrinol (Oxf). 1987;26:227-37.

[60] Martino E, Bartalena L, Mariotti S, Aghini-Lombardi F, Ceccarelli C, Lippi F, et al. Radioactive iodine thyroid uptake in patients with amiodarone-iodine-induced thyroid dysfunction. Acta Endocrinol (Copenh). 1988; 119:167-73.

[61] Nademanee K, Piwonka RW, Singh BN, Hershman JM. Amiodarone and thyroid function. Prog Cardiovasc Dis. 1989; 31:427-37.

[62] Martino E, Aghini-Lombardi F, Mariotti S, *et al.* Amiodarone iodine-induced hypothyroidism: risk factors and follow-up in 28 cases. *Clin Endocrinol* 1987;26:227–37.

[63] Martino E, Mariotti S, Aghini-Lombardi F, *et al.* Short term administration of potassium perchlorate restores euthyroidism in amiodarone iodine-induced hypothyroidism. *J Clin Endocrinol Metab* 1986; 63:1233–6.

[64] van Dam EW, Prummel MF, Wiersinga WM, *et al.* Treatment of amiodarone-induced hypothyroidism with potassium perchlorate. *Neth J Med* 1993;42:21–4

[65] Newman CM, Price A, Davies DW, Gray TA, Weetman AP. Amiodarone and the thyroid: a practical guide to the management of thyroid dysfunction induced by amiodarone therapy. *Heart* 1998;79:121–7.

[66] de Jong M, Docter R, van der Hoek H, *et al.* Different effects of amiodarone on transport of T4 and T3 into the perfused rat liver. *Am J Physiol* 1994;266:E44–9.

[67] Weetman AP. Hypothyroidism: screening and subclinical disease. *BMJ* 1997;314:1175–8.

[68] Amico JA, Richardson V, Alpert B, *et al.* Clinical and chemical assessment of thyroid function during therapy with amiodarone. *Arch Intern Med* 1984;144:487–90.

[69] Shukla R, Jowett NI, Thompson DR, *et al.* Side effects with amiodarone therapy. *Postgrad Med J* 1994;70:492–8.

[70] Martino E, Safran M, Aghini-Lombardi F, *et al.* Environmental iodine intake and thyroid dysfunction during chronic amiodarone therapy. *Ann InternMed* 1984;101:28–34.

[71] Trip MD, Wiersinga WM, Plomp TA. Incidence, predictability, and pathogenesis of thyrotoxicosis and hypothyroidism. *Am J Med* 1991;91:507–11.

[72] Newnham HH, Topliss DJ, Le Grand BA, Chosich N, Harper RW, Stockigt JR. Amiodarone-induced hyperthyroidism: assessment of the predictive value of biochemical testing and response to combined therapy using propylthiouracil and potassium perchlorate. Aust N Z J Med. 1988; 18:37-44.

[73] Harjai KJ, Licata AA. Amiodarone-induced hyperthyroidism: a case series and brief review of literature. Pacing Clin Electrophysiol. 1996;19:1548-54.

[74] van Beeren, HC, Bakker, O, Wiersinga, WM. Structure-function relationship of the inhibition of the 3, 5,3'-triiodothyronine binding to the alpha-1 and beta-1-thyroid hormone receptor by amiodarone analogs. Endocrinology 1996; 137:2807.

[75] Martino E, Aghini-Lombardi F, Mariotti S, Bartalena L, Braverman L, Pinchera a. Amiodarone: a common source of iodine-induced thyrotoxicosis. Horm Res. 1987; 26:158-71.

[76] Fradkin, JE. Iodide-induced thyrotoxicosis. Medicine 1983; 62:1.

[77] Harjai KJ, Licata AA. Effects of amiodarone on thyroid function. *Ann Intern Med* 1997; 126:63–73.

[78] Martino, E, Bartalena, L, Bogazzi, F, et al. The effects of amiodarone on the thyroid. Endocr Rev 2001; 22:240.

[79] Bogazzi F, Bartalena L, Brogioni S, *et al.* Color flow Doppler sonography rapidly differentiates type I and type II amiodarone-induced thyrotoxicosis. *Thyroid* 1997; 7:541–5.

[80] Leger AF, Massin JP, Laurent MF, *et al.* Iodine-induced thyrotoxicosis: analysis of eighty-five consecutive cases. *Eur J Clin Invest* 1984;14:449–55.

[81] Brennan MD, van Heerden JA, Carney JA. Amiodarone associated thyrotoxicosis (AAT): experience with surgical management. *Surgery* 1987;102:1062–7.

[82] Lambert, M, Unger, J, De Nayer, P, et al. Amiodarone-induced thyrotoxicosis suggestive of thyroid damage. J Endocrinol Invest 1990; 13:527.

[83] Brennan, MD, Erickson, DZ, Carney, JA, et al. Nongoitrous (type I) amiodarone-associated thyrotoxicosis: Evidence of follicular disruption in vitro and in vivo. Thyroid 1995; 5:177.

[84] Martino, E. Amiodarone iodine-induced hypothyroidism: Risk factors and follow-up in 28 cases. Clin Endocrinol 1987; 26:227.

[85] Newnham HH, Topliss DJ, Le Grand BA, Chosich N, Harper RW, Stockigt JR. Amiodarone-induced hyperthyroidism: assessment of the predictive value of biochemical testing and response to combined therapy using propylthiouracil and potassium perchlorate. Aust N Z J Med. 1988; 18:37-44.

[86] Bartalena, L, Grasso, L, Brogioni, S, et al. Serum interleukin-6 in amiodarone-induced thyrotoxicosis. J Clin Endocrinol Metab 1994; 78:423.

[87] Brennan MD, Erickson DZ, Carney JA, Bahn RS. Nongoitrous amiodarone-associated thyrotoxicosis: evidence of follicular disruption in vitro and in vivo. *Thyroid* 1995; 5:177–83.

[88] O'Sullivan, AJ, Lewis, M, Diamond, T. Amiodarone-induced thyrotoxicosis: left ventricular dysfunction is associated with increased mortality. Eur J Endocrinol 2006; 154:533

[89] Martino E, Aghini-Lombardi F, Mariotti S, *et al.* Amiodarone iodine-induced hypothyroidism: risk factors and follow-up in 28 cases. *Clin Endocrinol* 1987; 26:227–37.

[90] Bartalena, L, Bogazzi, F, Braverman, LE, Martino, E. Effects of amiodarone administration during pregnancy on neonatal thyroid function and subsequent neurodevelopment. J Endocrinol Invest 2001; 24:116.

[91] Harjai KJ, Licata AA. Amiodarone-induced hyperthyroidism: a case series and brief review of literature. *Pacing Clin Electrophysiol* 1996;19:1548–4.

[92] Bogazzi, F, Bartalena, L, Tomisti, L, et al. Glucocorticoid response in amiodarone-induced thyrotoxicosis resulting from destructive thyroiditis is predicted by thyroid volume and serum free thyroid hormone concentrations. *J. Clin. Endocrinol. Metab.* 2007; 92:556.

[93] Daniels, GH. Amiodarone-induced thyrotoxicosis. J Clin Endocrinol Metab 2001; 86:3.

[94] Uzan, L, Guignat, L, Meune, C, et al. Continuation of amiodarone therapy despite type II amiodarone-induced thyrotoxicosis. Drug Safe 2006; 29:231.

[95] Bogazzi, F, Bartalena, L, Cosci, C, et al. Treatment of Type II Amiodarone-Induced Thyrotoxicosis by Either Iopanoic Acid or Glucocorticoids: A Prospective, Randomized Study. J Clin Endocrinol Metab 2003; 88:1999.

[96] Bartalena L, Brogioni S, Grasso L, *et al.* Treatment of amiodarone-induced thyrotoxicosis, a difficult challenge: results of a prospective study. *J. Clin. Endocrinol. Metab.* 1996; 81:2930–3.

[97] Chopra, IJ, Baber, K. Use of oral cholecystographic agents in the treatment of amiodarone-induced hyperthyroidism. *J. Clin. Endocrinol. Metab.* 2001; 86:4707.

[98] Kurnik, D, Loebstein, R, Farfel, Z, et al. Complex drug-drug-disease interactions between amiodarone, warfarin, and the thyroid gland. *Medicine* (Baltimore) 2004; 83:107.

[99] Bartalena, L, Bogazzi, F, Braverman, LE, Martino, E. Effects of amiodarone administration during pregnancy on neonatal thyroid function and subsequent neurodevelopment. *J. Endocrinol. Invest.* 2001; 24:116.

[100] Rey E, Bachrach LK, Burrow GN. Effects of amiodarone during pregnancy. *Can. Med. Assoc. J.* 1987; 61: 75-77.

[101] Magee LA, Nulman I, Rovet JF, Koren G. Neurodevelopment after in utero amiodarone exposure. *Neurotoxicol. Teratol.* 1999. 21:261-265.

[102] de Wolf D, de Schepper J, Verhaaren H, Deneyer M, Smitz J, Sacre-smits L. Congenital hypothyroid goitre and amiodarone. *Acta Paediatr. Scand.* 1988; 77: 616-618.

In: Thyroid Hormones: Functions, Related Diseases and Uses ISBN: 978-1-60741-080-5
Editors: F. S. Kuehn, M. P. Lozada

Chapter XI

Effects of Secondhand Smoke on the Thyroid

Andreas D. Flouris*
Institute of Human Performance and Rehabilitation,
Centre for Research and Technology – Thessaly, Trikala, GR42100, Greece

Abstract

Experimental evidence for the physiological effects of secondhand smoke is limited although it affects millions of people globally and its prevalence is increasing, despite currently adopted anti-smoking measures. As early as adolescence, exposure to tobacco products increases the risk for developing cardiovascular disease (1) highlighting the necessity to understand the secondhand smoke effects on human health. Recent evidence demonstrated that a 1-hour secondhand smoke exposure to bar/restaurant levels is accompanied by statistically significant increases in triiodothyronine (T_3) and free thyroxine (fT_4) levels of healthy adult non-smokers (2). These increases of thyroid hormone levels effects affected metabolism with a 6% increase in resting energy expenditure and were not attributed to an anterior pituitary response (i.e., thyroid stimulating hormone secretion), but to the – probably short-term – effects of a different mechanism. Interestingly, further work in this area revealed that the same secondhand smoke exposure is accompanied by a decrease in gonadal hormones in both sexes as well as marked increases in thyroid hormone secretion and interleukin-1β production in men (3). The less pronounced alterations in thyroid hormone secretion of women suggested the involvement of estrogens which are known to influence serum total T_4 and T_3 concentrations by increasing the glycosylation of thyroxine-binding globulin – a protein heavily involved in T_4 and T_3 binding – and by slowing its clearance from the blood. Analogously, the statistically significant decrease in the T_3:fT_4 ratio following the secondhand smoke exposure in men as well as the inverse association between testosterone and T_3 suggested the involvement of androgens, which are known to decrease the glycosylation of thyroxine-binding globulin. These results were not limited

* e-mail: aflouris[at]cereteth.gr.

to extrathyroidial processes, as fT_4 levels were not significantly influenced by changes in the serum concentrations of binding proteins, reflecting purely functional thyroid state. Therefore, the observed effects of gonadal hormones may also indicate a down-regulating effect on thyroid gland hormonogenesis. Based on these results and data from chronic active smoking, it was suggested that chronic passive smoking (lifestyle incorporating frequent exposures to passive smoke) may have clinical implications such as thyroid and gonadal abnormalities particularly in males. In this light, this chapter reviews current knowledge on the effects of secondhand smoke on the thyroid in an attempt to unravel the underlying mechanisms associated with the increase in thyroid hormone secretion following exposure to secondhand smoke.

Introduction

It is beyond any doubt that both active and passive smoking generate adverse effects on human health (4-8). And yet, despite adopted measures, the prevalence rates of smoking are increasing (6, 7), primarily among young girls (1, 8). At present, more than half of American adult nonsmokers suffer daily passive smoking, while similar prevalence rates exist for Europe and China and global estimates include 700 million children and 50 million pregnant women (5, 9). Latest reports show that the global tobacco epidemic is worse today than it has been the past decades (6-8). Indeed, it may come as a surprise to some that the tobacco industry predicts a global expansion of the tobacco epidemic in the near future (7). This expansion is fuelled in part by the scarcity of human experimental studies assessing the acute passive smoking effects, permitting criticism (10) of the tobacco control movement with arguments that only chronic passive smoking increase the risk of cardiovascular disease and that there is no scientific basis for claims that brief, acute, transient passive smoking represent a significant acute cardiovascular health hazard to nonsmokers.

Effects on Thyroid Function

Metabolism is a vital physiological function providing for bioenergetics, body composition as well as byproduct removal, and is largely affected by perturbations in the body's internal and/or external environment (11). Active smoking has been repeatedly identified as a factor that alters normal metabolic status (12) and increases the occurrence of metabolic disorders (13). Resting energy expenditure (REE) – the primary indicator of human metabolism (14) – increases significantly with active smoking (15). This is attributed to an augmented neuroendocrine function through the activation of G protein-coupled beta-2 and beta-3 receptors in the sympathetic nervous system (16). Concomitantly, smoking alters normal thyroid hormone secretion by increasing triiodothyronine (T_3), free thyroxine (fT_4) and diminishing the thyroid stimulating hormone (TSH) levels (17-19). As a consequence, active smoking may have serious chronic clinical implications (12, 13) including body composition imbalance (20) and development of Grave's disease (21, 22).

The detrimental effects of active smoking are generally similar to those of passive smoking (23). This is partly supported by the fact that avoidance of passive smoking significantly minimizes the risk for developing metabolic-related disorders, such as Grave's disease (24). However, until recently there was a lack of experimental investigations on the effects of passive smoking on human metabolism. The majority of previous studies on passive smoking had been focused on the respiratory and cardiovascular systems and had mainly employed qualitative methods to establish passive smoking exposure (17, 25-28) which generates significant methodological limitations (29). Furthermore, several studies had dealt with excessively high passive smoke concentrations which have limited relevance and application for normal every-day environments (30).

The objective of a recent investigation in my laboratory was to experimentally assess the effects of 1-hour of passive smoking in a controlled simulated bar/restaurant environment on the metabolism and thyroid hormone levels in healthy non-smokers (2). Based on previous data showing stimulatory effects of active smoking on thyroid function (17-19), our hypothesis was that passive smoking would increase metabolism and thyroid hormone secretion.

In repeated-measures randomized blocks, eighteen (female=9) healthy individuals (25.3±3.1yrs, 174.0±10.1cm, 65.2±13.7kg) visited the laboratory on two consecutive days after a 12-hour overnight fast in both occasions. In the experimental session they were exposed to 1-hour of moderate passive smoking at a carbon monoxide concentration of 23±1ppm [concentrations previously reported for bar/restaurant environments (31)] in an environmental chamber, whereas in the control session participants remained in the same chamber for 1-hour breathing normal atmospheric air. In both sessions, cotinine serum and urine levels, REE, as well as concentration of T_3, fT_4 and TSH were assessed just prior to participants entered the chamber and immediately following their exit. Heart rate and blood pressure were tested in 10-minute intervals during all REE assessments. The results of the experiments showed that serum (9.6±5.4 vs. 23.2±7.9 ng/mL, $p<0.001$) and urine (6.0±1.4 vs. 13.6±4.2 ng/mL, $p<0.001$) cotinine levels were elevated following the exposure to passive-smoking. This was also the case for REE (1504.3±286.2 vs. 1584.9±296.8 kcal/day, $p<0.05$), T_3 (1.05±0.1 vs.1.17±0.1, $p<0.05$) and fT_4 (1.3±0.2 vs. 1.5±0.2 μIU/mL, $p<0.05$). No significant differences were detected for TSH, heart rate or blood pressure ($p>0.05$).

Overall, the results from this experiment demonstrated that a 1-hour passive smoking exposure to levels similar to those of bars/restaurants is accompanied by a significant increase in metabolism and thyroid hormone secretion of healthy non-smokers (2). These results were in line with our research hypothesis which was derived from previous data showing stimulatory effects of active smoking on thyroid function (17-19).

To our knowledge, this was the first study that directly investigated the effects of passive smoking on metabolism, demonstrating an increase in REE similar to that previously reported for active smoking (12). This confirms recent reports in the literature highlighting that the detrimental effects elicited by active smoking are equivalent to that of passive smoking (23). Based on the results of our experiment, it could be suggested that frequent exposure to passive smoke may be accompanied by significant alterations in metabolism which, in turn, may lead to malnutrition and abnormal changes in body composition (32). Moreover, the linear associations detected between REE and both serum and urine cotinine concentrations suggested that the effects of passive smoking on REE were dose-dependent. This was in line with reports on active smoking indicating that increases in energy expenditure are relevant to the total amount of smoke inhaled (15, 33).

The data obtained from this experiment also confirmed that environmental tobacco smoke generates significant disruption of the hypothalamic-pituitary-thyroid axis. We found that the exposure to passive smoke was accompanied by a significant increase in T_3 and fT_4 levels and a non-significant decrease in TSH. These findings were in line with previous results (18, 19), and provided support to the notion that the increases in T_3 and fT_4 seen in our study were not attributed to an anterior pituitary response (TSH secretion), but to a spontaneous (and probably short-term) thyroid gland dysfunction. It is unlikely that this thyroid dysfunction was nicotine-induced, given the absence of a linear relationship between T_3 and fT_4 with either serum or urine cotinine levels. This was also supported by previous findings from animal models that showed no effect of nicotine on serum T_3 and fT_4 (34). The notion of tobacco-induced alterations in normal thyroid function has been suggested by several other investigators reporting that chronic active smoking lowers the pituitary set-point with potentially beneficial effects on the thyroid gland (35). However, our findings suggested that single brief exposures to passive smoking in non-smokers may generate thyroid dysfunction resulting in mild increases in thyroid hormone secretion. Unfortunately, we were unable to identify the causative agent of the observed thyroid gland dysfunction based on the obtained data.

Although the increase in T_3 and fT_4 discussed in the previous paragraph would suggest an increase in heart rate and arterial blood pressure through a sympathetic activation, our data showed only a marginal and non-significant increase in these parameters. Such controversial findings have been reported several times in the literature thus far for both passive and active smoking, suggesting that low or moderate inhalation of tobacco smoke levels is unlikely to cause an increase in heart rate or arterial blood pressure (36).

It is important to note that the observed alterations in metabolism and hypothalamic-pituitary-thyroid axis in response to passive smoking did not arise from an extreme and/or prolonged exposure but from a comparatively brief exposure to a simulated bar/restaurant environment. The cotinine levels in both serum and urine suggest moderate passive smoking exposure (37) confirming a successful simulation of a bar/restaurant smoking environment. Further, the adopted randomized design provided credence to our findings suggesting that the reported physiological changes where indeed due to passive smoke. On the other hand, our results would be further strengthened by additional biochemical analyses, such as evaluation of catecholamines. In conclusion, this experiment demonstrated that a 1-hour passive smoking exposure to levels similar to those of bars/restaurants is accompanied by a significant increase in metabolism and thyroid hormone secretion of healthy non-smokers.

Effect of Gonadal Hormones

Experimental data (2-4, 36, 38-41) suggest that even brief exposures to secondhand smoke cause marked changes in thyroid hormone secretion, platelet aggregation, endothelial function, arterial pressure waveform, inflammatory markers, as well as other haemodynamic alterations involved in the development of ischemic heart disease. At least some of these effects appear to be more pronounced in males compared to females (40, 42), but the mechanism underlying this phenomenon has yet to be elucidated. To aid in the understanding of these phenomena, we conducted a randomized single-blind crossover study to investigate the sex-specific effects of a 1-hour exposure to secondhand smoke on gonadal and thyroid hormones, inflammatory cytokines and specific parameters of vascular function (3).

Twenty eight (women=14; age=26.4±4.4 years; height=171.63±10.28 cm; weight=64.83±13.12 kg) non-smoking adults underwent a 1-hour exposure to moderate secondhand smoke and a 1-hour control trial. To simulate a bar/restaurant environment, the carbon monoxide concentration of 23±1ppm was used (31). Serum and urine cotinine, gonadal and thyroid hormones, inflammatory cytokines, heart rate, and arterial blood pressure were assessed prior to exposure and immediately after in both trials. Results showed that testosterone ($P=0.019$) and progesterone ($P<0.001$) in men, and 17β-estradiol ($P=0.001$) and progesterone ($P<0.001$) in women were significantly decreased following secondhand smoke. In men, secondhand smoke was accompanied by increased fT_4 ($P<0.001$), T_3 ($P=0.020$), and decreased T_3: fT_4 ratio ($P=0.033$). In women, significant secondhand smoke-induced change was observed only in fT_4 ($P=0.010$), with considerable sex variation in fT_4 and T_3 and a decrease in luteinizing hormone ($P=0.026$) and follicle-stimulating hormone ($P<0.001$). Following secondhand smoke, interleukin-1 beta ($P=0.001$) and systolic blood pressure ($P=0.040$) was increased in men but not women (3).

To the author's knowledge, that was the first study to directly investigate sex-specific differences in the effects of secondhand smoke on gonadal and thyroid hormones, inflammatory markers and parameters of vascular function. Our results suggested that a moderate secondhand smoke exposure is accompanied by a decrease in gonadal hormones in both sexes as well as marked increases in thyroid hormone secretion and interleukin-1 beta production in males. This sexual dimorphism in the effects of secondhand smoke on thyroid hormone secretion and interleukin-1 beta production is also associated with a significantly increased systolic blood pressure following exposure to secondhand smoke in males as compared to females.

The lower T_3:fT_4 ratio following the secondhand smoke exposure suggests inhibited extrathyroidal T_4 deiodination to T_3, resulting in larger amounts of unbound hormone which is available for uptake into cells and interaction with nuclear receptors, as well as a smaller circulating hormone storage pool. In turn, this may be due to a lower circulation of binding proteins or interaction of binding proteins with fT_4 and T_3 (43). Although these factors were not directly investigated in our experiment, the absence of significant change in the T_3:fT_4 ratio following the secondhand smoke exposure in females suggests the involvement of estrogens. The latter significantly influence serum total T_4 and T_3 concentrations by increasing the glycosylation of thyroxine-binding globulin – a protein heavily involved in T_4 and T_3 binding – and by slowing its clearance from the blood (43). Ergo, it is attractive to postulate that the observed association between 17β-estradiol and T_3:fT_4 ratio in the entire sample as well as the negative association between 17β-estradiol and fT_4 in females reflected an increase in thyroxine-binding globulin concentration. In turn, this increase in hormone binding reduces fT_4 concentration by increasing the clearance of thyroxine. Analogously, the statistically significant decrease in the T_3:fT_4 ratio following the secondhand smoke exposure in males as well as the inverse association between testosterone and T_3 suggest the involvement of androgens, which are known to decrease the glycosylation of thyroxine-binding globulin (43). Yet, it is important to also consider that the present results are not limited to extrathyroidial processes, as fT_4 levels are not significantly influenced by changes in the serum concentrations of binding proteins, reflecting purely functional thyroid state (44). Therefore, the observed effects of gonadal hormones may also indicate a down-regulating effect on thyroid gland hormonogenesis.

The observed effects of secondhand smoke on thyroid hormone secretion may also reflect the involvement of circulating inflammation markers – and particularly interleukin-1 beta – which have been shown to influence the hypothalamic-pituitary-adrenal axis (45, 46). Interleukin-1 beta inhibits differentiated thyroid cell functions (47) including human thyroid cell adenylate cyclase and thyroglobulin release (45, 46). Consistent with this notion is the finding that interleukin-1 beta in our experiment demonstrated significant secondhand smoke-induced changes only in males, reflecting an anti-inflammatory effect of estrogens which well-supported by previous research (48). The present secondhand smoke-induced increase in interleukin-1 beta supports a small number of previous investigations reporting an increase of circulating inflammation markers including white blood cell count, C-reactive protein, homocysteine, fibrinogen (41) and leukocyte counts accompanied by an activation of the immune cells (49). In fact, recent evidence suggested that neutralizing interleukin-1 beta in mice reduced secondhand smoke-induced inflammation in lung cells (50). While tumor necrosis alpha and interleukin 6 were also increased following the secondhand smoke exposure in our study, these changes did not reach statistical significance.

The significantly increased systolic blood pressure following the secondhand smoke exposure in males compared to females confirms the findings of our earlier study (40) that used similar secondhand smoke exposure levels and duration. Sexual dimorphism in the effects of tobacco smoke has also been reported for branchial flow-mediated dilatation (51) as well as for intimamedia thickness (52). The increase in vascular tone observed in our experiment may be due to the confirmed smoke-induced sympathetic nervous system activation (53). Given the significant effect of thyroid hormone regulation on the sympathetic nervous system (54), it is not surprising that one of the parameters associated with systolic blood pressure in our study was the T_3:fT_4 ratio. On the other hand, our regression analysis demonstrated that gonadal hormones were also associated with systolic blood pressure. The negative link between both major gonadal hormones examined herein (i.e., 17β-estradiol and testosterone) and systolic blood pressure confirms their well-known cardioprotective role against the noxious effects of secondhand smoke (40, 55, 56). Concomitantly, the observed link between systolic blood pressure and tumor necrosis alpha supports a recent study proposing a link between secondhand smoke-induced increase in tumor necrosis alpha and cardiovascular alterations leading to atherogenesis (57). Active cigarette smoking has also been associated with an imbalance in the production of tumor necrosis alpha and soluble tumor necrosis receptors, leading to a relative excess of tumor necrosis alpha (58). This may also explain the minor secondhand smoke-induced increase in tumor necrosis alpha in our experiment.

It is important to note that, as in the experiment introduced in the earlier section of this chapter, the current alterations in gonadal and thyroid hormone secretion, inflammatory markers and systolic blood pressure in response to secondhand smoke pertain to acute changes and did not arise from an extreme and/or prolonged exposure. The reported cotinine levels suggested a moderate and brief secondhand smoke exposure (37), confirming a successful simulation of a bar/restaurant smoking environment. The adopted design did not influence our results as no differences were detected between participants performing the experimental trial first or second in sequence. It is concluded that a 1-hour secondhand smoke exposure to levels similar to those of bars/restaurants is accompanied by a decrease in gonadal hormones in both sexes as well as marked increases in thyroid hormone secretion, interleukin-1 beta production and systolic blood pressure in males.

Concluding Remarks

This chapter reviewed current knowledge on the effects of secondhand smoke on the thyroid in an attempt to unravel the underlying mechanisms associated with the increase in thyroid hormone secretion following exposure to secondhand smoke. Based on the results from the two experiments conducted in my laboratory as well as data from chronic active smoking, it can be suggested that chronic passive smoking (lifestyle incorporating frequent exposures to passive smoke) may have clinical implications such as thyroid and gonadal abnormalities particularly in males.

References

[1] Flouris AD, Faught BE, Klentrou P. Cardiovascular disease risk in adolescent smokers: evidence of a 'smoker lifestyle'. J Child Health Care. 2008;12(3):217-27.

[2] Metsios GS, Flouris AD, Jamurtas AZ, Carrillo AE, Kouretas D, Germenis AE, et al. A brief exposure to moderate passive smoke increases metabolism and thyroid hormone secretion. J Clin Endocrinol Metab. 2007 Jan;92(1):208-11.

[3] Flouris AD, Metsios GS, Jamurtas AZ, Koutedakis Y. Sexual dimorphism in the acute effects of secondhand smoke on thyroid hormone secretion, inflammatory markers and vascular function. Am J Physiol Endocrinol Metab. 2008 Feb;294(2):E456-62.

[4] Raupach T, Schafer K, Konstantinides S, Andreas S. Secondhand smoke as an acute threat for the cardiovascular system: a change in paradigm. Eur Heart J. 2006 Feb;27(4):386-92.

[5] U.S. Department of Health and Human Services. The Health Consequences of Involuntary Exposure to Tobacco Smoke: A report of the Surgeon General. Atlanta, GA: U.S. Department of Health and Human Services, Centers of Disease Control and Prevention, Coordinating Center for Health Promotion, National Center for Chronic Disease Prevention and Health Promotion, Office on Smoking and Health. 2006.

[6] Substance Abuse and Mental Health Services Administration. Results from the 2006 National Survey on Drug Use and Health: National Findings (Office of Applied Studies, NSDUH Series H-32, DHHS Publication No. SMA 07-4293). Rockville, MD.; 2007.

[7] Mackay J, Eriksen M. The tobacco atlas. Geneva, Switzerland: World Health Organization; 2008.
[8] Warren CW, Jones NR, Peruga A, Chauvin J, Baptiste JP, Costa de Silva V, et al. Global youth tobacco surveillance, 2000-2007. MMWR Surveill Summ. 2008;57:1-28.
[9] Eisner MD. Passive smoking and adult asthma. Immunol Allergy Clin North Am. 2008 Aug;28(3):521-37, viii.
[10] Siegel M. Is the tobacco control movement misrepresenting the acute cardiovascular health effects of secondhand smoke exposure? An analysis of the scientific evidence and commentary on the implications for tobacco control and public health practice. Epidemiol Perspect Innov. 2007;4:12.
[11] Muller MJ, Bosy-Westphal A, Kutzner D, Heller M. Metabolically active components of fat free mass (FFM) and resting energy expenditure (REE) in humans. Forum Nutr. 2003;56:301-3.
[12] Walker JF, Kane CJ. Effects of body mass on nicotine-induced thermogenesis and catecholamine release in male smokers. Sheng Li Xue Bao. 2002 Oct 25;54(5):405-10.
[13] Kapoor D, Jones TH. Smoking and hormones in health and endocrine disorders. Eur J Endocrinol. 2005 Apr;152(4):491-9.
[14] Poehlman ET. A review: exercise and its influence on resting energy metabolism in man. Med Sci Sports Exerc. 1989 Oct;21(5):515-25.
[15] Collins LC, Walker J, Stamford BA. Smoking multiple high- versus low-nicotine cigarettes: impact on resting energy expenditure. Metabolism. 1996 Aug;45(8):923-6.
[16] Grassi G, Seravalle G, Calhoun DA, Bolla GB, Giannattasio C, Marabini M, et al. Mechanisms responsible for sympathetic activation by cigarette smoking in humans. Circulation. 1994 Jul;90(1):248-53.
[17] Knudsen N, Bulow I, Laurberg P, Perrild H, Ovesen L, Jorgensen T. High occurrence of thyroid multinodularity and low occurrence of subclinical hypothyroidism among tobacco smokers in a large population study. J Endocrinol. 2002 Dec;175(3):571-6.
[18] Fisher CL, Mannino DM, Herman WH, Frumkin H. Cigarette smoking and thyroid hormone levels in males. Int J Epidemiol. 1997 Oct;26(5):972-7.
[19] Ericsson UB, Lindgarde F. Effects of cigarette smoking on thyroid function and the prevalence of goitre, thyrotoxicosis and autoimmune thyroiditis. J Intern Med. 1991 Jan;229(1):67-71.
[20] Bray GA. Reciprocal relation of food intake and sympathetic activity: experimental observations and clinical implications. Int J Obes Relat Metab Disord. 2000 Jun;24 Suppl 2:S8-17.
[21] Holm IA, Manson JE, Michels KB, Alexander EK, Willett WC, Utiger RD. Smoking and other lifestyle factors and the risk of Graves' hyperthyroidism. Arch Intern Med. 2005 Jul 25;165(14):1606-11.
[22] Bartalena L, Marcocci C, Tanda ML, Piantanida E, Lai A, Marino M, et al. An update on medical management of Graves' ophthalmopathy. J Endocrinol Invest. 2005 May;28(5):469-78.
[23] Barnoya J, Glantz SA. Cardiovascular effects of secondhand smoke: nearly as large as smoking. Circulation. 2005 May 24;111(20):2684-98.

[24] Cheng AC, Pang CP, Leung AT, Chua JK, Fan DS, Lam DS. The association between cigarette smoking and ocular diseases. Hong Kong Med J. 2000 Jun;6(2):195-202.

[25] Zhang X, Shu XO, Yang G, Li HL, Xiang YB, Gao YT, et al. Association of passive smoking by husbands with prevalence of stroke among Chinese women nonsmokers. Am J Epidemiol. 2005 Feb 1;161(3):213-8.

[26] Lee CH, Ko YC, Goggins W, Huang JJ, Huang MS, Kao EL, et al. Lifetime environmental exposure to tobacco smoke and primary lung cancer of non-smoking Taiwanese women. Int J Epidemiol. 2000 Apr;29(2):224-31.

[27] McGhee SM, Adab P, Hedley AJ, Lam TH, Ho LM, Fielding R, et al. Passive smoking at work: the short-term cost. J Epidemiol Community Health. 2000 Sep;54(9):673-6.

[28] McGhee SM, Hedley AJ, Ho LM. Passive smoking and its impact on employers and employees in Hong Kong. Occup Environ Med. 2002 Dec;59(12):842-6.

[29] Kawachi I. More evidence on the risks of passive smoking. Bmj. 2005 Feb 5;330(7486):265-6.

[30] Tikuisis P, Buick F, Kane DM. Percent carboxyhemoglobin in resting humans exposed repeatedly to 1,500 and 7,500 ppm CO. J Appl Physiol. 1987 Aug;63(2):820-7.

[31] Jo WK, Oh JW, Dong JI. Evaluation of exposure to carbon monoxide associated with passive smoking. Environ Res. 2004 Mar;94(3):309-18.

[32] Agarwal R. Smoking, oxidative stress and inflammation: impact on resting energy expenditure in diabetic nephropathy. BMC Nephrol. 2005 Nov 22;6:13.

[33] Perkins KA, Sexton JE. Influence of aerobic fitness, activity level, and smoking history on the acute thermic effect of nicotine. Physiol Behav. 1995 Jun;57(6):1097-102.

[34] Colzani R, Fang SL, Alex S, Braverman LE. The effect of nicotine on thyroid function in rats. Metabolism. 1998 Feb;47(2):154-7.

[35] Belin RM, Astor BC, Powe NR, Ladenson PW. Smoke exposure is associated with a lower prevalence of serum thyroid autoantibodies and thyrotropin concentration elevation and a higher prevalence of mild thyrotropin concentration suppression in the third National Health and Nutrition Examination Survey (NHANES III). J Clin Endocrinol Metab. 2004 Dec;89(12):6077-86.

[36] Otsuka R, Watanabe H, Hirata K, Tokai K, Muro T, Yoshiyama M, et al. Acute effects of passive smoking on the coronary circulation in healthy young adults. Jama. 2001 Jul 25;286(4):436-41.

[37] Benowitz NL. Biomarkers of environmental tobacco smoke exposure. Environ Health Perspect. 1999 May;107 Suppl 2:349-55.

[38] Sidorkewicz N, Carrillo AE, Metsios GS, Flouris AD, Jamurtas AZ, Koutedakis Y. Resting energy expenditure response following environmental tobacco smoke exposure. Med Sci Sports Exerc. 2006;38(5):S457-8.

[39] Flouris AD, Metsios GS, Carrillo AE, Jamurtas AZ, Koutedakis Y, Tzatzarakis MN, et al. Effects of passive smoking on resting and exercising humans. Can J Appl Physiol. 2005;30:S28.

[40] Mahmud A, Feely J. Effects of passive smoking on blood pressure and aortic pressure waveform in healthy young adults--influence of gender. Br J Clin Pharmacol. 2004 Jan;57(1):37-43.

[41] Panagiotakos DB, Pitsavos C, Chrysohoou C, Skoumas J, Masoura C, Toutouzas P, et al. Effect of exposure to secondhand smoke on markers of inflammation: the ATTICA study. Am J Med. 2004 Feb 1;116(3):145-50.

[42] Perkins KA. Individual variability in responses to nicotine. Behav Genet. 1995 Mar;25(2):119-32.

[43] Ekins R. The free hormone hypothesis and measurement of free hormones. Clin Chem. 1992 Jul;38(7):1289-93.

[44] Mendel CM, Weisiger RA, Jones AL, Cavalieri RR. Thyroid hormone-binding proteins in plasma facilitate uniform distribution of thyroxine within tissues: a perfused rat liver study. Endocrinology. 1987 May;120(5):1742-9.

[45] Rasmussen AK, Diamant M, Blichert-Toft M, Bendtzen K, Feldt-Rasmussen U. The effects of interleukin-1beta (IL-1beta) on human thyrocyte functions are counteracted by the IL-1 receptor antagonist. Endocrinology. 1997 May;138(5):2043-8.

[46] Rasmussen AK, Kayser L, Feldt-Rasmussen U, Bendtzen K. Influence of tumour necrosis factor-alpha, tumour necrosis factor-beta and interferon-gamma, separately and added together with interleukin-1 beta, on the function of cultured human thyroid cells. J Endocrinol. 1994 Nov;143(2):359-65.

[47] Rasmussen AK, Feldt-Rasmussen U, Bendtzen K. The effect of interleukin-1 on the thyroid gland. Autoimmunity. 1993;16(2):141-8.

[48] Simoncini T, Maffei S, Basta G, Barsacchi G, Genazzani AR, Liao JK, et al. Estrogens and glucocorticoids inhibit endothelial vascular cell adhesion molecule-1 expression by different transcriptional mechanisms. Circ Res. 2000 Jul 7;87(1):19-25.

[49] Anderson R, Theron AJ, Richards GA, Myer MS, van Rensburg AJ. Passive smoking by humans sensitizes circulating neutrophils. Am Rev Respir Dis. 1991 Sep;144(3 Pt 1):570-4.

[50] Castro P, Legora-Machado A, Cardilo-Reis L, Valenca S, Porto LC, Walker C, et al. Inhibition of interleukin-1beta reduces mouse lung inflammation induced by exposure to cigarette smoke. Eur J Pharmacol. 2004 Sep 13;498(1-3):279-86.

[51] Celermajer DS, Adams MR, Clarkson P, Robinson J, McCredie R, Donald A, et al. Passive smoking and impaired endothelium-dependent arterial dilatation in healthy young adults. N Engl J Med. 1996 Jan 18;334(3):150-4.

[52] Gariepy J, Denarie N, Chironi G, Salomon J, Levenson J, Simon A. Gender difference in the influence of smoking on arterial wall thickness. Atherosclerosis. 2000 Nov;153(1):139-45.

[53] Hausberg M, Mark AL, Winniford MD, Brown RE, Somers VK. Sympathetic and vascular effects of short-term passive smoke exposure in healthy nonsmokers. Circulation. 1997 Jul 1;96(1):282-7.

[54] Polikar R, Burger AG, Scherrer U, Nicod P. The thyroid and the heart. Circulation. 1993 May;87(5):1435-41.

[55] Malkin CJ, Pugh PJ, Jones RD, Jones TH, Channer KS. Testosterone as a protective factor against atherosclerosis--immunomodulation and influence upon plaque development and stability. J Endocrinol. 2003 Sep;178(3):373-80.

[56] Simoncini T, Mannella P, Genazzani AR. Rapid estrogen actions in the cardiovascular system. Ann N Y Acad Sci. 2006 Nov;1089:424-30.

[57] Yuan H, Wong LS, Bhattacharya M, Ma C, Zafarani M, Yao M, et al. The effects of second-hand smoke on biological processes important in atherogenesis. BMC Cardiovasc Disord. 2007;7:1.

[58] Glossop JR, Dawes PT, Mattey DL. Association between cigarette smoking and release of tumour necrosis factor alpha and its soluble receptors by peripheral blood mononuclear cells in patients with rheumatoid arthritis. Rheumatology (Oxford). 2006 Oct;45(10):1223-9.

Index

#

A

B

C

D

G

H

I

J

K

L

M

N

Q

R

T

U

V

W

X

Y

Z